This

s

Immunology

A Textbook

Immunology

A Textbook

C V Rao

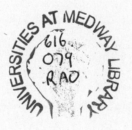

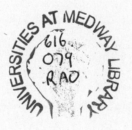

Alpha Science International Ltd.

Harrow, U.K.

C V Rao
Department of Zoology
St. Xavier's College
Mumbai, India

Copyright © 2005
First reprint 2006
Second reprint 2006

Alpha Science International Ltd.
Hygeia Building, 66 College Road
Harrow, Middlesex HA1 1BE, U.K.

ISBN 1-84265-255-9

Printed in India

Dedicated to
My Daughter
Ramya,
An Enthusiastic Student

Preface

I decided to come out with a textbook version of my previous book titled "AN INTRODUCTION TO IMMUNOLOGY," which was published in 2002. After receiving feedback about the book from a large majority of undergraduate students, I decided to tone down the contents of most of the chapters so that undergraduate students find it easier to understand. At the end of each chapter, exercises are suggested for the benefit of students and to know the depth of answering the questions.

I have made a humble attempt to make this textbook as simple as possible by covering important aspects of immunology without neglecting current status of developments. I am sure that this book will enthuse and invigorate interest in undergraduate students who are novice to the subject of immunology. I am confident that this book would help in understanding the basics and concepts of immunology and stimulate research interest in some students who would take up research as a career.

The textbook has twenty-two chapters, and I hope reading them will be interesting to the students.

C V RAO

Acknowledgments

First of all I would like to express my deep gratitude to Mr. Vidyut Sonde, a student of mine, who has custom designed and drawn almost all diagrams on the computer under my guidance with his ingenuity. Any success that this book might achieve will be due to his fine illustrations, which I owe to Vidyut. Secondly, I would like to thank Mr. Alain D' Souza, a student of mine, for helping me in preparing the manuscript and the overall page layouts as required by the publisher and proofreading of galleys as well as page proofs. I would also like to thank my colleagues, student fraternity and other teachers for their valuable suggestions to write this textbook. A special thanks to my family who stood by me while I was working on this book.

I would like to express my gratitude to the Principal for providing the laser printer facility in the office so that my task became easy to take the printout of this book. I would like to thank Mr. Bipin and Mr. Albert of the college office for helping me in taking out the print-outs.

I am especially grateful to the many immunologists who were kind enough to send their original articles and publications when I requested them. It is these original research papers and articles that make the study of immunology interesting and up-to-date.

I would also like to thank Narosa Publishing House, New Delhi for accepting to publish this textbook.

Finally, I would like to apologize, in advance for any errors that may have occurred in the text, and express my heartfelt embarrassment. Any comments or criticisms from readers would be greatly appreciated. They can be directed to Editor, Narosa Publishing House Pvt. Ltd., 22 Daryaganj, Delhi Medical Association Road, New Delhi 110 002.

C V RAO

Contents

Preface   *vii*

Acknowledgments   *ix*

1. Introduction   **1**

Origin of Immune System in Invertebrates   4

Immune System in the Beginning   4

Origin of Vertebrate Immune System   7

Two Parts of the Immune System   8

Exercise   12

2. Innate Immunity   **13**

Non-Immunological Surface Protective Mechanisms (Anatomical Barriers)   14

Antimicrobial Peptides in Mammalian System   15

Immunogenic Innate Immune Response (Physiologic Barrier)   16

Innate Immune Response against Blood Group Antigens   17

Innate Immune Response through Alternate Pathway of Complement   17

Macrophage   18

Endocytosis   19

Phagocytosis   20

Chemokines   21

Interferons in Innate Immune Response   21

Natural Killer Cells (NK Cells) in Innate Immune Response   22

Contribution of T-Cells Bearing γδ T-Cell Receptors to
Innate Immune Response   22

CD5-B cell in Innate Immune Response   22

Inflammatory Response as Barrier   22

Mast Cells and their Role in Innate Immunity   24

Mechanism of Innate Immune Recognition   25

Control of Effector Cytokines by Innate Immune System   26

Exercise   26

3. Acquired Immunity   **27**

Naturally Acquired Passive Immunity   27

Artificially Acquired Passive Immunity   28

Naturally Acquired Active Immunity   29

Artificially Acquired Active Immunity   29

Acquired Immune Memory   31

Specificity of Acquired Immunity   32
Co-Stimulatory Molecules of Acquired Immune Response   32
Cells Involved in Immune System   33
Antigen Presenting Cells   36
Factors Affecting Immune System   36
Nutrition and Immunity   37
Exercise   38

4. Cells and Organs of Immune System   **39**
Cells of the Immune System   40
B–Lymphocytes   40
T–Lymphocytes   42
Null Cells   43
Mononuclear Phagocytes   43
Granulocytes   45
Neutrophils   45
Eosinophil   47
Basophil   47
Mast Cells   48
Dendritic Cells   48
Organs of the Immune System   49
Primary Lymphoid Organs   49
Thymus   49
Bone Marrow   50
Lymphatic System   51
Secondary Lymphoid Organ   52
Lymph Node   52
Spleen   53
Mucosal Associated Lymphoid Tissue (MALT)   54
Functions of IEL   55
Lamina Propria T Cells (LP T Cells)   56
Functions of LP T Cells   57
Coordinated Functions of the Intestinal Mucosal Immune System   58
Cutaneous Associated Lymphoid Tissue   60
Exercise   62

5. Antigens or Immunogens   **63**
Types of Antigens   63
General Properties of Antigens   64
Role Played by Biological System in the Immunogenicity   67
Adjuvants   68
Antigenic Determinants or Epitopes   69
Haptens   69
Superantigens   71
Exercise   71

6. Major and Minor Histocompatibility Complex   **72**
Inheritance of HLA System, Location and Functions   73

Structure of MHC Molecules   75
Peptide Interaction with MHC Molecule   78
Genetic Polymorphism of Class I, II and III MHC Molecules   79
Cellular Distribution and Regulation of MHC Expression   80
MHC and Immune Responsiveness   81
MHC and Susceptibility to Infectious Diseases   81
Minor Histocompatibility (H) Antigens   82
Identification of Minor H Antigens and their Genes   83
Exercise   84

7. Antibodies (Immunoglobulins)   **85**
Immunoglobulin Structure and Function   85
Antigenic Determinants on Immunoglobulins   90
Immunoglobulin Classes   92
Immunoglobulin G (γ Globulin G or IgG)   92
Immunoglobulin M (γ-Globulin M or IgM)   93
Immunoglobulin A (γ-Globulin A or IgA)   94
Immunoglobulin E (γ-Globulin E or IgE)   97
Immunoglobulin D (γ-Globulin D or IgD)   97
Exercise   100

8. Antigen-Antibody Interactions   **101**
Precipitin Reactions   103
Immunodiffusion (Ouchterlony Technique)   103
Radial Immunodiffusion (Mancini Method)   105
Rocket Immunoelectrophoresis   105
Two-Dimensional Immunoelectrophoresis   106
Counter Current Immunoelectrophoresis   108
Immunoelectrophoresis   109
Agglutination Reaction   110
Coomb's Test   111
Complement Fixation Test   112
Radioimmunoassay (RIA)   114
Enzyme Linked Immunosorbent Assay (ELISA)   116
Immunofluorescence   116
Western Blotting   119
Experimental Assessment of Humoral Immunity   119
Direct Hemolytic Plaque Assay   119
Elispot Assay   120
Exercise   121

9. Immunoglobulin Genes—Organization and Expression   **122**
Genetic Model for Immunoglobulin Structure   123
Organization of Immunoglobulin (Ig) Genes   124
Gene Rearrangements in Variable Region   126
Mechanism of Variable Region DNA Rearrangements   128
Allelic Exclusion   131
Generation of Antibody Diversity   131

Expression of Ig Genes   138
Regulation of Ig Gene Transcription   139
Exercise   141

10. B-Cell and T-Cell Maturation, Activation and Differentiation   **142**
B-Cell Maturation, Activation and Differentiation   142
B-Cell Maturation   143
Bone Marrow Microenvironment   143
Ig – Gene Rearrangements and Formation of Pre-B Cell Receptors   143
Selection of Immature Self-reactive B Cells   145
B-Cell Activation and Proliferation   146
Overview of the Major Pathways of BCR Signaling   149
Role of Btk in B Cell Development and Signaling   150
B-Cell Coreceptor Complex   150
Role of T_H Cells in Humoral Response   151
Formation of T and B Cell Conjugate   151
B-Cell Differentiation   153
T-Cell Maturation, Activation and Differentiation   155
T-Cell Maturation   156
Discrete Stages in Early T Cell Development   156
The Role of the Thymic Environment in Early T Cell Development   159
Thymic Selection of the T Cell Repertoire   160
T Cell Activation   162
TCR Coupled Signal Transduction   162
Redox Signaling Mechanism in T Cell Activation   162
IL-2 Signaling and the Activation of Proliferation of T Cells   167
Co-stimulation in T Cell Responses   167
Altered Peptide Ligands as Antagonists or Partial Agonists   169
T Cell Clonal Anergy   169
Evidence for Transcriptional Repression in Anergy   169
Superantigen-induced T Cell Activation   170
Differences in Costimulatory Signals among Antigen Presenting Cells   171
γδ T Cells and their Function   171
Exercise   172

11. T-Cell and B-Cell Receptors   **173**
Structure of T-Cell Receptor   173
TCR Multigene Families   174
T-Cell Receptor Complex (TCR – CD3)   178
T Cell Accessory Membrane Molecules   179
Ternary TCR-Peptide-MHC Complex   180
B-Cell Receptors   183
Exercise   188

12. Antigen Processing and Presentation   **189**
Self-MHC Restriction of T Cells   190
Cytosolic Pathway of Antigen Presentation   191
Endocytic Pathway of Exogenous Antigen Presentation   193
Exercise   195

13. Effector Responses of Cell-Mediated and Humoral Immunity   **196**
Effector Response of Cell-Mediated Branch   196
Properties of Effector T cells   197
Cell-Mediated Direct Cytotoxic Response   198
Cytotoxic T Lymphocytes (CTLs)   198
NK Cell-Mediated Cytotoxicity   200
Antibody-Dependent Cell-Mediated Cytotoxicity (ADCC)   201
Delayed-Type Hypersensitivity   202
Detection of Cell-Mediated Immunity   202
Effector Response of the Humoral Branch   204
Detection of Humoral Immune Response   205
Regulation of Immune Effector Response   206
Immunological Memory   210
Factors Controlling the Long-term Survival of Memory Cells   212
Requirement for Cell-Cell Communication   212
Exercise   213

14. Cytokines   **214**
General Properties of Cytokines   215
Functions of Cytokines   216
Cytokines that Stimulate Haematopoiesis   216
Cytokines that Mediate Innate Immunity   218
The Role of Chemokines in Infectious Diseases   222
Cytokines that Regulate Lymphocyte Activation, Growth and Differentiation 223
Cytokines that Regulate Immune Mediated Inflammation   228
Cytokine Related Diseases   232
Exercise   233

15. Complement System   **234**
The Complement Components   234
Classical Complement Pathway   235
Alternative Complement Pathway   237
Lectin Pathway of Complement   237
Consequences of Complement Activation   241
Evasion of Complement—Mediated Damage by Microbes   243
Complement Deficiencies   243
Exercise   244

16. Vaccines   **245**
Active Immunization through Designing Vaccines   246
Vaccines from Whole Organisms   247
Polysaccharide Vaccines   249
Outer Membrane Protein Vaccines   251
Vaccines in the Form of Toxoids   252
Vaccines from Recombinant Vectors   252
DNA as Vaccines   254
Vaccines from Synthetic Peptides   256
Exercise   259

17. Immune Response to Infectious Diseases   **260**
   Viral Infection and Immunity   260
   Cell-Mediated Immune Response against Virus   261
   Viral Strategies of Immune Evasion   264
   Immune Response against Bacterial Infection   267
   Immune Response against Protozoan Parasites   270
   Immune Response against Helminthine Parasites   273
   B-cell Effector Mechanisms against Chronic Infections   275
   Exercise   276

18. Hypersensitivity   **277**
   Type I-IgE-Mediated Hypersensitivity   278
   Allergens   279
   Basophils and Mast Cells   281
   Mechanism of IgE-Mediated Degranulation   282
   Mediators of Type I Reactions   282
   Consequences of Type I Reactions   284
   Passive Transfer Anaphylaxis   285
   Cutaneous Anaphylaxis   285
   Localized Anaphylaxis   286
   Infantile Eczema or Atopic Dermatitis or Allergic Eczema   288
   Late Phase Reaction   288
   Detection of Type I Hypersensitivity   289
   Treatment of Type I Hypersensitivity   289
   Type II Hypersensitivity or Antibody Mediated Cytotoxic Hypersensitivity   290
   Type III-Immune Complex Mediated or Antibody-Antigen Complex
       Mediated Hypersensitivity   291
   Type IV-Delayed Type Hypersensitivity or T_{DTH} Mediated Hypersensitivity   294
   Type V-Stimulatory Hypersensitivity   297
   Exercise   297

19. Transplantation Immunology   **298**
   Immunology of Graft Rejection   299
   Methods of Graft Rejection   299
   Precautions against Graft Rejection   300
   Methods for Tissue Typing   301
   Graft Versus Host Disease or (Reaction) (GVHD)   302
   Mechanism of Graft Rejection   304
   CD40 in Allograft Rejection   306
   Tissue and Organ Transplantation   307
   Immunosuppressive agents   308
   Strategies to Induce Graft Acceptance or Tolerance by Manipulating CD40   310
   Specific Immunosuppressive Therapy during Transplantation   311
   Immunology of Tolerance   313
   Tolerance in Tetraparental (Allophenic) Mice   314
   Non-Autoreactive Nature of Positively Selected T Cells   315
   APL (Altered Peptide-Ligand) Concept: Nature of Selecting Antigens   317

The Adaptation Concept: Nature of the Immature T Cells 318
Anergy Concept: Nature of APC 319
Active Termination of T Cell Immune Response 322
Exercise 324

20. Immunology of Tumors **326**
Clinical Evidence of Immune Response in Malignancy 326
Tumor Antigens 327
Tumor Antigens Recognized by T- Lymphocytes 328
Tumor Antigens Defined by Xenogenic Antibodies 333
Immune Response to Tumor Antigens 334
Immunological Surveillance 336
Immune Therapy of Cancer 337
Evasion of Immune Response by Tumors 343
Exercise 344

21. Autoimmune Diseases **345**
Organ-Specific Autoimmune Diseases 345
Diseases Mediated by Direct Cellular Damage 346
Diseases Mediated by Stimulating or Blocking Antibodies 347
Systemic Autoimmune Diseases 348
Insight into Mechanism of Autoimmune Disease based on Clinical Findings 349
Autoantibodies to T Cell Receptors 352
Cell and Nuclear Penetration by Autoantibodies 352
Treatment of Autoimmune Diseases 352
Experimental Therapeutic Approach 353
Exercise 354

22. Immunodeficiency Diseases **355**
Phagocytic Deficiencies 355
Defective Phagocytic Functions 358
Humoral Deficiencies 359
Cell -mediated Deficiencies 360
Combined Immunodeficiencies 361
Exercise 363

Glossary **364**
Index **386**

Chapter 1

Introduction

- ■ Origin of Immune System in Invertebrates
- ■ Immune System in the Beginning
- ■ Origin of Vertebrate Immune System
- ■ Two Parts of the Immune System

Every organism in its lifetime is constantly being attacked by disease causing germs. In response to this organism have evolved a strategy to tackle these organisms and overcome disease collectively called as *immune system*. The word "immune"(Lt.: *immunis* meaning "exempt") implies freedom from a burden: an organism, which develops immunity to a specific infecting agent, will remain free of infection by that agent life long. The study of the immune system is called *immunology*.

The immune system works by the principle of learning process, where the first encounter with a bacterial, fungal, protozoan or viral pathogen leads to an infection, often accompanied by disease symptoms. The immune system helps in recovering from the infection, and after recovery, the individual usually remains free of that disease forever. The immune system has learned to recognize this specific pathogen as a foreign infecting agent; should it attack again, it will be rapidly killed. Immune response to various disease-causing organisms and the strategies developed by these organisms to evade the immune system and survive in a host are given in detail in *Chapter 17*.

The most basic requirement of any immune system is *recognition*. The system must be able to distinguish the cells, tissues and organs that are a legitimate part of the host body, i.e. "*self*" from foreign things, called "*non-self*", that might be present. The second job is to eliminate those non-self invaders, which are often dangerous bacteria or viruses. In addition, the immune system can recognize, and usually eliminate "altered self"-cells or tissues that have been changed by injury or disease such as cancer. Most immunologist would agree that the immune systems of mammals, such as humans, have the most sophisticated mechanism both for recognition and eliminating invaders. When such discrimination fails, it leads to *autoimmune diseases*; most severe ones are fatal. Details are dealt in *Chapter 21*. The recognition of foreign invader is only the first step of the immune system's attack; it must be followed by, steps that will kill and eliminate the invader. Thus immune system carried out two types of activities: *recognition process* directed against the invader and *destructive responses* that follow from the recognition and allow the system to mount an attack against the invader. Precise recognition is the function of *lymphocytes* while destruction is carried out both by lymphocytes and by cells called *macrophages* and *neutrophils*.

Consider an example, when a person gets wounded, within minutes after the blood stops flowing, the immune system begins its work to eliminate undesirable microbes introduced through the wound. Already on the scene (quick to arrive) are phagocytic white blood cells, known as macrophages. These cells not only engulf and destroy any invading microbes but also release proteins that activate other parts of the immune system and alert other phagocytes that they may be needed. This fast response of immune system is called *innate or natural immunity* because the cells that execute it are already active in the body before an invader appears. All animals possess a defensive mechanism of this kind, which is believed to be the most ancient form of immunity (Chapter 2). Another component of innate immunity is known as *complement system.* It is composed of more than 30 proteins in the blood, which work in succession like cascade, to identify and destroy invaders. This has been dealt in greater details in *Chapter 15.*

Innate immunity usually suffices to destroy invading microbes. If it does not, vertebrates rely on another response: *acquired immunity (Chapter 3).* The soldiers of acquired immunity are the specialized white blood cells called lymphocytes that function together as an army against the invaders. Moving through the blood and lymph glands, lymphocytes are normally at rest, but they become active and multiply if they encounter specific molecules called antigens that are associated with the invading organisms. Lymphocytes are of two classes-B and T. B-lymphocytes secrete antibodies-defensive proteins that bind to antigens and help to eliminate them. The human body usually contains more than 100 billion B-lymphocytes, each of which secretes an antibody that is different from most of the others. It has been dealt in greater details in *Chapter 10.* T lymphocytes serve a variety of purposes; they recognize and kill cells bearing non-self molecules on their surface or the cells infected by virus, bacteria or any intracellular parasites. Cytotoxic T cells and NK cells help in killing the infected cells thereby getting rid of the pathogen. They also mount an immune reaction on cancerous cells and kill them too. Cytotoxic T cells and NK cells also bind to cells to which already the antibody molecule is bound and they kill the antibody bound cell, which is called antibody dependent cell-mediated cytotoxicity. This property of T cells is dealt in greater detail in Effector responses of T cells in *Chapter 13.*

Acquired immunity also has a hall mark trait called immunologic memory, which arises from the DNA based mechanisms that allows the body's lymphocytes to recognize diverse antigens even though each lymphocyte recognizes only one type of antigen. Essentially, each encounter with an invading germ stamps a genetic "blueprint" on to certain T and B-lymphocytes. The next time these cells encounter that same invader or its antigen, they use the blueprint in such a way that the response occurs faster and more powerfully than it did the first time. This is what is referred as immunologic memory, which makes familiar booster shots, or immunizations given to the children. It is dealt in greater details in *Chapter 13.*

The injection of any foreign macromolecule (except pure DNA, Carbohydrates like starch and glycogen, pure lipids or fats and homopolymer chain of peptides of aliphatic amino acids) into an animal elicits the formation of both antibodies and immune cells that specifically bind to that substance. The substance that provokes antibody or lymphocyte formation, or is recognized by an antibody or lymphocytes, is called an *antigen.* The details of qualities of an antigen and what qualifies to be an antigen are dealt in *Chapter 5.* Just simply encountering the antigen by the lymphocyte does not suffice to develop an immune response. The antigen needs to be recognized by the T cells, which occurs through interaction of class I or class II MHC molecule with the T cell receptor. Class I or class II MHC molecules carry in their groove processed antigen in the form of micropeptide and this processing takes place within an antigen presenting cell or a target cell infected by the virus or pathogen. The mechanism of antigen processing and presentation to T cells by the target cells as well as by the antigen presenting cells is dealt in greater details in *Chapter 12.*

During the development of cell-mediated and humoral immune response against an antigen, there is effective communication or talk going on between different types of cells involved in immune response.

Phagocytes on encountering the antigen get activated and start secreting certain chemical messengers called cytokines, which warn and trigger the T lymphocytes to wake up from inactive state and recognize the antigen. T cells in turn recognize the processed antigen presented by the phagocytes or the antigen presenting cells. When the processed antigen is presented to T helper cells, they undergo stimulation and activation and start secreting varied kinds of cytokines. Some of these cytokines are not only essential for the T cells themselves to proliferate but also stimulate another arm of the immune response i.e. humoral response to develop. The details of the cytokines and their role in immune response are given in *Chapter 14.*

The humoral response develops from another kind of lymphocyte called B cells. These cells are also capable of recognizing the antigen on their own but for the great majority of antigens they need T helper cell assistance to undergo activation and proliferation. The maturation, activation, and differentiation of B cells are given in greater details in *Chapter 10.*

The activated mature B lymphocyte undergoes differentiation to form plasma cells and starts secreting different classes of antibodies, which are specific for antigenic epitopes. The details of different classes of antibodies and their physico-chemical properties are given in detail in *Chapter 7.* These antibodies are secreted into the body fluid and they freely circulate. In the bargain, whenever these antibody molecules encounter an antigen against whose epitopes they have been produced they immediately react and form antigen-antibody complex and get rid of the antigen from the body. The mechanism of antigen-antibody interactions and the techniques used for the study of antigen-antibody interactions are dealt in *Chapter 8.*

Most wonderful aspect of the immune system is its ability to produce antibodies and receptors of different specificities against different types of antigens. The whole mechanism of production of antibodies and the appropriate receptors for encountering the antigen rests on the genetic milieu of the B and T lymphocytes. The genes responsible for the production of antibodies and the receptors are capable of undergoing rapid gene rearrangements so that at any given time some of the permutation and combination of these gene rearrangements produce productive proteins responsible for the immunoglobulin or receptor formation. The details of gene rearrangements for the production of antibodies is given in *Chapter 9* and the details of gene rearrangement for the production of T cell and B cell receptors to recognize the antigen is given in *Chapter 11.*

Immune system in an individual consists of many structurally and functionally diverse organs and tissues that are widely distributed throughout the body. These organs belong to two groups, primary lymphoid organs and secondary lymphoid organs. The primary lymphoid organs provide appropriate microenvironment for lymphocyte maturation, whereas, secondary lymphoid organs trap antigens and provide sites where mature lymphocytes can interact effectively with that antigen. The detail of this complicated system, which prepares cells to defend in our body, is given in *Chapter 4.*

The immune system also prevents tissue transplantation between individuals. This is because every vertebrate individual has a unique set of molecule called major and minor histocompatibility complex on the surface of the cells (*details are given in Chapter 6*). The immune system recognizes those cells as self, but grafted cells from other individuals, even of the same species, are seen as foreign and are killed, or rejected. Inhibition of this rejection reaction is necessary when grafts are attempted between non-related individuals. Without special treatment, the only transplants that are accepted without a rejection reaction are those from an identical twin and immunologically privileged sites like cornea. It is covered in greater details in *Chapters 19.*

The immune system also has other abilities besides the recognition and killing of invading pathogens. It can kill cancer cells, and in experimental animals at least, it can protect the body against certain tumors. This forms a different chapter altogether, which is dealt in greater detail in *Chapter 20.*

As a consequence of immune reaction in the body once in a while an individual may develop severe reactions with respect to a particular antigen, which has entered second time into the same individual, whose body had activated T lymphocytes and circulating antibody against that antigen at higher level. In such cases individual shows certain reactions called as *allergy or hypersensitivity*. Details are given in *Chapter 18*.

If one has to understand immune system, one needs to answer some key questions. How does the immune system recognize different types of pathogens? How does it discriminate foreign matter from endogenous material, self from non-self? How does it translate the information of recognition of a foreign invader into a killing reaction? How does it learn, so that the second attack by the same invader is repulsed so much faster than the first? Answers to some of these questions are partly known for instance how recognition develops, but it is not well known how the system avoids reacting with the self-components. This has been dealt in greater details with recent evidences and concepts in *Chapter 17*.

Finally, the importance of an immune system and the fine tuned balance between various effector mechanisms involved in the immune system could be understood only when these systems fail. This can be understood that from studying various immuno deficiency diseases and the fatalities associated with these immunodeficiency diseases. Details of this are given in *Chapter 22*.

ORIGIN OF IMMUNE SYSTEM IN INVERTEBRATES

In 1882 a Russian zoologist named Elie Metchnikoff took a stroll along the beach in Messina, a town on Sicily northeastern coast. While walking on the beach he had collected a tiny transparent larva of starfish, he pierced the little creature with a rose thorn while returning to his cottage. When he examined the larva next morning, he saw minute cells covering the thorn as though they are going to engulf it. He immediately recognized the significance of this process. The cells covering the thorn were attempting to defend the larva by ingesting the invader, which is called as phagocytosis. Phagocytosis is in fact a fundamental mechanism by which creatures throughout the animal kingdom defend themselves against infection. From this work of Metchnikoff the birth of cellular immunology began. For his work in this field he shared the 1908 Nobel Prize in medicine with Paul Ehrlich the proponent of the importance of humoral immune response in immunity.

The starfish is an invertebrate animalcule that has remained unchanged since its appearance at least 600 million years ago. Metchnikoff thought that the phagocytic response shown by the cells of starfish larva is not much different than it would have been in the earth's primordial sea tens of millions of years before the first living things with backbones (vertebrates) appeared. Metchnikoff visualized that the host defense systems of all modern animals have their roots in countless creatures that have populated this planet since life began. From this idea yet another branch of science was born i.e., *comparative immunology*. This gives us insight and enables us to understand from a different perspective one of the most complex of all evolutionary creations: the immune systems of humans and other higher mammals. This discipline also gives insights into nature of evolution of invertebrates and vertebrates. The invertebrates make up more than 90 percent of all the earth's species. Moreover, comparative immunology has led scientists to uncover several immune related substances that seem to show some promise for human use.

Immune System in the Beginning

The immune system of higher vertebrate's i.e., mammals can be broken down into two components: innate and acquired. The latter includes immunologic memory as a significant distinguishing characteristic from the invertebrates. Many different agents, as you know mediate the immune response, macrophages and other phagocytic cells, B and T lymphocytes, antibodies and a multitude of other participating proteins. The major question that bothers comparative immunologist is how often these features or similar ones appear in other individuals and the ancient group of organisms? It is observed that many groups of organisms belonging to different classes show similarity in certain elements of immunity. Other features are unique to higher vertebrates but bear intriguing similarities to invertebrate host defense systems. These similarities are important from the evolutionary point of view, which suggest that the invertebrate mechanisms are precursors of the corresponding ones in the vertebrates. This shows that the immune system of the other mammals and humans evolved from more ancient creatures over hundreds of millions of years.

Host defense system must have originated since the advent of life with protozoans on this earth. Protozoans are single cell life forms, which go back to 2.5 billion years and they accomplish every physiological function in just one cell. The process of phagocytosis at least in part shown by protozoans during respiration, excretion, digestion and defense is almost similar to the phagocytosis shown by phagocytic cells in humans. In the animal kingdom, from starfish to humans, phagocytic cells travel through a circulatory system or fluid filled body cavity or coelom (starfish). In metazoans, which do not possess body cavity and circulatory system (sponges), the phagocytic cells patrol the tissues and surrounding spaces by wandering through them. Similar feature is observed in higher organisms like mammals, where macrophages do the same.

Another fundamental aspect of the immune system is its ability to distinguish between self and the non-self, which also dates back to early history of life on earth. Some protozoans are colonial forms (live in colonies); thousands of them will live in one colony. In such condition they must be able to recognize one another, thus it is very likely that they should have this ability to recognize each other to live together. Even the sponges, one of the oldest and simplest metazoans can distinguish self from non-self: its cells can attack graft from other sponges. This rejection response shown by sponges and jellyfishes is not similar to that found in vertebrates. In vertebrates, because of immunologic memory, if one graft from a donor is rejected, a second response for the graft from the same donor will be much quicker than the first one. In sponges and jellyfish, however, the second response of rejection is no faster than the first. The results suggest that the memory component of the immune system of vertebrates is missing in the invertebrates. This conclusion is supported by experimental evidence from starfish and other higher invertebrates, which also lack immunologic memory.

Two other important components of the vertebrate immune system i.e., complements and lymphocytes are also missing from invertebrates, but for both these components invertebrates seem to have analogues. Several phyla of invertebrates including various insects, crabs and worms, in place of complements are known to possess *prophenoloxidase* (proPO) system. Like the complement system, proPO is activated by a series of enzymes and a cascade of reaction ends with the conversion of proPO to the fully active enzyme *phenoloxidase*, which plays a role in encapsulating foreign objects. Recent discoveries have shown that proPO system serves other purposes as well, such as, blood coagulation and killing of microbes.

The other component of the immune system i.e., lymphocytes and an antibody based humoral immune system is lacking in invertebrates. Nevertheless, they do have lymphocyte like cells, which are found in earthworms-which probably appeared 500 million years ago. Most significantly almost all invertebrates have molecules that appear to be functioning like antibody molecules and may be their forerunners. These protein molecules are called as *lectins,* which can bind to sugar molecules on cells, thereby making the cells sticky and causing them to agglutinate (clump). Lectins are ubiquitous and they might have evolved quite early since the origin of life, because they are found in plants, bacteria and vertebrates, in addition to invertebrates.

The exact role of lectins in immune response is not well known, but they are known to play a part in tagging invading organisms, which are probably covered with different types of carbohydrate molecules. Lectins isolated from invertebrates such as, earthworms, snails and clams are known to participate in coating the foreign particle and hence enhance phagocytosis. Chemical constitution of lectins, vary from species to species in the animal kingdom due to variation in carbohydrate moieties of each type of lectin. It is observed that the lectins isolated from the flesh fly *(Sarcophaga peregrina)* and from the sea urchin are related to a family of vertebrate proteins called *collectins*. Collectins play an important role in innate immune response in humans by coating over the microbes; they make them accessible for phagocytosis and also in the activation of immune cells or complements.

Invertebrates do not have antibodies in their immune system, but molecules resembling antibodies have been detected. The antibody like molecules have characteristic structure called Ig (immunoglobulin) fold. The Ig fold probably evolved during the metazoan evolution and is involved in recognition of self and the non-self. The fold might have been originally a pattern recognition molecule involved in identification of self. The same molecule, later, might have evolved into an antigen recognition molecule by setting the stage for the emergence of true immunoglobulins. Ig molecules belong to immunoglobulin superfamily. A protein called *haemolin* isolated from the haemolymph of moths is a member of immunoglobulin superfamily. Like lectins, it binds to microbial surfaces and participated in their removal. Such immunoglobulin superfamily molecules have been detected in many invertebrates. These observations suggests that antibody like immune response took its origin in invertebrates and became a true antibody based response in vertebrates immune defense mechanisms.

Precursors of immune regulation

In the evolution of animal organization it appears that, higher vertebrates have conserved not only many aspects of host defense mechanisms found in invertebrates but also the control signals involved in immune system. The cells involved in immune response are known to release different types of protein factors called *cytokines*, which are responsible for stimulation or inhibition of other cells involved in the immune system to bring in a coordinated effort to curtail infection. Some of the cytokines involved in immune regulation include interferons (IFNs), interleukins (IL) and tumor necrosis factor (TNF). Beck and Habicht during their extensive work on invertebrate cytokine system, hypothesized that invertebrate immune system should also possess interleukin-1 (IL-1) or similar molecule for several reasons. First and the foremost, IL-1 regulates some of the primitive mechanism of vertebrate immunity. Second, the structure and the function of IL-1 are similar in many vertebrates belonging to different groups. This suggests that the IL-1 might have evolved from a common precursor right from invertebrates to vertebrates by conserving certain genes. Most important of all, the macrophages, which produce IL-1 on encountering the antigen, are ubiquitous throughout the animal kingdom.

Beck and Habicht in their investigation on invertebrate immune system found a molecule resembling IL-1 in the coelomic fluid of Atlantic starfish. This molecule behaved like IL-1 in many respects: its physical, chemical and biological properties were the same as compared to vertebrate IL-1. It could stimulate the vertebrate immune cells, which respond to vertebrate IL-1. Antibodies against vertebrate IL-1 are also capable of recognizing this molecule. Subsequently they have found that many invertebrates possess molecules similar to vertebrate cytokines. Beck has found molecules resembling IL-1 and IL-6 in the tobacco hornworm. Worms and tunicates (ascidians) carry substances similar to IL-1 and TNF.

As shown in the illustration (Fig. 1.1), the invertebrate cytokines seems to perform functions similar to those found in vertebrates. Beck and Habicht found cells called coelomocytes in starfish, which are similar to macrophages that produce IL-1. Cooper and Raftos together with Beck and Habicht showed

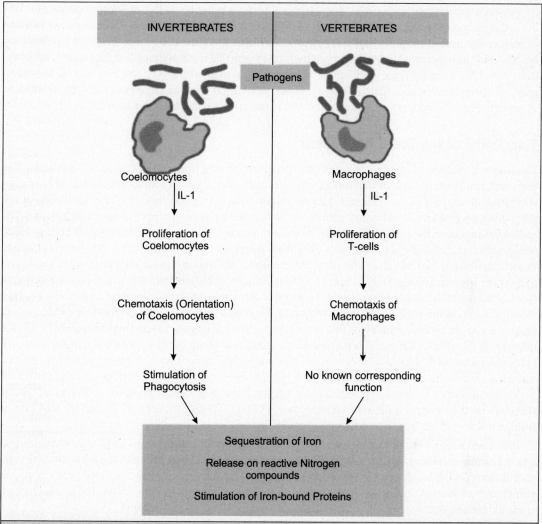

Fig. 1.1 Release of cytokine can stimulate many functions in invertebrates and vertebrates, which are almost similar in functions.

that IL-1 stimulates coelomocytes to engulf and destroy the invaders similar to the response shown by vertebrate macrophages against the invaders. Therefore, it appears that cytokines orchestrate much of their host defense response in invertebrates as vertebrate cytokines do in innate immune response.

ORIGIN OF VERTEBRATE IMMUNE SYSTEM

If we try to trace the vertebrate ancestry, some 500 million years ago the ancestors of all the jawed vertebrates appeared on this earth in the primitive seas. Some of the earliest known fossils of jawed vertebrates belonged to a group called placoderms. Placoderms took their origin from early jaw less vertebrates (lampreys and hagfish). Transition is the key for evolution, where new creatures evolve from the pre-existing ones with advanced characters and better adaptation to suit the new environment. It is likely that during this experimentation of nature in the vertebrate evolution that the simultaneous evolution of multicomponent of adaptive immune system took place. It is hard to imagine how such evolutionary success could have occurred in creatures with immune system that were anything less than usually effective. Litman and his team has been working on immune system of sharks and its relatives, one of the oldest group of vertebrates, perhaps 450 million years since their origin. They observed that the adaptive immune system of elasmobranchs (sharks, skates and rays) is as effective and efficient as in human beings.

Two Parts of the Immune System

The adaptive immune responses consist of two basic components, called humoral and cell-mediated. The humoral component is made of B-lymphocytes or B cells, which produce antibodies that bind to foreign substances or antigens such as potential harmful bacteria, bacterial toxins and viruses in the blood stream. Antibodies are also known as immunoglobulins; humans have five major types of immunoglobulins. The antibodies produced by a single B cell are of same type and bind to a specific antigen. B cells produce antigen binding (antibody like) receptors, which are projected on their membrane. Antigens on binding to these antibodies like receptors stimulate the B cells to undergo proliferation and produce antibodies against the antigen. Human body is known to have billions of B-lymphocytes, which produce different types of antibodies against different antigens. It is this incredible diversity among antigen receptors of the B-lymphocytes gives such a vast range of humoral immune response. This diversity of production of antigen receptors by B-lymphocytes lies in its genes and its ability to mutate (hypermutability). On the other hand, the cellular immunity is carried out by a different group of cells, termed T lymphocytes or T cells. In contrast to B cells, T cells do not produce antibodies; rather they recognize antigens bound to a molecule, known as class I and class II MHC (major histocompatibility complex) on the surface of different kinds of cells. To recognize this molecule the T lymphocytes are equipped with special type of receptors on their surface called T cell receptors (TCRs). Typical functions of T cells are rejection of foreign tissue graft, killing of tumor cells, cytotoxicity etc.

Individual specific immune response relies on the types of immunoglobulins and T cells receptors that can recognize specific antigens. Although humoral and cell mediated immune response are different, they interact during building an immune response against a pathogen. For example T helper cells help in recognition of foreign antigen and building B cell response against it. Any failure in this mechanism leads to immune deficiency as in AIDS (acquired immune deficiency syndrome).

Litman and his team found that, to some extent there seems to be similarity in the immune system of elasmobranchs and humans. As in humans, these fishes have spleen, which is the source of B-lymphocytes and when immunized with antigens, their B cells respond by producing antibodies. The similarities between humans and elasmobranchs have also been observed in cellular immunity. Like in humans, sharks and skates also possess thymus, in which T cell undergo maturation and T cells of sharks also have T cell receptors. Recent work of Litman and Rast showed that, as in humans, diversity in these receptors arise from the same type of genetic mechanisms that gives rise to antibody diversity. They also observed that skin grafted from one shark to another ultimately results in rejection, which is over a period of weeks but not quickly as in humans.

Besides similarities, there are significant differences in the immune system of cartilaginous fishes and humans. For e.g. Cartilaginous fishes have four different classes of immunoglobulins, of which only IgM class of antibody is common between humans and sharks. Furthermore, these shark antibodies lack the ability to recognize exquisitely specific antigens of bacteria with subtle differences. In addition shark antibodies lack the capacity of human antibodies to bind more and more strongly to an antigen during the course of a prolonged immune response, which is an added advantage in humans for fighting infections.

A receptor for every antigen

Litman and his team have been working on horned sharks for elucidating their humoral immune system. They observed in this shark, like in all vertebrates, the diversity in antigen receptor is genetic. Specifically, each antibody's antigen receptor is formed through the interaction of two peptide chains called as heavy and light. The basic antibody molecule has two antigen binding (receptor) sites. The binding ability of the receptor to antigen will depend on the sequence of amino acids at the site. The specific gene segments located in the B cell nucleus, known as antibody genes produce the receptor proteins for antigens. There are three types of gene segments, **V** segment or variable, **D**-diverse and **J**-joining. All the three gene segments encode the amino acids sequences in the heavy chains, whereas light chains are specified by V and J only. A fourth type of gene segment, designated as C (constant), determines the class of antibody.

V, D, J and C gene segments are located on the same chromosome in humans in clusters. For Ex. Some 50 functional V, 30 D, six J and 8 C elements in a single location occupying a million nitrogenous base pair sequences of the DNA ladder. When, an antibody is being produced by a B cell, various cellular mechanisms ensure the recombination of single V, D, and J segments adjacent to a C segment in a multistep process. The recombination of these gene segments determines the antigen binding characteristics of the antibody. This recombination of V, D, J elements in humans, is an important factor in antigen receptor diversity (Fig. 1.2)(See Chapter 9 for more details).

In sharks, too, the antibody gene segments are organized in clusters. However, heavy chain cluster in sharks, contains only one V segment, two Ds, a single J and a single C. There are more than 100 such clusters distributed on different chromosomes in sharks. When, a B cell produces an antibody in sharks, only the four gene segments (V, D1, D2 and J) from a single cluster are recombined and the C segment is already linked to J. The recombination of V, D1, D2 and J elements found in one cluster in shark could be the probable reason why sharks immune system does not have great diversity of antigen receptors (Fig. 1.2). Of course, there are hundreds of different antibody gene clusters spread over several different chromosomes of sharks. Furthermore, neither sharks nor mammalian immune system rely on recombinatorial diversity to generate many different antibodies. In fact, in cartilaginous fishes, two other significant mechanisms exist for fostering this diversity; they are termed junctional diversity and inherited diversity.

The junctional diversity occurs when the V and D or D and J segments come together. At the point where the junction occurs, where two segments unite, before fusion, several base pairs of DNA are removed and new ones are introduced in a random manner. This localized alteration leads to change in amino acid sequence, which is the characteristic of the antigen receptor. For this reason, the real advantage lies in the extra D gene segment in shark antibody producing system. With four different gene segments, there are three places where this diversity can occur, i.e., between V and D1, D1 and D2, and D2 and J. Due to which, millions of different variants of antibody molecules are produced, each possessing different receptor structure, created by each cluster. On the other hand, and D segments and D and J. Therefore, junctional diversity leads to somewhat less variation in mammals. This ability to generate many different antibodies will give protection against vast array of foreign invaders. But in practice it may take a long time to generate enough antibodies, select the best ones, expand their numbers and then deal with the invading pathogen. There is a possibility of loosing a race against the infectious agent.

In order to prevent the host from losing the race, body relies on a separate mechanism, which rapidly selects the blue print of the antibody needed at that time. This blue print is first expressed by one B cell

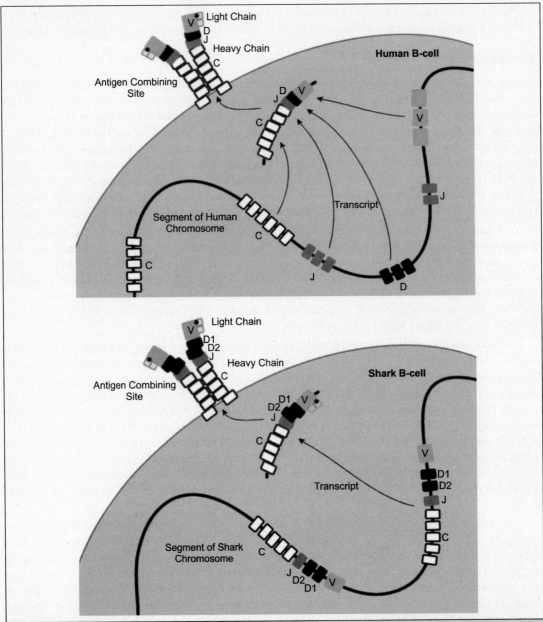

Fig. 1.2 Comaparison of human and shark antibody gene system. Note the differences in the arrangement of the gene segments that recombine to produce antigen receptors. A simplified version of formation of heavy chain molecule that makes up the part of the receptor is shown, which is an IgM antibody common between humans and sharks. In humans the gene segments that come together are scattered along a relatively long length of one chromosome. In sharks the gene segments are already next to one another on any one of several chromosomes.

among the body's billions. Elasmobranchs on the other hand, rely on inherited diversity. This is the most distinctive feature of the shark immune system, which allows the animals to avoid depending on a chance occurrence. In sharks, greater percentage of gene clusters in every cell is inherited with their V, D1, D2 and J gene segments, which are already pre-joined entirely or partially. In such gene clusters, there is limited chance or none at all for junctional diversity. Combinatorial, junctional and inherited forms of diversity are not only the diversity producing mechanisms; there also exists other mechanism in the two types of gene clusters, i.e. mutation. It occurs at a very high frequency in the antibody genes of higher vertebrates and is directed at altering the characteristics of the antigen receptor sites of the antibodies, i.e. hyper-variable region. One interesting comparative observation of human and shark humoral immune system is that 450 million years of evolution has added relatively little changes to the antibody molecule that the protein structure of shark and human antibodies are very similar. Moreover, the V, D and J sequences of gene segments that encode the antibody protein are similar. The evolutionary process has only radically altered the way these gene segments that specify antibodies are organized; especially it has laid greater emphasis on junctional and inherited diversity in sharks.

Comparative cellular immune response

T cells and antibodies both have receptors that are specified by the similar genes. The basic mechanism of gene segment rearrangement that produces antibody molecules with varied diversity also creates T cell receptors. Unlike antibody molecule, T cell receptor is found only on the cell's surface and is responsible for recognition of foreign substance bound to the special protein molecule (MHC) on a different cell surface. The affinity for foreign molecule shown by the T cell receptor is relatively low in comparison to some antibodies. The T cell receptor molecule does not show mutation in the same manner as antibodies. Litman and his colleagues recently found that all four classes of mammalian T cell antigen receptors are also found in skates and sharks. Extensive characterization of one of the T cell receptors of sharks showed it to be complexly diversified as its human equivalent. This indicates that in contrast to antibody gene organization, T cell receptor gene seem to have undergone limited changes since the time of evolution of sharks some 450 million years ago. Recent studies have also shown that genes belonging to different clusters responsible for immune system have undergone various types of recombination with one another during evolution. With hundreds of clusters and plenty of genome, recombination between various clusters may have been a very efficient way of generating novel gene clusters. It is possible, with the help of modern available molecular biology techniques such as PCR, that many more receptors in the shark immune system will be discovered in future.

In shark, the peculiar redundancy of different immune receptor gene clusters and the groupings of essentially identical V, D1, D2 and J segments repeated over and over again on various chromosomes, which shows recombination affords a means for rapidly evolving new families of receptor molecules. In mammalian system the gene segments are isolated to a single chromosome, and there is hardly any redundancy, which means the opportunity for this type of recombination is remote. Furthermore, the hallmark of the mammalian immune system i.e., the existence of multiple gene segments as Vs, Ds and Js due to duplication appears to come at the time of introduction and retention of significant numbers of nonfunctional genetic elements. On the other hand, in elasmobranchs nonfunctional elements are uncommon or probably lost quickly from the genome.

As surviving representatives of a very ancient line of vertebrate evolution, sharks and skates and their relations may be our only remaining link to the distant origins of T and B cell immunity. In addition to this, immune system that is found in other vertebrates is summarized in Table 1.1.

Table 1.1 Comparison of immune features in vertebrates

Immune features	Agn	Chon	Ost	Anu	Rep	Ave	Mam
Non-self recogntn.	P	P	P	P	P	P	P
Immune memory	P	P	P	P	P	P	P
MHC	A	A	P	P	A	P	P
IgM	1	1, 5	4, 5	5, 6	5	5	5
IgG	A	A	A	P	P	P	P
IgA, IgE, IgD	A	A	A	A	A	A	P
Secondary response	A	A	A	P	P	P	P
Thymus	A	P	P	P	P	P	P
Spleen	A	P	P	P	P	P	P
Bone marrow	A	A	A	P	P	P	P
Lymph nodes	A	A	A	P	P	P	P

P = Present; A = Absent; IgM (1= monomer; 4= tetramer; 5= pentamer; 6= hexamer)

Exercise

1. Give a brief account of (5 marks each):
   (a) Immune system of invertebrates
   (b) Immune system of vertebrates
2. Give a comparative account of invertebrate and vertebrate immune system (20 marks)
3. Write a comparative, illustrated account of shark and human immunoglobulin gene and immune system (20 marks)

Chapter 2

Innate Immunity

- Non-immunological Surface Protective Mechanisms (Anatomical Barriers)
- Antimicrobial Peptides in Mammalian System
- Immunogenic Innate Immune Response (Physiologic Barrier)
- Innate Immune Response Against Blood Group Antigens
- Innate Immune Response through Alternate Pathway of Complement
- Interferons in Innate Immune Response
- Natural Killer Cells (NK Cells) in Innate Immune Response
- Contribution of T-cells Bearing γδT-cell Receptors to Innate Immune Response
- Mast Cells and their Role in Innate Immunity
- Mechanism of Innate Immune Recognition
- Control of Effector Cytokines by Innate Immune System

Resistance to certain infection is a natural phenomenon and it is called innate immunity, it is called first line of defense. The mechanism of its development is not known. Innate immunity may be species specific, race specific or individual specific.

Species specific innate immunity

Human beings are naturally resistant to *Distemper virus*, which causes 30-50% deaths in dogs. Birds are immune to tetanus, which is fatal to human beings. Birds are also immune to anthrax, because of their high body temperature, which inhibits the growth of the pathogen.

Individual specific innate immunity

Some differences in individuals of same species occur with regard to susceptibility for certain infections. For e.g., individuals of heterozygous trait of sickle cells anemia, thalassemia and deficiency of glucose-6-phosphate dehydrogenase are resistant to some type of malaria. Individuals of blood group O and B are more resistant to small pox than those of blood group A.

A number of innate defense mechanisms are operative non-specifically against a large number of microorganisms. They are:

1. Mechanical barriers (Surface protective mechanisms).
2. Antagonism of indigenous flora.

3. Microbicidal substances of the body fluids and those liberated by damaged cells.
4. Phagocytosis by macrophage.

Immunity at body surfaces

This is also called as first line of immune response because it occurs on body surfaces and prevents various types of diseases. There are two types of surface protective mechanisms, namely, non-immunological and immunological.

Non-immunological Surface Protective Mechanisms (Anatomical Barriers)

This occurs at skin surface, gastrointestinal tract, urinogenital tract, mammary gland and respiratory tract.

The Skin: It acts as a major barrier to various invading microorganisms. On the surface of the skin dense population of resident bacterial growth occurs which is regulated by low pH due to the presence of sebum, desiccation, desquamation etc. If any of these properties are altered due to various environmental factors, its protective properties are reduced and infection through skin may occur. Those who stand in water for long hours are prone to fungal infection in the sodden part of the skin. Infection in groin and axilla are generally high because of relatively high pH and humidity in the area.

Gastrointestinal tract: The resident flora of bacteria of gastrointestinal tract plays an important role in control of potential pathogens but also for the digestion of some food like cellulose in herbivores. In addition, the natural development of the immune system depends on continuous antigenic stimulus provided by intestinal flora. The flora of the digestive tract normally acts competitively against potential invaders through mechanisms that supplement the other physical defenses of this system. In the mouth flushing action of the saliva stimulate streptococci to produce peroxides. In the stomach, the gastric juices maintain sufficiently low pH to have bactericidal and viricidal action. Some food substances such as milk, buttermilk and curd are potent buffers.

In the intestine, the resident bacterial flora ensures that the pH is sufficiently low and the anaerobic condition is maintained. The intestinal flora is also influenced by the diet, for e.g. Milk fed animals show colonization of intestine largely by lactobacilli, which produce large quantities of lactic acid and butyric acid. These acids inhibit the colonization of intestine by pathogenic E. coli. The antibacterial and antiviral lysozymes are synthesized in the gastric mucosa and in macrophages within the intestinal mucosa. As a result it is found in large quantities in intestinal fluid. Macrophages can migrate through the intestinal wall and may be active for a short time within the lumen.

Urinogenital tract: In the lumen of the urinogenital tract, the flushing action of the urine and maintenance of low pH provide adequate protection. In adult women, vaginal wall is lined by squamous epithelium composed of rich amount of glycogen. When these cells desquamate, they provide a substrate for lactobacilli that in turn generate large quantities of lactic acid, which protects the vaginal passage against invasion. Glycogen storage in the vaginal epithelium is stimulated by estrogen and thus occurs only in adult women. Because of this, vaginal infections tend to be most common before puberty and after menopause.

Mammary gland: In the mammary gland, flushing action of milk prevents invasion by some potential pathogens, while milk itself contains bacterial inhibitors, which are called lactenins. The lactenins include complement, lysozymes, and the iron binding protein lactoferrin and the enzyme lactoperoxidase. The lactoferrin competes with bacteria for iron and therefore, render it unavailable for their growth. It also enhances respiratory activity in neutrophils. Lactoperoxidase and thiocyanate ions of milk in the presence of exogenous hydrogen peroxide get activated and lactoperoxidase reacts on thiocyanate and converts it into bacteriostatic sulfur dicyanide. Some bacteria are resistant to this pathway because they can reduce thiocyanate ions. IgA has the ability to enhance the activity of lactoperoxidase. The phagocytic cells released into the mammary gland in response to irritation caused by sucking stimulus may also contribute to antimicrobial resistance not only through their phagocytic action but also by producing lactoferrins, hydrogen peroxide, and lysosomal peroxidase.

Respiratory tract: The respiratory tract provides unhindered access of air to the alveoli and it differs from other systems, because of its intimate contact with the interior of the body. The air entering the respiratory tract is largely deprived of any suspended particles by turbulence that directs the particles on to the mucous covered walls, where they adhere. This turbulence filter removes particles as small as 5 μm before they reach the alveoli. A layer of mucous covers the wall of the upper respiratory tract, produced by goblet cells and provided with antiseptic properties through its content of lysozymes and IgA. This mucous layer is continuously produced and moves up in the respiratory tract and reaches the pharynx where, it is swallowed. Particles smaller than 5μm that can by pass this mucous layer reach the alveoli are phagocytosed by alveolar macrophages.

In spite of all these protective anatomical barriers, there are some organisms, which have evolved various strategies to escape these defense mechanisms and invade the body through mucous membrane surface. For example, *influenza* virus which causes flu in humans is known to have surface molecules that enable it to attach itself to cells in mucous membrane, thereby preventing it from getting swept away by the mucous secretion of ciliated epithelial cells. Adherence of bacteria to the mucous membrane is facilitated by hair like projections on bacterial cell wall called fimbriae or pili, which interact with certain glycoproteins or glycolipids expressed on the mucous membrane of the some epithelial cells. Therefore, some tissues are susceptible to bacterial invasion. For example, mucous membrane epithelial lining of the urinogenital tract is susceptible to infection by *gonorrhea*, which has surface projections that allows it to attach to mucous membrane lining of UG tract.

Antimicrobial Peptides in Mammalian System

The cells of many animals produce various antimicrobial substances that act as endogenous, natural antibiotics or disinfectants. These antimicrobial substances are micropeptides that contain fewer than 100 amino acids. Most of these peptides are zwitterions or amphipathic, therefore carry net positive charge while reacting and manifest themselves as α-helical or β-sheet in membrane like environment. The epithelial lining of GI tract, respiratory and genitourinary tracts produce some of these peptides. Others are produced together with the glandular secretions that moisten and lubricate these systems. Antimicrobial peptides are also produced in abundance by the phagocytes and other cells, which kill the microbial invaders. The expression of antimicrobial peptides can be inducible or constitutive or both.

β-Sheet Peptides

These constitute mainly *defensins*, which exist in two forms, namely, α and β forms.

α-Defensins

There are six known human α-defensins (hADs), of which four of them belong to neutrophil α-defensins (HNP 1-4), exclusively produced by neutrophils or polymorphonuclear cells. Human a defensin (hAD-5) and hAD-6 are produced constitutively by secretory *Paneth* cells found within small intestinal crypts. hAD-5 is expressed constitutively in the vagina and ectocervix. In the endocervix, endometrium and fallopian tube the concentrations of hAD-5 peaks during the secretory phase of the menstrual cycle. This suggests that expression is modulated by hormonal factors.

β-defensins

Human β-defensin (hBD-1) is synthesized in the loop of Henle, distal tubules and collecting tubules of the kidney. High concentrations of hBD-1 are also found in the vagina, cervix, uterus and fallopian tubes. Human urine contains various isoforms of hBD-1 containing 36-47 amino acid residues at a concentration of 10-100µg/l. Similar hBD-1 isoforms have been identified in the plasma and vaginal secretions, where they are bound to macrocarriers. An hBD expressed by pulmonary epithelia and submucosal glands (hBD-2) was detected in the airway surface fluid of human lung. The fully processed peptide had broad spectrum, salt-sensitive antibacterial activity and showed synergy with lysozyme and lactoferrin.

Cathelicidins

Cathelin is an acronym of cathepsin L inhibitor and cathelin-containing precursor of antimicrobial peptides. They are called Cathelicidins. Cathelicidins are found to be active against Gram-negative and Gram-positive organisms including, *Pseudomonas aeruginosa* and it is presumed that it acts synergistically with lactoferrin and lysozyme.

Protegrins

They are broad-spectrum antimicrobial peptides produced by neutrophils, where they are stored as cathelin containing precursors.

Granulysin

It is found in granules of human cytolytic T lymphocytes and natural killer cells. These peptides belong to saposin like protein family. Acting in combination with perforins it is known to gain access to the intracellular compartment of microorganisms and kill them. The combination of Granulysin and perforin may equip T cells to kill many intracellular pathogens.

Histatins

These are small, histidine-rich, human salivary proteins that display moderate activity against *Candida albicans* at acidic pH, under relatively low ionic strength. The antifungal mechanisms of action of histatins are presently unclear.

Secretory leukoprotease inhibitor (SLPI)

SLPI was found to be active against *Aspergillus fumigatus* and *C. albicans*-acting preferentially against metabolically active fungal cells. SLPI also exhibits antimicrobial activity against various skin-associated microorganisms. LPS and lipotechoic acid from Gram-positive bacterial cell walls was fund to induce SLPI synthesis in murine macrophages.

Immunogenic Innate Immune Response (Physiologic Barrier)

In this immune response following categories of innate responses occur in an individual.

Antibodies against blood group antigens

Alternate pathway of complement system

Macrophages

Interferons

Natural killer cells

γδ T cells

CD5-B cells

Mast cells

Innate Immune Response against Blood Group Antigens

Presence of natural antibodies or Isohaemagglutinins against human blood groups is an innate response. Since the evolution of mankind these blood group antigens are present in human beings and against each antigen, human body naturally possess antibodies so as to prevent contamination of blood by opposite blood group through blood transfusion. Body mounts a violent immune response against opposite blood group once it is sensitized against it. This helps in the maintenance of uncontaminated blood in each individual. The antibodies against the opposite blood group are present in an individual since birth. Immunity of isohemagglutinins is shown in Table 2.1.

Table 2.1　Immunity shown by isohemagglutinins of blood group

Blood Group	Antibody	Antigen
A	B	A
B	A	B
AB	None	AB
O	A and B	None
Rh^+	None	DD or Dd
Rh^-	D	None

Innate Immune Response through Alternate Pathway of Complement

It is a first line of defense shown by alternative pathway of complement. Some surface proteins of microbes activate it in the absence of specific antibodies. Unlike the classical pathway, which depends on antigen-antibody complex formation to start the reaction it is an immediate response to counter the microbial infection. The reaction cascade is shown in the Fig. 2.1. **C3** complement is abundant in plasma and it is capable of spontaneous cleavage to produce **C3a** and **C3b**. Most of the **C3b** is inactivated by hydrolysis, but some of it reacts with the host cell membrane or the membrane of the pathogen through thioester bond. **C3b** bound in this manner is able to attract and bind factor **B**, which is cleaved into **Bb** and **Ba**, by serum protease factor **D**. **Bb** remains bound to **C3b** and **Ba** is released. Host cells are unaffected by the binding of **C3b**, **Bb** on their membrane as they express the membrane proteins **Decay Accelerating Factor** (DAF) and **membrane co-factor of proteolysis** (MCP) and also favor binding of factor **H** from serum. DAF and factor **H** displaces **Bb** from **C3b**, while MCP and factor **H** catalyzes the cleavage of bound **C3b** by factor **I** to produce inactive **C3bi**.

Microbial cells lack the protective proteins MCP and DAF, and factor **H**. Consequently **C3b, Bb** complex formed on the surface of the microbes is not dissociated and acts as active **C3/C5** convertase of classical complement pathway. Microbial cells also favor the binding of a positive component of the alternative pathway known as Properdin or factor **P**, which facilitates activation by binding to **C3b, Bb** complexes and stabilizing them, preventing their dissociation by factor **H** and subsequent cleavage by factor **I**. The stabilized **C3b, Bb** complex then acts in the same manner as **C3/C5** convertase of classical pathway and converts large number of **C3** molecules to **C3b**, which coat the adjacent surface and bind **C5**, inducing its cleavage and initiating lytic pathway. Once initiated, the alternative pathway can promote its own feed back regulation with bound **C3b** binding more **B** molecules, increasing the **C3/C5** convertase activity on the pathogens surface. This causes opsonization of bacterial cell membrane resulting in alteration of membrane property, ultimately leading to death of bacteria (Fig. 2.1).

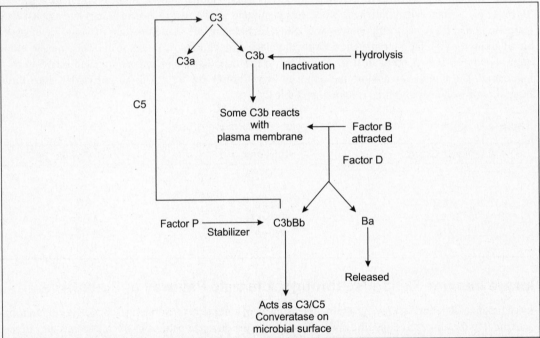

Fig. 2.1   A schematic representation of involvement of alternative pathway of complement in destruction of bacterium as an innate immune response.

Macrophage

The major function of macrophage is phagocytosis and endocytosis. Both these processes are yet another important innate immune mechanisms, which are internalization processes not only brings in different types of molecules into the cells but also differ in their actions in several ways.

Endocytosis

In this process macromolecules are internalized from the extracellular fluid through the receptors to which extracellular molecules bind and the plasma membrane undergoes inward folding together with molecule bound to receptor and create a exocytic vesicle (Fig. 2.2).

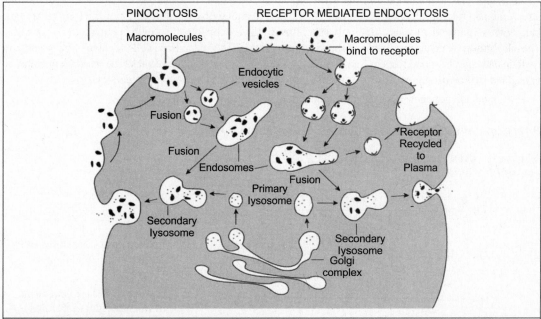

Fig. 2.2 A diagrammatic representation of process of receptor mediated endocytosis and non-receptor mediated phagocytosis

Endocytosis may occur in two ways: pinocytosis and receptor mediated endocytosis. In both cases endocytic vesicle formed is approximately 0.1μm in diameter. Pinocytosis is a nonspecific membrane invagination process at the site of extracellular molecule in proportion to their extracellular concentration. In receptor-mediated endocytosis, macromolecules are selectively internalized after binding to membrane receptors.

The endocytic vesicles fuse with the acidic chambers of lysosomes called *endosomes* in the cytoplasm. The acidic environment inside the endosomes facilitates dissociation of macromolecular bonds with their receptors. The dissociated receptors are returned back to the cell surface and the free molecules inside the endosomes are subjected to degradation by fusion of endosomes with *primary lysosomes*. The fusion results in the formation of *secondary lysosomes*.

Primary lysosomes originated from the Golgi complex and they are filled with large number of lytic enzymes, including proteases, nucleases, hydrolases and lipases. In the secondary lysosomes the macromolecules are digested by the lytic enzymes which, eventually thrown out of cell or utilized by the cell.

Phagocytosis

It involves ingestion of particulate matter including whole pathogenic microorganisms. In this process the plasma membrane of phagocytic cells extends over the particulate matter enclosing a *phagosome* or vesicle (Fig. 2.2). These vesicles are comparatively 10 to 20 times larger than the endocytic vesicles. Extension of plasma membrane in the form of pseudopodia over macromolecule involves cytoplasmic streaming and microfilaments, which do not take part in endocytosis. Another major difference between phagocytosis and endocytosis is that only specialized cells are capable of showing phagocytosis, whereas, virtually almost all cells are capable of showing endocytosis. The specialized cells capable of phagocytosis include neutrophils, monocytes in free circulation and macrophages in the tissues. The particulate material entrapped in phagosome with lysosomes and processed in a similar manner as endocytosis.

(1) Oxygen dependent, (2) Oxygen independent.

Reactions of the oxygen dependent mechanisms

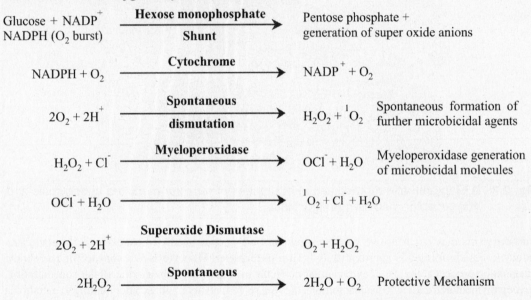

$$Glucose + NADP^+ \xrightarrow[\text{Shunt}]{\text{Hexose monophosphate}} \text{Pentose phosphate} + \text{generation of super oxide anions}$$
NADPH (O_2 burst)

$$NADPH + O_2 \xrightarrow{\text{Cytochrome}} NADP^+ + O_2$$

$$2O_2 + 2H^+ \xrightarrow[\text{dismutation}]{\text{Spontaneous}} H_2O_2 + {}^1O_2 \quad \text{Spontaneous formation of further microbicidal agents}$$

$$H_2O_2 + Cl^- \xrightarrow{\text{Myeloperoxidase}} OCl^- + H_2O \quad \text{Myeloperoxidase generation of microbicidal molecules}$$

$$OCl^- + H_2O \longrightarrow {}^1O_2 + Cl^- + H_2O$$

$$2O_2 + 2H^+ \xrightarrow{\text{Superoxide Dismutase}} O_2 + H_2O_2$$

$$2H_2O_2 \xrightarrow{\text{Spontaneous}} 2H_2O + O_2 \quad \text{Protective Mechanism}$$

From the circulating monocytes, macrophages mature continuously and migrate into tissues throughout the body. They are found in large numbers in connective tissue, liver and spleen. They are large phagocytic cells play a key role in all phases of host defense. Macrophages on their surface possess receptors for microbial constituents, immunoglobulins and complements, by which they engulf the opsonized particles. When pathogens cross an epithelial barrier, phagocytes in the sub-epithelial connective tissue with three important consequences recognize them. The first is the trapping, engulfment and destruction of pathogen by tissue macrophages, which therefore provide an immediate innate immune response. This response is sufficient to prevent infection. Intracellular killing takes place by two independent mechanisms:

Oxygen dependent mechanisms

With the formation of phagosome, there is a dramatic increase in activity of the hexose monophosphate (HMP) shunt, increased glycolysis and increased oxygen consumption, with an exaggerated formation of hydrogen peroxide, lactic acid and a subsequent fall in pH, which is a prerequisite for optimal functioning of hydrolytic enzymes. All this activity termed as *respiratory burst*. HMP shunt generates NADPH, which is ultimately utilized to reduce molecular oxygen bound to cytochrome, causing a burst of oxygen consumption. As a result oxygen is converted to superoxide anion (O_2*), hydrogen peroxide, singlet oxygen ($^1O_2$) and hydroxyl radicals (OH*), all of which are powerfully microbicidal agents. In addition to this, the combination of peroxides, myeloperoxidase and halide ions constitute a potent halogenating system capable of killing bacteria and viruses.

Oxygen independent mechanism

Lysozymes and lactoferrins as well as certain cationic proteins act as bacteriostatic substances, which are oxygen independent and function under anaerobic conditions. Finally, hydrolytic enzymes digest the killed organisms and the degraded products are released to the exterior.

For microbe to become pathogenic, it must devise strategies to avoid engulfment by phagocytes. Many extracellular bacteria coat themselves with a thick polysaccharide capsule that is not recognized by any phagocyte receptor molecule. The second important effect of interaction of tissue phagocytes with pathogens is the secretion of cytokines by the phagocytes. It is presumed that the pathogen induces cytokine secretion by binding to the same receptors used for engulfment.

Chemokines

They belong to a family of closely related proteins, which are released by monocytes in response to infection. They are also called *monokines*. They are not only released by macrophages but also by fibroblasts, epithelial cells (endothelial and keratinocytes) and smooth muscle cells. The chemokines act as chemoattractants for phagocytic cells, recruiting macrophages and neutrophils from blood to sites of infection. They are also known as *intercrines*. The chemokines fall into two categories, α and β distinguished by minor differences in structure and acting on different cell types. α-chemokines promote neutrophil migration, while β-chemokines promotes the migration of monocytes. (For details refer to Chapter 14).

IL-8 is α-chemokine and human macrophage chemoattractant and activating factor (MCAF) and other chemokines may promote the infiltration into tissues of other cell types including effector T-cells. Both IL-8 and MCAF activate their respective target cells, so that not only neutrophils and macrophages are brought to the potential sites of infection, but also in the process they are armed to deal with any pathogen they may encounter.

Interferons in Innate Immune Response

Interferons (IFN) are produced by variety of cells due to infection by viruses. They are proteins known to interfere with viral replication hence the name interferons. There are three different types of interferons, namely IFN-α, IFN-β and IFN-γ respectively. IFN-α consists of family of several closely related proteins, is synthesized by leukocytes upon exposure to viruses. Fibroblasts and many other cell types as a response to viral infection synthesize IFN β. Effector T- cells produce IFN-γ and it appears mainly after induction of the adaptive immune response (acquired immunity). IFN-α and β bind to a common receptor on cells and trigger the synthesis of several hosts cells proteins that contribute to the inhibition of viral regulation.

The second effect of interferons in host defense is to increase expression of the MHC (Major histocompatibility complex) class I complex and TAP transporter proteins, enhancing the ability of virus-infected cells to present viral peptides to CD8-T cells. Unlike interferon γ, however, interferon α and β do not induce synthesis of MHC class II proteins. The third property of interferons is the activation of natural killer cells.

Natural Killer Cells (NK Cells) in Innate Immune Response

NK cells are capable of killing certain lymphoid tumor cell lines *in vitro* without prior immunization or sensitization. NK cells function in host defense in the early phases of infection with several intracellular parasites, particularly herpes virus and *Listeria monocytogenes*. IFN-α, β and IL-12 are capable of increasing NK cell activity by 20 to 110 fold. IL-12 in synergy with the monokine-tumor necrosis factor α (TNF-α) can also elicit production of large amounts of interferon γ by NK cells, which plays a key role in controlling some infections before T-cells have been activated to produce this cytokine. Virus infected cells are made susceptible to NK cell killing by either of two mechanism. First, some viruses inhibit all host protein synthesis, so that enhanced class I MHC protein synthesis induced by interferon is selectively blocked in infected cells, which is recognized by NK cells. Second, some viruses, prevent export of class I MHC molecule to the membrane surface, which is recognized by NK cells and these cells are killed. There is also evidence that introduction of new peptides into self-MHC class I is detected by NK cells. This would allow infected cell to be detected even when MHC expression is not altered by infection.

Contribution of T-cells Bearing $\gamma\delta$T-cell Receptors to Innate Immune Response

In many species $\gamma\delta$T-cells are found in surface epithelia. Each epithelium has a homogeneous population of $\gamma\delta$T-cells. It is postulated that these cells recognize a self-protein that is expressed by infected but not normal cells in the epithelium. The infected cell is killed by $\gamma\delta$T-cells to prevent spread of infection. Candidate targets are MHC class 1B molecules, peptides of heat shock proteins or heat shock proteins themselves. Heat shock proteins are proteins expressed selectively by stressed cells, such as cells that are infected.

CD5-B Cell in Innate Immune Response

They form a separate lineage of B-cells marked by the cell surface proteins CD5 and produce antibodies to common bacterial proteins. These CD5-B cells are analogous to epithelial $\gamma\delta$T-cells. They arise very early in ontogeny of B-cells and are self replicating in the periphery. They are the predominant lymphocytes in the peritoneal cavity. CD5-B cells produce T-cell independent immune response and produce antibodies against polysaccharide antigens of bacteria. The predominant antibody produced is IgM type. And there is no class switching or somatic hyper mutation of immunoglobulin gene of variable region. This response appears within 48 hr of exposure to antigen, which is too soon for generation of antigen specific T- cells.

Inflammatory Response as Barrier

It is yet another innate immune mechanism, which involves complex sequences of events that occur collectively at the site of infection and tissue injury caused by the microbes. The series of events that involve in inflammatory response are vasodilation, increased capillary permeability and extravasation of phagocytes (Fig. 2.3).

1. **Vasodilation:**   At the site of injury, generally blood vessels show increase in diameter, especially the arteries carrying the blood toward the site of infection. On the other hand, blood vessels (veins)

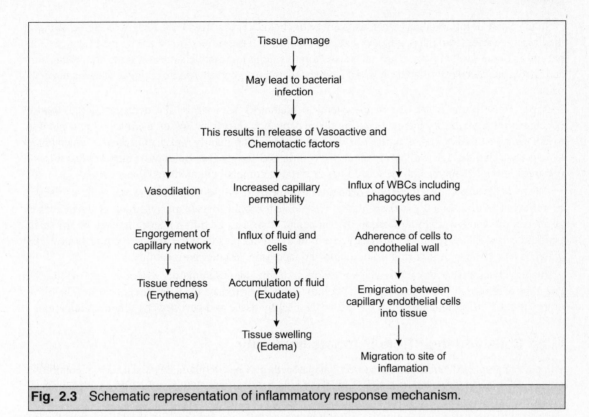

Fig. 2.3 Schematic representation of inflammatory response mechanism.

carrying blood away from the site constrict resulting in engorgement of capillaries with blood. The engorged capillaries are responsible for tissue redness or *erythema* and increased tissue temperature. Increased blood supply increases O2 tension at the site of infection and increased temperature acts as hindrance for microbial growth. This prevents spreading of infection.

2. **Increased capillary permeability:** This mechanism facilitates influx of fluids and defense cells such as, neutrophils and monocytes from the engorged capillaries into the tissue at the site of infection. The fluid that accumulates has higher protein content than the intravascular fluid (i.e., blood plasma). The accumulation of fluid contributes to the tissue swelling or edema.

3. **Extravasation of phagocytes:** From the blood capillaries *extravasation* or *diapedesis* of phagocytes into the tissue is facilitated by increased capillary permeability. The emigration of phagocytes from the intravascular space to extravascular space involves complex series of events. First, adherence of the phagocytic cells to the endothelial lining of the blood vessels called *margination.*

Second, emigration of phagocytes between the endothelial lining into the tissue is called as extravasation. Finally, the migration of phagocytes to the site of infection is called *chemotaxis.* Extensive phagocytic activity at the site of infection results in release of certain lytic enzymes and thereby localized tissue damage. This results in accumulation of dead cells, digested material and fluid, which forms a substance called *pus.*

In the event of inflammatory response variety of chemical mediators play a key role. Some of these mediators are released by the damaged cells in response to tissue injury, some are derived from several plasma enzymes systems, some are generated from invading microorganisms and some are products of activated white blood cells (neutrophils and monocytes) and macrophages participating in the inflammatory response.

Acute phase proteins are one of the chemical mediators released by the damaged tissue, whose concentration dramatically increases during tissue damaging infections. When the liver is damaged due to any parasitic or microbial infection, C-reactive protein predominantly makes its presence, which binds to C-polysaccharide, cell wall component of bacteria and fungi. This binding, results in clearance of pathogen through complement-mediated lysis or through complement mediated phagocytosis.

Histamine is also known to be one of the principal mediators of inflammatory response. It is released by variety of cells in response to tissue injury. Histamine is capable of causing vasodilation and increased permeability. Another important group of compounds that acts as inflammatory mediators are small peptides called *kinins* found in an inactive form in the blood plasma. One among them is *bradykinin*, which is also capable of inducing vasodilation and increased vascular permeability.

Increased vascular permeability and vasodilation during the inflammatory response also enables the enzymes of blood clotting mechanism to leak into tissue. They induce the formation of fibrin. The fibrin clots surround the injured area from the rest of the healthy tissue and prevents the spread of infection.

Mast Cells and their Role in Innate Immunity

Almost a century ago, Paul Ehrlich proposed that mast cells may help to maintain the nutrition of connective tissues and coined the term "mastzellen" i.e. well fed cells, because their cytoplasm is stuffed with prominent granules. Several years late Elie Metchnikoff suggested that mast cells are phagocytic and therefore contribute to host defense. At present, it is clear that mast cells can phagocytose and kill bacteria but the phagocytic efficiency of mast cells appears to be much less than the macrophages. It has been demonstrated *in vitro* that mast cells can process bacterial and other protein antigens and can function as antigen-presenting cells via mechanism that are dependent on MHC class I or class II. In addition to these properties, mast cells are exceedingly good at initiating inflammation. In Th2-cell associated responses, mast cells bind IgE antibodies via FcεRI receptors on the cells' surfaces. Aggregation of FcεRI by contact of cell-bound IgE with multivalent antigen has several effects:

* The rapid extracellular release of histamine, proteoglycans, proteases from the cytoplasmic granules
* Synthesis and secretion of leukotrienes and prostaglandins
* Synthesis and release of diverse array of cytokines

Mast cells can also be activated to release proinflammatory mediators and cytokines in response to activation by IgG-dependent mechanisms. These products can result in bronchoconstriction, increased gastrointestinal motility, changes in blood vessel tone, and increased vascular permeability and immunoregulatory effects. Malaviya and his co-workers showed three major mast cell functions, such as, clearance of virulent strain of *Klebesiella pneumoniae* from the lung*s* or peritoneal cavity of mice; mast cells can reduce the mortality associated with experimental intraperitoneal infection; and evidence was provided that the TNF-α that is released by mast cells, due to contact with bacteria is important in generation of influx of neutrophils. Bacterial products including LPS (lipopolysaccharide) and at least one fimbrial adhesin can directly induce the release of some mast cell products. Pathogens may also activate mast cells indirectly via activation of complement system

The innate immune system is believed to have predated the adaptive or acquired immune response on several grounds. First, innate host defense mechanisms are found in all multicellular organisms, whereas adaptive immunity is found only in vertebrates. Second, innate immunity can distinguish self from non-self perfectly, a condition not observed in adaptive immune response. Third, the receptors used in innate immune system are ancient in their lineage, whereas adaptive immune response uses the same gene family responsible for antibody and T-cell receptor production, which belongs to Ig gene superfamily.

Mechanism of Innate Immune Recognition

The evolution of immune system has taken place under tremendous selection pressure imposed by pathogens. The problem with recognizing pathogens is their enormous ability to undergo mutation and molecular heterogeneity. To cope with this, all multicellular organisms have developed the ability to recognize invading microbes and to eliminate them efficiently without causing any damage to self.

Firstly the innate immune system should recognize molecular structures that are shared by large groups of pathogens and therefore must represent molecular patterns rather than structures. Secondly these molecular patterns should be highly conserved molecules, which are byproducts of microbial metabolism and are not subjected to antigenic variability. Pathogens are unable to change these products because they are essential for pathogenicity and the survival of the microbes. Any attempt to change them will render the microbe non-pathogenic or kill it. Finally the most crucial part is the immune recognition, which helps in destruction of target, for which the structures or patterns that are recognized should be absolutely different from self-antigens.

The invariant molecular structures that are found in many pathogens that meet the requirements mentioned in the previous paragraph represent the main targets of innate immune recognition. They are called as *pathogen associated molecular patterns* (**PAMPs**). Some of the PAMPs that stimulate the innate immune responses are:

1. Lipopolysaccharides and teichoic acids are shared by all Gram – ve and Gram + bacteria.
2. The unmethylated CpG sequences are characteristic of bacterial DNA and not found in mammalian DNA.
3. Double stranded RNA is characteristic of RNA viruses. None of these structures are found in host organisms and all of them are shared by large groups of pathogens and they are absolutely essential for the microbes.

The host organisms have developed a set of receptors that can recognize PAMPs, it is indicative of presence of pathogens in the body. These receptors have broad specificity so that they can recognize wide variety of ligands, as long as ligands share a common molecular pattern. They are called as *pattern recognition receptors* (**PRRs**). PRRs are different from clonally selected antigenic receptors of T and B-lymphocytes. Their specificities are germ line encoded and they arise over a long course of time due to selection pressure exerted by pathogens. PRRs are strategically expressed on cells that are first to encounter pathogens during infection. They are present in the membrane of surface epithelia, monocytes, macrophages, neutrophils and antigen presenting cells (APCs). Recognition of pathogens, specifically by their PAMPs through PRRs results in the activation of various types of innate immune responses. The families of molecules that are involved in recognition process belong to various categories.

Control of Effector Cytokines by Innate Immune System

A variety of pathogens may infect an individual, and these pathogens are eliminated by different means. Therefore, a number of distinct effector mechanisms have evolved, which are used against different types of pathogens.

The innate immune system cannot only discriminate self from non-self but can also discriminate between different pathogens. This helps in mounting an effective immune response through the synthesis of particular effectors. Different effector cells of innate immune response include, macrophages, NK cells, mast cells, basophils, eosinophils, epithelial cells, and NK-T cells. Major effectors produced by these cells are listed in Table 2.3. These cytokines are expressed early in an infection and they determine the effector type of the acquired immune response. IL-12 and IFNγ (type 1 cytokines) induce the differentiation of T cells into Th1 and effector cells, whereas cytokine IL-4 and IL-10 (type 2 cytokines) induce the Th2 differentiation.

Table 2.2　Major effector cytokines and their cell sources during innate immune response

Cell Type	Effector cytokine	Effector response
Macrophage	IL-2	Th$_1$
Macrophage	IL-10	Th$_2$
NK cells	IFNγ	Th1, IgG2
Mast cells, Basophils	IL-4	Th2, IgG1, IgE
Eosinophils	IL-5	IgE
Epithelial cells, Macrophages	TGFβ	IgA
NK-T cells	IL-4	Th2, IgG1, IgE

Source:　R. Medzhitov and C.A. Janeway Jr. *Curr. Opinion in immunology*, **9:** 4-9 (1997).

Exercise

1. What is innate immunity? Give detailed account of immunogenic (physiologic) innate immune response. (20 marks)
2. Give an account of role played by any three of the following with respect to innate immunity (20 marks). (One each could be asked for 5 to 8 marks).
   (a) Antibodies against blood group antigens
   (b) Alternate pathway of complement
   (c) Macrophage
   (d) Interferon
   (e) Natural killer cells
   (f) $\gamma\delta$T cells and CD5 B-cells
   (g) Mast cells
3. Write a note on role played by surface protective (first line of defence) mechanisms in innate immunity. (10 marks)
4. Write a note on role played by (8 to 10 marks each)
   (a) Antimicrobial peptides in innate immunity
   (b) Inflammatory response in innate immunity
5. Explain the mechanism of innate immune recognition (15 marks)

Chapter 3

Acquired Immunity

- Naturally Acquired Passive Immunity
- Artificially Acquired Passive Immunity
- Naturally Acquired Active Immunity
- Artificially Acquired Active Immunity
- Acquired Immune Memory
- Specificity of Acquired Immunity
- Co-stimulatory Molecules of Acquired Immune Response
- Cells Involved in Immune System
- Antigen Presenting Cells
- Factors Affecting Immune System
- Nutrition and Immunity

☐ ☐

Acquired immunity is also called as adaptive immune response usually develops following a natural or artificial stimulation of the antibody producing mechanism. By natural stimulation means it is imparted by the infection through microorganisms and contracting a disease and recovering from it. This will usually result in a long lasting immunity to another attack of the same organisms. It reflects the presence of a functional immune response that is capable of specifically recognizing and selectively eliminating foreign antigens of microbial or tissue origin. Acquired immunity can be of active or passive type, which can be schematically represented as follows: (Fig 3.1.)

Naturally Acquired Passive Immunity

This occurs on account of transplacental transfer of antibodies (IgG) from mother to fetus and it lasts for nearly six months after birth. Maternal antibodies to diphtheria, streptococci, tetanus, rubella, mumps, rubeola and poliovirus provide protection to developing fetus through passive immunity. Secretory antibodies (IgA) present in mother's milk also provide local immunity in gastrointestinal tract of the breast fed infants. Human colostrum is rich in macrophages and lymphocytes. These macrophages can process antigens and the lymphocytes are of T cell type, which can survive in the intestine of suckling infant for some time, and are capable of penetrating the intestinal wall to reach mesenteric lymph nodes. These cells (T- cells) can transfer cell-mediated immune response.

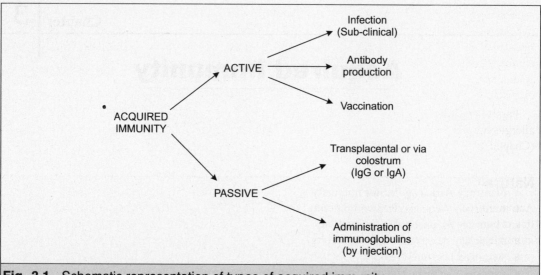

Fig. 3.1 Schematic representation of types of acquired immunity

Artificially Acquired Passive Immunity

Administering specific antibodies (immunoglobulins) or serum containing specific antibodies or sensitized lymphocytes from an individual who possesses specific immunity to a particular pathogen achieves this. For example, an individual who gets wounded is immediately administered with horse antiserum to tetanus toxin, if the individual has not been immunized against tetanus toxin. The preformed horse antibodies against toxin of *Clostridium tetani* neutralize the toxin produced at the site of wound. Routine passive immunization is done against botulinum, diphtheria, hepatitis, measles and rabies (Table 3.1). Protection against snakebites and black widow spider is provided by passive immunity by injecting horse antivenin. Usually, antibodies against a pathogen or its antigens or toxin are raised in a suitable animal by repeated injection of suitable antigen. The serum or purified immunoglobulin from the plasma is used as therapeutic measure in treatment of the diseases caused by the infective agent or as a prophylactic measure to prevent infection in individuals who are likely to suffer from the disease. For ex. anti-tetanus, anti-diphtheria, and anti-cholera antibodies are obtained by immunizing horse with corresponding toxoid. In

Table 3.1 Common substances used for passive immunization

Disease causing germ or Antigen	Antibody/Antiserum
Rabies	Pooled human γ globulin
Measles	Pooled human γ globulin
Hepatitis A and B	Pooled human γ globulin
Botulinum	Horse antitoxin
Diphtheria	Horse antitoxin
Tetanus	Horse antitoxin OR pooled human γ globulin
Snake venom	Horse antivenin
Black widow spider	Horse antivenin

such therapy, since immunoglobulins of animal origin are used, the patient is always at the risk of developing hypersensitivity against these foreign proteins of animal origin. Therefore, at present human voluntary blood donors are being used for the production of antiserum against tetanus, diphtheria etc. Antibodies of equine origin (horse) for non-infectious conditions are also available: antivenins against black widow spider, snake poisons. Human immunoglobulin to the Rh factor is widely used to prevent hemolytic disease.

Passive immunization should only be given when necessary because in certain individuals it leads to allergic complications due to pre-sensitization. This has been dealt in greater detail in Hypersensitivity (Chapter 18)

Naturally Acquired Active Immunity

Active immunity is acquired by natural infections caused by bacteria and viruses. In majority of cases this occurs by sub-clinical infections, which remain unnoticed. There are many advantages of active immunity over passive immunization, mainly because the individual's immune system is stimulated to produce antibodies as well as cellular immune response against the pathogen or antigen. Antibody production takes place through humoral immune response and T-cells help in cellular immune response as well as in immunologic memory to boost the response incase of subsequent exposure to the same antigen. Antibodies formed as a result of active immunity are longer lasting as compared to passively acquired immunoglobulins.

Artificially Acquired Active Immunity

Artificial active immunization is usually obtained by vaccination or in case the organisms, which produce potent exotoxins, by administration of toxoid.

Vaccines are killed or live attenuated microorganisms, which is done by heat killing or growing them in unnatural hosts or aging them in culture or treating the microorganisms with detergents etc. The toxoids are the preparations of toxins, which are inactivated by certain chemical treatment and some modification in toxin property is brought about so as to make it non-toxic. At the same time toxoid will retain antigenic potency and thus like toxin can induce antitoxin (antibody) formation. Therefore, they are used for artificial immunization to protect against toxic effects brought about by the infection of certain strain of bacteria.

The commonly used toxoid vaccines are

Diphtheria and tetanus, Cholera toxin B subunit in combination with killed *Vibrio cholera* organisms.

Bacterial polysaccharides as vaccines

Many bacterial polysaccharides have strong antigenicity. Hence, they are used in the preparation of vaccines. For e.g. *Hemophilus influenzae type B, Meningococcus, Pneumococcus*.

Commonly used Killed vaccines are

Bacterial vaccines: Typhoid, cholera, plague, and pertussis.

Viral vaccines: Rabies, hepatitis B, and influenza, poliomyelitis (Salk vaccine).

The pathogen is inactivated by heat or by chemicals, hence it is no longer capable of replicating in the host. During inactivation process, it is critically important to maintain the structures of epitopes on surface antigens. Heat inactivation generally leads to protein denaturation, which may lead to alteration in epitope structure and failure in immune recognition. Chemical inactivation with formaldehyde has met with success. Sabin vaccine and pertussis (Whooping cough) vaccines are produced by formaldehyde treatment. In the case of killed vaccines repeated booster doses are often needed to maintain the immune status of the host, where as attenuated vaccines generally require only one dose to induce long lasting immunity. Killed vaccines predominantly induce humoral immune response, whereas attenuated vaccines induce cell mediated as well as humoral immune response.

In rare instances, where quality control procedures were not properly followed while producing killed vaccines led to complications in the host. For example, due to inadequate treatment of pathogens by formaldehyde paralytic polio from Salk vaccine and pertussis from pertussis vaccine were caused in the host. Otherwise, killed vaccines are very safe and cause less complication.

Live attenuated vaccines

Bacterial: BCG (Bacille, Calmette, Guerin) a live attenuated *Mycobacterium bovis* for tuberculosis, Ty21a-live oral attenuated mutant typhoid bacilli.

Viral: Live vaccinia virus for small pox, rubella, measles, mumps, yellow fever, polio (Sabin vaccine).

Live attenuated vaccines have advantage over killed preparation of vaccines because, attenuated vaccines mimic natural behavior of the organisms without causing disease. The immunity developed against the attenuated vaccines is superior because actively multiplying organisms provide sufficient antigen supply. The immune response occurs at the site of natural infection, where the attenuated organisms under go multiplication. Modifying the conditions under which an organism grows brings about attenuation. The conditions could be higher temperature, anaerobic environment, and chemical constitution of growth medium. For e.g. in 1908 Calmette and Guerin at the Pasteur institute added bile to the culture medium of virulent strain of *Mycobacterium tuberculosis*. It resulted in attenuation of virulence of the bacteria. The same organism, BCG (Bacille, Calmette, and Guerin) is widely used today for immunization of tuberculin-negative individuals; it may also exhibit a reasonable degree of protection against Mycobacterium leprae. Attenuation by cold adaptation of influenza and other respiratory viruses seem to have yielded good results. The organisms can grow at the lower temperatures of 32-34°C of the upper respiratory tract, but fail to produce disease at 37°C in the lower respiratory tract because, of its inability to replicate. Sabin vaccine for polio was obtained by growing poliovirus in monkey kidney epithelial cells. The vaccine for measles contains a strain of rubella virus that was attenuated by growing in duck embryo cells and later in human diploid cell lines.

Table 3.2 CDC recommended (1995) vaccination schedule for infants and children.

Age	Vaccination
Birth to 2 months	Hepatitis B, BCG
2 months	Diphtheria-Pertussis-Tetanus (DPT), Poliomyelitis-oral polio vaccine (OPV), Haemophilus influenzae type b (Hib)
4 months	DPT, OPV, Hib
6-18 months	Hepatitis B, OPV
12-15 months	DTP, Varicella zoster (VZV), Measles, Mumps, Rubella (MMR)
4-6 years	DPT, OPV, MMR
11-12 years	Diphtheria-Tetanus, VZV

*Sabin vaccine consists of 3 attenuated strains of poliovirus.

The Sabin oral polio vaccine consists of three strains of attenuated polioviruses. These viruses colonize intestinal area and induce protective immunity against all the three virulent strains of poliovirus. Sabin vaccine induces production of secretory IgA, IgM and IgG class of antibodies. Unlike other vaccines, Sabin vaccine requires three times administration at definite intervals. Because, the three strains of attenuated viruses interfere with each other's replication in the intestine. Generally with first time immunization, one strain will predominate in its growth, thereby inducing immunity against that strain. In the second immunization, immunity generated by the previous strain will limit the growth of the previous predominant strain. This results in one of the remaining two strains to predominate and induce immunity. Finally, with the third immunization, immunity to all the three strains is obtained.

One of the reasons for multiple immunization schedules is because of presence of maternal antibodies in the infants, which were gained passively through placenta or mothers milk. For example, passively acquired maternal antibodies bind to epitopes on the DPT vaccines, thereby blocking adequate immune activation. Therefore, this vaccine must be given several times to achieve adequate immunity. Passively acquired maternal antibodies also interfere with MMR vaccine, because it is not given before 12-15 months of age. In the developing countries, measles vaccine is given at 9 months of age, because 30-50% of children in these countries contract the disease before 15 months of age.

Recombinant vaccines

Recombinant DNA technology is also being used for production of attenuated viruses such as influenza, hepatitis, Herpes etc. Here viral genome is trimmed to remove virulence coding segment of the gene and only replication and protein coat coding gene is allowed to remain. In addition to this many mutations in the viral genome are introduced so as to prevent it from reverting to virulent state by reverse mutations. An ingenious approach is to use a viral genome to carry the genes of another virus that cannot be grown successfully or it is deadly. Large DNA viruses such as vaccinia can act as carriers for one or many foreign genes in its chromosome (DNA) while retaining infectivity for animal and cultured cells. The proteins encoded by these genes are appropriately expressed with respect to glycosylation and secretion by the infected cells. A wide variety of genes such as influenza virus hemagglutinin, vesicular stomatitis virus glycoprotein, HIV-I gp120, herpes simplex virus glycoprotein D, and Hepatitis surface antigen (HbsAg) have been successfully expressed through recombinant vaccinia virus vector and these products are called as subunit vaccines, which are at present in use (refer to Chapter 16).

There is always limitation to use attenuated vaccines. A very small number of individuals develop encephalitis following measles vaccine, however, the danger of developing the disease from natural infection is more severe. There is a possibility of attenuated virus reverting to its virulent form (this can be avoided by having more mutations introduced in the DNA of the virus). For preservation purpose cold storage is a must, which is a problem faced by tropical countries. Live attenuated vaccines are not administered to the patients suffering from immunodeficiency or undergoing steroid or undergoing other immunosuppressive drug treatment and for those undergoing radiotherapy.

Acquired Immune Memory

When an individual makes an antibody against an infectious agent it is obvious that this infectious agent is ubiquitous in the environment and one likely to encounter it again and again. The immune mechanism alerted by the first contact with antigen leaves behind some immune memory system in the bone marrow of the individual. This would enable the response to any subsequent exposure to be faster and greater in magnitude. Individuals rarely suffer from such diseases as measles, mumps, chicken pox, whooping cough etc., until and unless the earlier response was suppressed. The first contact with the infectious agent sets in some information and imparts memory, so that the body is effectively prepared to repel any later invasion by that organism and a state of immunity is established. For e.g. when tetanus toxoid is injected into a rabbit, after several days the antibodies can be detected in the blood of the rabbit, these antibodies reach a peak and then fall. After some resting period, the animal is given second injection of the same toxoid. Within two to three days the antibody in the blood rises steeply to reach much higher values than were observed in the primary response. This secondary response is characterized by a more rapid and more abundant production of antibodies resulting from the turning up or priming of the antibody forming system. This is possible only due to the presence of immune memory cells, which were primed earlier for antibody production. For further details refer to Chapter 13.

Specificity of Acquired Immunity

In an individual establishment of immune memory or immunity by one organism does not confer protection against another unrelated organism. For example after the attack of measles we develop immunity to it but not against jaundice, polio or mumps, for which we will be still susceptible. Therefore it is said that acquired immunity develops specificity and the immune system can specifically differentiate between two organisms. In an experiment, discriminatory power of acquired immune response was demonstrated, where rabbits were immunized with tetanus toxoid and they developed immune memory for that antigen but not against influenza and vice versa. The reason for this type of response lies in the ability of the recognition sites of the antibody molecules to distinguish between antigens; antibodies made against toxoid will only bind to it and not the pathogen.

The ability to recognize and distinguish one antigen from the other can be extended further, where an individual should be able to recognize self and non-self (foreign). The failure to recognize self would lead to autoimmune disease, which would lead to various complications. Burnet and Fenner postulated that those circulating body components, which were able to reach the developing lymphoid system during the perinatal period, would some way make the immune system realize that as self. A permanent unresponsiveness or immune tolerance would result so that when immunological maturity is reached, there would normally be an inability to respond to self-components.

Co-stimulatory Molecules of Acquired Immune Response

As noted earlier in Chapter 2 acquired immunity does not occur independent of innate immunity. The phagocytic cells play a crucial role in non-specific immune response are intimately involved in activation of the adaptive immune response. The endogenous signals induced by PAMPs (*Pathogen associated molecular patterns*) recognized by PRRs (*Pattern recognition receptors*) are responsible for induction of adaptive immune response. The signals induced by PAMPs can be grouped into following three categories.

1. Signals that mediate inflammatory response, including IL-1, tumor necrosis factor α (TNFα), IL-6, type I interferons (IFNs) and various other chemokines.
2. Signals that function as co-stimulators of T cell activation, namely B7.1 and B7.2 are included in this group.
3. Signals that control the induction of effector functions; these include IL-4, IL-5, IL-10, IL-12, transforming growth factor β (TGFβ) and IFNγ.

All inflammatory cytokines can be induced by different types of pathogens and can stimulate multiple effector functions of innate immunity and also have generalized effects on the adaptive immunity. Type

I IFNs (α and β) are induced by viruses are capable of upregulation of class I MHC expression, thus increasing the efficiency of presentation of viral antigen to the cytotoxic T cells. IL-1, TNFα and chemokines direct the migration of antigen specific lymphocytes along with other cells such as macrophages, monocytes and neutrophils to the site of infection either by inducing the expression of adhesion molecules on endothelial cells (IL-1 and TNFα). IL-6 induces terminal differentiation of B-lymphocytes into Ig producing plasma cells.

In the beginning, when all the animals took origin, responses induced by PRRs upon recognition of pathogen consisted of similar defense mechanisms, such as phagocytosis, production of antibacterial peptides etc. However, when vertebrates evolved into different phyla, these responses were retained, but over time acquired new functions as well. One of these functions was to induce the expression of co-stimulatory molecules on the membrane of APCs (Antigen presenting cells), another was to facilitate pathogens uptake and degradation. The latter functions was further modified to present the degraded molecules of pathogens in the form of MHC bound antigens to the receptors on T cells. Thus, the presence of pathogen is recognized by the APCs through binding of one of the PAMPs of pathogen to PRRs and the specific antigens derived from the pathogen are presented by the same AP through a processing mechanisms and presentation of antigen specific to that pathogen. This whole mechanism ensured that the T cells should receive both signals necessary for activation only if the antigen recognized by the TCR (T cell receptor) is derived from the pathogen that initially induced the co-stimulatory activity.

A variety of pathogen products have been shown to be able to induce the expression of co-stimulatory molecules, such as B7.1 and B7.2: bacterial DNA, viral RNA, membrane of *mycobacterium*, porins from *Neisseria*, LPS, mannans, glycans etc. Each of these substances induces co-stimulatory molecules on all effector cells. Because, self-antigens lack PAMPs, they cannot induce co-stimulatory activity and therefore T cells specific for self-antigens normally cannot be activated. This way, the non-clonal innate immune response controls self/non-self discrimination in the adaptive immune response by regulating the expression of co-stimulatory molecules.

This also means that the innate immune system actually controls the activation of all acquired immune responses, although in some cases, such as, graft rejection, which is induced by APCs bearing non-self MHC molecules and co-stimulatory capacity, this control may not be obvious.

Cells Involved in Immune System

Two major groups of cells are involved in generation of an effective immune response: *lymphocytes and antigen presenting cells* (APCs). Lymphocytes possess antigen binding surface receptors and they belong to one of the many types of WBCs. They are produced in the bone marrow during leukopoiesis and later released into free circulation in blood and lymph system. Lymphocytes reside in various lymphoid organs, which includes thymus, spleen, lymph nodes, Peyer's patch, foetal liver, and bone marrow. Lymphocytes are the key to mediate immunologic attributes of specificity, diversity, Immune memory, self and non-self recognition. They belong to two major populations- B lymphocytes (B cells) to initiate humoral immune response and T-lymphocytes (T cells) to initiate cell mediated immune (CMI). A brief description of both the types is given Chapter 4.

B- lymphocyte

They are produced in bone marrow and reside there or in spleen and mature until they are ready to be dispatched for duty. When they are released into free circulation they possess a unique antigen binding receptor on their membrane (Fig. 3.2), which belongs to immunoglobulin or antibody superfamily. Hence it is called as Ig receptor. The Ig receptor is a glycoprotein resembling antibodies in structure. It consists of two identical heavy chains and two identical light chains of polypeptides. Two light chains are attached to heavy chain by disulfide bonds and the heavy chains are in turn held together by disulfide bond. The carboxyl terminal end of both light and heavy chains are not free but the aminoterminals of each pair of heavy and light chain has a cleft within which antigen binds. When a newly formed B lymphocyte encounters an antigen through its

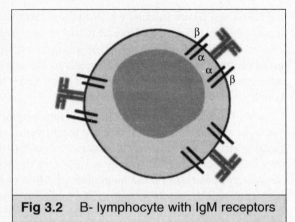

Fig 3.2   B- lymphocyte with IgM receptors

specific Ig receptor on its membrane, the cell is activated and begins to divide rapidly giving rise to memory B cells and effector B cells or plasma cells or plasmablasts.

The memory B cells continue to express Ig receptor on their membrane as the original parent naive B cells. Plasma cells loose Ig receptor from their membrane and grow into large size with large number of rough endoplasmic reticulum in their cytoplasm and start producing antibodies, which are released into free circulation to counter the antigen. Antibodies constitute the effector molecules of humoral immunity.

T-lymphocytes

They are also produced by stem cells during leukopoiesis in the bone marrow. Unlike B cells, they leave bone marrow and migrate to thymus and mature there. During the maturation process in the thymus, T cells express unique antigen binding receptors on their membrane, which also belongs to Ig superfamily. They are called T cell receptors (TCRs). Unlike Ig receptors of B cells, which can readily recognize antigen on their own TCRs cannot recognize antigens on their own, but will need a antigen-presenting molecule called major histocompatibility complex (MHC) situated on antigen presenting cells (APCs). When a newly formed T cells encounters an antigen presented on MHC by APC, it will undergo activation and starts dividing as well as differentiate into memory T cells and various effector T cells.

T cells constitute two major sub-populations: *T helper* (T_H) and *T cytotoxic* (T_C) cells, which play a different role in immune response. A third population of T cells called *T suppressor* (T_S) cells is also known but recent evidences indicate that they are not much different from T_H and T_C cells and their lineage is from T_C cells. The T_H cells possess CD4 glycoprotein on their membrane and T_C cells possess CD8 (Fig. 3.3). Other aspect of T lymphocytes and their lineage is dealt in greater detail in Chapter 10. In this chapter a brief account of T lymphocytes is given.

T_H cells specifically recognize through TCR antigen presented by class II MHC molecule, by APC. T_H cell gets activated on establishing contact with antigen and becomes an effector cell that secretes various growth factors or cytokines. The cytokines play an important role in activating other effector cells of immune system, which includes B cells, T_C cells, macrophages and other cells that participate in immune response. T_H cell derived cytokines also help in differentiation of other sub-population of T lymphocytes such as T_C cells, when they encounter and antigen presented by MHC class I molecule, which is present on all the cells of the body. An antigen may be presented on class I MHC molecule, when a cell is bearing an intracellular parasite or bacteria or virus. Under the influence of T_H cell, T_C cells under go differentiation

Nutrition and Immunity

It is well documented that malnutrition leads to immunodeficiency. Generally the infants and aged individuals suffer from immune deficiency and nutritional deficiency. This leads to impaired immune response, which is observed in over populated countries or the population affected by famine and migration. Immune system is repressed in person going through psychological depression. During early months of pregnancy, malnutrition in mother will have severe effects on developing child's immune system. Recent studies have shown that there is definite change in the histology of lymphoid tissue, number and function on lymphoid cells and the production of humoral antibodies when the fetus develops in the malnourished mother. Immunological changes occurring in malnourished individuals can be classified into following types:

1. Morphological and histological changes in the immune system organs
2. Changes in T-lymphocyte function
3. Changes in the function of B-lymphocytes
4. Altered function of polymorphonuclear cells
5. Changes in complement function
6. Changes in the function of other factors involved in immune response

1. Morphological and histological changes in the immune system organs   The lymphoid tissue such as thymus, spleen, lymph nodes and bone marrow, show remarkable changes in histology. Protein malnutrition is known to severely affect the thymus function and its structure. It shows reduction in size depletion of lymphocytes, loss of cortico-medullary architecture and degeneration of Hassal's corpuscles. In the lymphnodes and spleen, similar changes are observed in the thymus dependent areas. Malnourished status of mother may possibly lead to poor development of thymus and the thymus dependent lymphoid organs.

2. Changes in the T-lymphocyte function   The humoral and cell mediated immune responses are T-cell dependent. It has been observed that T-cells form rosette with sheep red blood cells (SRBC's) and they are enumerated in the peripheral blood. During malnourishment, T-cells fail to form rosettes with SRBC's. Various studies have shown that protein malnourishment leads to lymphopenia (decreased lymphocytes), which is due to improper differentiation cortico-medullary region of thymus and decreased levels of thymus hormone in protein malnourished individuals.

Lymphocyte blast transformation and lymphocyte-mediated cytotoxicity seemed to be abrogated in malnourished individuals. During protein malnourishment there is decrease in delayed cutaneous hypersensitivity reaction following antigen challenge, which will return to normal on nutrition supplementation.

3. Changes in the function of B-lymphocytes   There is no remarkable change in B-lymphocyte status during malnutrition. On the contrary to T-lymphocytes and their response during malnutrition, B-lymphocytes show elevated response of immunoglobulin production and are probably a response to infection. However, T-cell dependent immune response will be poor because stimulation of certain B-cells for the production of antibody is T-cell dependent for certain antigens. Such antigens would cause repeated infection in a malnourished individual and they will lack memory T- cells.

Decreased secretory IgA (sIgA) on mucosal surfaces in malnourished individuals is of significance. Since sIgA plans an important role in innate immune response of mucosal surface against primary infection through gastro-intestinal tract. Decrease in secretory IgA may be due to decrease in IgA bearing cells or due to lowered turnover of sIgA components.

4. Altered function of polymorphonuclear cells   In the malnourished individuals, neutrophil after phagocytosis does not show respiratory burst and the activity of hexose monophosphate shunt does not rise. The chemotactic migration and intracellular digestion of bacteria and fungi is remarkably reduced.

5. Changes in complement function   During malnutrition, many of the complements produced by the liver are significantly reduced especially when protein deficiency occurs. It has been well documented that undernourished children show reduced levels of C3, C1, C2 and C5 complements and decreased cytolytic activity. Not only classical complement pathway but also alternative pathway is affected due to malnutrition.

6. Changes in the function of other factors involved in immune system   The non-specific host responses such as lysozymes in saliva, tears and other secretions are very low when an individual is malnourished. Decreased mucous secretion and metaplasia of mucous epithelia during malnutrition also influence susceptibility to infection. Production of interferon and other lymphokines is reduced during nutritional deficiency.

Exercise

1. Give a detailed account of acquired immune response. (20 marks)
2. Explain: (10 marks each)
    (a) Passive acquired immunity
    (b) Active acquired immunity
    (c) Co-stimulatory molecules of acquired immune response
    (d) The role of T and B lymphocytes in acquired immune response
    (e) The role of antigen presenting cells in acquired immune response
    (f) The factors that affect the immune system
3. With examples write a note on: (5 marks each)
    (a) Artificially acquired passive immunity
    (b) Artificially acquired active immunity
4. Write notes on: (5 marks each)
    (a) Naturally acquired active and passive immunity
    (b) The role of B-lymphocytes in acquired immunity
    (c) The role of T-lymphocytes in acquired immunity
    (d) Signals that pre-mediate acquired immune response

Chapter 4

Cells and Organs of Immune System

- Cells of The Immune System
- Mononuclear Phagocytes
- Neutrophils
- Basophil
- Dendritic Cells
- Primary Lymphoid Organs
- Bone Marrow
- Secondary Lymphoid Organ
- Spleen
- Functions of IEL
- Functions of LP T Cells
- Cutaneous Associated Lymphoid Tissue
- Null Cells
- Granulocytes
- Eosinophil
- Mast Cells
- Organs of the Immune System
- Thymus
- Lymphatic System
- Lymph Node
- Mucosal Associated Lymphoid Tissue (MALT)
- Lamina Propria T Cells (LP T Cells)
- Coordinated Functions of The Intestinal Mucosal Immune System

❏ ❏

Immune system of an organism consists of several structurally and functionally different organs and tissues that are widely dispersed in the body. On the basis of functions, these organs are classified into two types: the primary lymphoid organs- that provide appropriate environment for lymphocyte maturation, the secondary lymphoid organs that trap antigens and make it available for mature lymphocytes, which can effectively deal with these antigens. These organs are richly supplied with blood vascular and lymphatic system, so that they are not only provided with nutrition but also from them cells responsible for immune response and the cytokines that elaborate the immune response are carried to other parts of the body. Among the cells that play an important role in the development of the immune response are leukocytes, which are transported to different parts of the body through blood and lymph. Of these cells only lymphocytes posses the characters such as diversity, specificity, memory and self and non-self recognition, which are key features of the immune response. All the other cells are responsible for elaboration of immune response by playing various other roles such as, activation of lymphocytes, antigen presentation, phagocytosis etc. In this chapter, the properties of various cells of immune system and the lymphoid organs is dealt.

CELLS OF THE IMMUNE SYSTEM

As mentioned earlier, the lymphocytes are the chief cells of the immune system, because they have a major role to play during an immune response.

Lymphoid Cells

In the total white blood count of a normal human blood 20-40% of cells will belong to lymphocytes and in the lymph 99%. In a normal human, there are about $10^{10} - 10^{12}$ lymphocytes. The lymphocytes continuously circulate in the blood and lymph and they have the capability to migrate into the tissue spaces and lymphoid organs. The lymphocytes are broadly classified on the basis of functions and cell membrane components into three types: B cells, T cells and null cells. All three forms are non-phagocytic, motile cells can be distinguished by specially prepared monoclonal antibodies against their markers, otherwise morphologically they are indistinguishable. Since they are small, they are also called as small lymphocytes. B and T lymphocytes that have not come in contact with antigen are called naive or resting or unprimed cells. The naive cells have short life span and when they come in contact with an antigen they are activated and triggered by certain cytokines to undergo proliferation or mitosis. As they progress through the different phases of cell cycle they enlarge and become lymphoblasts, which measure up to 15μm diameter. The lymphoblasts proliferate and finally differentiate into effector cells or into memory cells. The main function of effector cells is to encounter antigen and eliminate it from the body. The effector cells have short life span of few days to few weeks. Plasma cells are one of the effector cells, which have B cells lineage. They have large amount of cytoplasm containing concentric array of rough endoplasmic reticulum and many Golgi vesicles, indicating the active role of protein synthesis and secretion. The effector cells of T cell lineage are called T_H cells and T-cytotoxic cells. Some population of T and B – lymphocytes undergo differentiation into memory cells. It is the persistence of this population of cells, which is responsible for life long immunity observed for many pathogens.

Monoclonal antibodies against membrane specific proteins have enabled identification of several types of cell markers on different types of lymphocytes at different stages of development. These specific membrane molecules are called cluster of differentiation (CD). Each time a new molecule is identified on the lymphocyte by a monoclonal antibody, it is compared with the existing CD designated molecules; if it is a newly discovered molecule, it is given new CD number and nomenclature. Table 4.1 lists some common CD molecules found on human lymphocytes.

The two major populations of lymphocytes, B – lymphocytes (B cells) and T – lymphocytes (T cells)- are briefly described here.

B – LYMPHOCYTES

They mature within the bone marrow of mammals and in Bursa of Fabricius in birds hence the name B – lymphocytes. They leave the bone marrow by expressing a unique antigen binding receptor mIgM. This receptor is a membrane bound antibody molecule. When a naive B cell encounters a antigen molecule through its receptor, the cell gets activated and begins to divide rapidly; the progeny derived from these B cells differentiate into memory B cells and effector B cells or plasma cells. The memory B cells have a long life span and they continue to express membrane bound antibody with the same specificity as the original parent B cell. Plasma cells do not possess membrane bound antibody, instead they start producing the antibody molecules within their cytoplasm and secrete enormous amounts of antibody, which is the major effector molecule of humoral immunity. It is estimated that a single plasma cell can secrete as much as 2000-antibody molecules per second. The plasma cells last only for few days.

The receptors other than the antibody molecules found in the B cell membrane are as follows:

- B220 or CD45: It is the earliest marker of the B lymphocytic lineage. First it appears during the maturation of Pre-B cells, remains throughout the life span of the B cell and functions as signal transducer.
- Class II MHC molecule: It endows B cells with antigen presenting property.
- CR1 (CD35) and CR2 (CD21): These are receptors for certain complements
- FcγRII (CD32): It serves as a receptor for the Fc region of IgG
- B7: It serves as a co-stimulatory molecule that interacts with CD28 on T_H cells.

Other important B cell membrane receptors are discussed in Chapter 12.

The interaction of antigen with the membrane bound antigen of the naive B cell, together with T cell and macrophage interaction, induces clonal selection of B – lymphocytes. During this selection process, the B – lymphocyte divides repeatedly and differentiates, over a period of 4 to 5 days and produces sufficient population of plasma cells and memory cells (Fig. 4.1). All clonal progeny of plasma cells secrete antibody molecules with same antigen binding specificity.

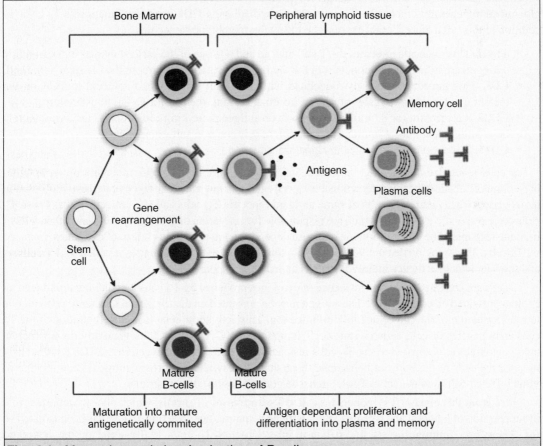

Fig. 4.1 Maturation and clonal selection of B cells

T – LYMPHOCYTES

These lymphocytes derive their name from their site of maturation in the thymus. They also arise from the hematopoietic stem cells in the bone marrow and later migrate to the thymus gland to mature. Like B – lymphocytes, T cells also have a membrane bound antigen receptor, which is structurally different from immunoglobulin, but it does share some common structural features with immunoglobulin molecule. This receptor is called **T cell receptor (TCR)**, which can only recognize the antigen being presented by a cell membrane bound protein called **major histocompatibility complex (MHC)**. When a naive T cell encounters an antigen on its receptor through a MHC molecule, the T cell gets activated and proliferates and differentiates in to memory T cells and various other effector T cells. Thus the fundamental difference between the humoral and cell mediated immune response is that the B cells are capable of binding to soluble antigens, whereas the T cells can bind only to antigens displayed on self cells (APCs, virus infected cells, cancer cells and grafts) complexed with MHC. The T cell system has evolved to eliminate these altered self-cells, which are a threat to the normal functioning of body.

There are two well defined subpopulations of T cells, which in addition to expression of TCR, they also express on their membrane one or the other of two membrane molecules called CD4 and CD8. The T cells are accordingly called as **T helper (T_H) and T cytotoxic (T_C) cells**. T cells displaying **CD4 glycoprotein** generally function as T_H cells and those displaying **CD8** generally function as T_C cells. In addition to this, all mature T cells express the following membrane molecules:

- **Thy-1,** This molecule indicates the T cell lineage and it is one of the earliest marker expressed first during maturation of T lymphocytes in the thymus and remains throughout the life span of the cell.
- **CD3,** This molecule is closely associated with TCR and it is situated adjacent to TCR on the membrane. It helps in transfer of certain information in to the cell for signal transduction.
- **CD28,** It is receptor for B7 molecules present on antigen presenting cells. It plays an important role in co-stimulation during immune recognition of self and non self-component.
- **CD45,** It is a molecule involved in signal transduction.

T_H cells recognize and interact with antigen presented on class II MHC molecule on an antigen-presenting cell. Following this interaction the T_H cells gets activated and undergoes extensive proliferation to give rise to many daughter cells of same antigenic specific T_H cells called as effector cells. These T_H cells secrete specific cytokines, which are responsible for activation of B cells, T_C cells and other cells of immune response. The type of immune response depends on the change in pattern of cytokines produced by T_H cells. The cytokine that activates only T cytotoxic cells and macrophages is called **T_H1** response, and the one, which, activates mainly B cells is called **T_H2** response.

T_C cells are activated under the influence of cytokines produced by T_H cells and on interaction with an antigen presented on class I MHC. The antigen may be presented on the surface of an altered self-cell due to transformation of the cell or due to viral infection. This activation, results in differentiation of the T_C cells into an effector cell, called cytotoxic T lymphocytes (CTL). The CTLs generally do not secrete many cytokines as compared to the T_H cells instead they exhibit cytotoxic activity. CTLS continuously monitor the cells of the body and eliminate those that, display altered surface antigens (tumor cells) or virus infected cells and the cells of foreign tissue graft (Allograft or xenograft).

There is another class of T lymphocytes called **T-suppressor (T_S) cells**, which play an important role in suppression of humoral and cell-mediated immune response, but no actual T_S cell has been isolated so far. Therefore, immunologists are still not sure, whether T_S cells really exist or the observed immunosuppression is simply the result of suppressive activity of T_H and T_C cell subpopulations.

NULL CELLS

These are small group of peripheral blood cells, which do not possess membrane molecules that distinguish T and B cell lineages. They lack the ability of immunologic memory and specificity, because they fail to display the antigen binding receptors of either the T or B cell lineage. **Natural killer (NK)** cells belong to this group. They are large, granulated lymphocytes and constitute 5 to 10% of the peripheral blood lymphocytes in humans. The natural killer cells show cytotoxic activity against tumor cells in the absence of any previous immunization with the tumor. The NK cells can interact with tumor cells in two different ways. In some cases NK cells will interact with tumor cells directly in a nonspecific antibody independent manner and in some NK cells express CD16 molecule as the Fc receptor for the IgG molecule. Therefore, NK cells show antibody dependent cytotoxicity against tumor cells, because they can interact with tumor cells, which are bound by the tumor specific IgG antibodies. The mechanism of cytotoxicity and cell killing by NK cells is discussed in Chapter 11.

MONONUCLEAR PHAGOCYTES

It consists of **monocytes** in circulating fluid and **macrophages** in the tissues. Monocytes circulate in the bloodstream for about 8 hrs, during which time they enlarge and migrate into tissue spaces to differentiate into specific tissue macrophages. This process involves several changes in monocyte, such as cell enlarges five to ten folds, intracellular organelles increase in both number and complexity and it acquires increased phagocytic ability, secretes higher levels of lytic enzymes, and produces variety of cytokines. Some take up permanent residence in certain tissues, which are called fixed macrophages and other remain motile and are called free or wandering macrophages. Free macrophages move about by amoeboid movement and the fixed macrophages show certain properties and functions, which are specific to the tissue in which they reside. For ex.

- **Kupffer cells** in the liver
- **Alveolar macrophages** in the lung
- **Histiocytes** in the connective tissue
- **Osteoclasts** in the bone
- **Mesangial cells** in the kidney
- **Microglial cells** in the brain

For the macrophages, phagocytosis of particulate antigen serves as an initial stimulus for activation. However, the activity of the macrophages is further enhanced by cytokines secreted by the T_H cells, by bacterial cell wall, C3b component of complement, IgG bound to macrophage Fc receptor and the mediators of inflammatory response. One of the potent activator of macrophages is the interferon gamma (IFNγ) secreted by activated T_H cells (Fig. 4.2).

Activated macrophages show greater phagocytic activity than compared to resting ones. Activated macrophages secrete certain cytokines, one of them is responsible for activation of T cells, i. e. IL-1 and cytotoxic proteins that help them to eliminate a broad range of pathogens, such intracellular bacteria, tumor cells and virus infected cells. Factors secreted by activated macrophages are as follows:

- **Interleukin 1 (IL-1)**   Induces activation of T_H cells following the interaction with antigen-MHC complexes. It promotes inflammatory response and fever.
- **Hydrolytic enzymes**   Promote inflammatory response.
- **Complement proteins**   Promote elimination of pathogens and are responsible for inflammatory response.

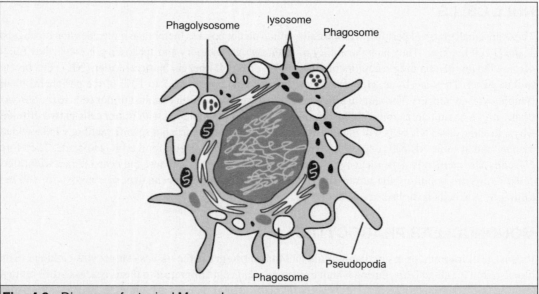

Phagolysosome   lysosome   Phagosome

Phagosome   Pseudopodia

Fig. 4.2 Diagram of a typical Macrophage.

- **Interferon alpha (IFN-α)**   It confers antiviral property to cells by activating cellular genes.
- **Tumor necrosis factor alpha (TNF-α)**   Kills tumor cells.
- **Interleukin 6 (IL-6), GM-CSF, G-CSF, M-CSF**   All these act as growth factors and help in hematopoiesis.

Activated macrophage serve as antigen presenting cells by expressing higher levels of class II MHC molecules on their surface and presenting the antigen through the MHC to T_H cells. Activated macrophages phagocytose exogenous antigens such as whole microorganisms, cellular debris, dead and injured cells, insoluble particles, and activated clotting factors. Macrophages are capable of chemotaxis and get attracted toward antigenic substances or antigen-antibody complexes. The molecules toward which the macrophage was attracted will attach itself to the molecule and develop protrusions around it called pseudopodia. The pseudopodia surround the membrane bound material and fuse to form a vacuole called phagosome, which is then taken into the cytoplasm (Fig. 4.3).

The phagosome in the cytoplasm of the macrophage moves toward the **lysosome** to form a **phagolysosome**. The lysosomes contain many lytic enzymes, hydrogen peroxide, peroxides, oxygen free radicals, which digest the ingested material. The digested material is then thrown out by a process called **exocytosis**. Besides this macrophage membrane also possesses receptors of antibody and certain complement components. Antibodies or the complement components bound to the particulate antigen readily adhere to the macrophage membrane through their respective receptors, which are then phagocytosed. The antibody and complement component thus serve as **opsonins** and the process by which particulate antigens are rendered more susceptible to phagocytosis is called **opsonization**.

Some microorganisms can survive and multiply in the cytoplasm of the macrophage by resisting lysis through prevention of fusion of lysosome and phagosome. These pathogens then multiply within the phagosome. For. ex. *Lysteria monocytogenes, Mycobacterium leprae, Mycobacterium tuberculosis, Mycobacterium avium, Neisseria gonorrhoea* and *Candida albicans*. Some pathogens escape from the

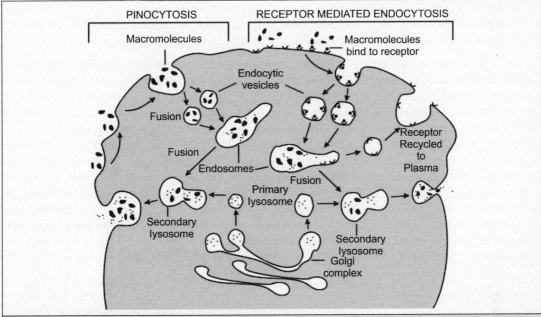

Fig. 4.3 Diagram showing the process of phagocytosis or endocytosis and antigen processing by the macrophage.

phagosome and multiply within the cytoplasm of the infected macrophages and inhibit the production of class I or II MHC thereby preventing the mechanism of antigen presentation by MHC molecule. This is how these pathogens avoid immune recognition (Details are given in Chapter 18).

GRANULOCYTES

On the basis of cellular morphology and cytoplasmic staining property the granulocytes are classified into three types, namely, neutrophils, eosinophils and basophils. First of all these cells have granulated cytoplasm but their nuclear characteristics and the cytoplasmic staining property with respect to acidic and basic stains differ remarkably.

NEUTROPHILS

They are predominant among the white blood corpuscles and they are produced in the bone marrow. They have a multilobed nuclei and a granulated cytoplasm that stains with both acid and basic dyes. Therefore, it is often called polymorphonuclear cells or leukocyte for its multilobed nucleus (Fig. 4.4). After their production in the bone marrow, they are released into the peripheral blood, where they circulate for 7 to 10 h before they migrate into the tissue where they have 3-day life span. Whenever there is infection, there is a transient increase in the population of neutrophils, which is called leukocytosis, because bone marrow releases more than the usual number of neutrophils. Neutrophils are generally the first cells to arrive at the site of inflammatory reaction. Neutrophils are capable of entering the tissue spaces or the site of infection by penetrating through the wall of the blood vessel and the phenomenon is called extravasation. This process involves several steps (Fig. 4.5):

- The neutrophil first adheres to the endothelial wall of the blood vessel.
- Penetrate the wall of the blood vessel through the gap between adjacent endothelial cell lining
- Penetrate the vascular basement membrane, moving out into the tissue spaces.

There are number of chemotactic factors that are responsible for the accumulation of neutrophils at the site of inflammation. The chemotactic factors such as IL-1, IL-8, and transforming growth factor β, are the cytokines secreted by activated macrophages, and several cytokines secreted by activated T_H cells are all responsible for neutrophil infiltration into infected area. Neutrophils also show phagocytosis like macrophages, except that they contain lytic enzymes and bactericidal substances within primary and secondary granules (Fig. 4.4). The azurophilic granules are larger and denser, and are a type of lysosomes containing lytic enzymes, peroxidase and various hydrolytic enzymes. The secondary granules contain lactoferrin, collagenase and lysozymes. Both primary and secondary granules fuse with phagosome, whose content is then subjected for digestion. Neutrophils also employ both Oxygen-dependent and oxygen-independent pathways to generate antimicrobial substances as in the case of macrophages. Neutrophils exhibit a larger respiratory burst than macrophages, therefore, they are able to generate more reactive oxygen species and reactive nitrogen intermediates. Neutrophils have receptor for Fc region of IgE antibody, therefore they are capable of showing antibody mediated cytotoxic reaction against the

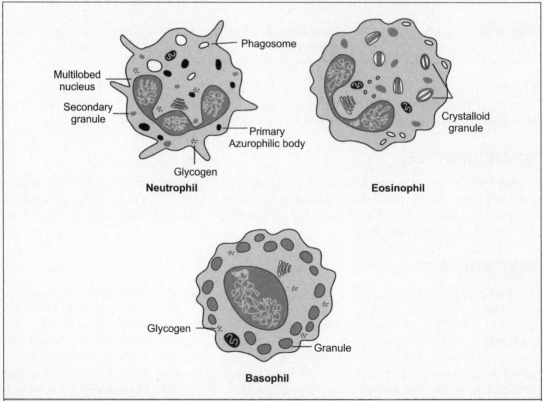

Fig. 4.4 Diagrammatic sketches of the granulocytes. Note the difference in the shape of the nucleus and the shape and size of the cytoplasmic granules.

parasites. They respond to NCF (neutrophil chemotactic factor secreted by the mast cells, sensitized against the parasite (Fig. 4.5).

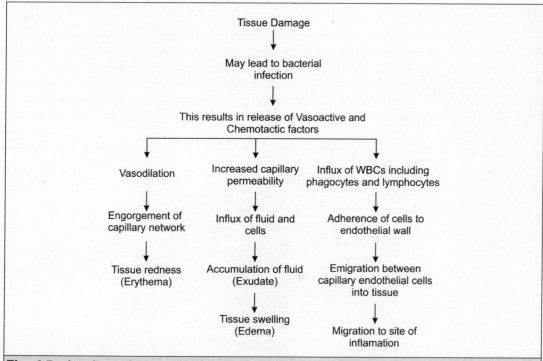

Tissue Damage

↓

May lead to bacterial infection

↓

This results in release of Vasoactive and Chemotactic factors

Vasodilation → Engorgement of capillary network → Tissue redness (Erythema)

Increased capillary permeability → Influx of fluid and cells → Accumulation of fluid (Exudate) → Tissue swelling (Edema)

Influx of WBCs including phagocytes and lymphocytes → Adherence of cells to endothelial wall → Emigration between capillary endothelial cells into tissue → Migration to site of inflamation

Fig. 4.5 A schematic representation of process of extravasation and immune response generated against a parasite by neutrophil and eosinophil.

EOSINOPHIL

They are also mobile like neutrophils and show phagocytosis as well as extravasation (Fig. 4.5) from the blood vessels to tissue spaces. Their major role is the defense against parasitic organisms. They are known to secrete basic proteins, sulfotransferases and sulfatases, which are stored in the form of eosinophilic granules in their cytoplasm (Fig. 4.4). These secretions are known to cause damage to the parasitic membrane. They also have Fc receptor for IgE and show antibody dependent cell-mediated cytotoxic reaction against parasites. They respond to ECF (Eosinophil chemotactic factor) secreted by mast cells sensitized against the parasite.

BASOPHIL

They are nonphagocytic granulocytes responsible for release of various pharmacologically active mediators found in their cytoplasmic granules. (Fig. 4.4) Release of these substances leads to various degrees of allergy in certain people. It also plays a major role in type I hypersensitive reaction. Antigen sensitized IgE molecules bind to basophils through their Fc receptor and stimulate the release of pharmacological mediators, which exert biological effects on the surrounding tissue. The principal effects are vasodilation and smooth muscle contraction. They play major role in certain allergic reactions.

MAST CELLS

The precursors of the mast cells are produced in the bone marrow and are released into the blood stream. The precursor cells remain undifferentiated in the blood and differentiate only on entering the tissue. They are found in almost all parts of the body along with the endothelial cells of the blood vessels as well as the mucosal epithelial tissue. They also store pharmacologically active mediators in their cytoplasm as granules and release these mediators by degranulation when an antigen specific IgE molecule binds to the Fc receptor on the membrane of the mast cells (See Fig. 4.6). Like basophils, they also play a major role in allergic reactions.

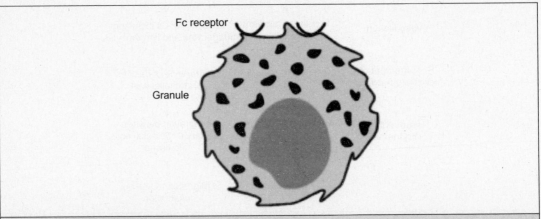

Fc receptor

Granule

Fig. 4.6   Diagrammatic presentation of a mast cell.

Mast cells can be divided into subsets based on the types of proteases contained in their exocytotic granules. This division also correlates roughly with their tissue distribution; mast cells from lung mucosa (M_T) produce *tryptase*, whereas those isolated from skin (M_{TC} or connective tissue mast cells) produce combination of *chymase* and tryptase.

DENDRITIC CELLS

These cells get their name because of membranous long processes projecting out from their membrane, resembling the dendrites of nerve cells. They process antigen and present it to T_H cells on the class II MHC attached to their membrane. Dendritic cells are classified on the basis of their location:

- Langerhans cells: These are found in the epidermal layer of the skin and mucous membrane
- Interdigitating dendritic cells: They are found in the T cell areas of secondary lymphoid tissue and the thymic medulla
- Interstitial dendritic cells: found in most of the organs like, heart, lungs, liver, kidney and gastrointestinal tract.
- Blood dendritic cells: They are circulating cells, which constitute about 0.1% of the blood leukocytes and those in the lymph. They are also called as veiled cells.

In each of these locations, the dendritic cells show morphologic and functional differences. In all these locations, the dendritic cells have the ability to express high levels of class II MHC and B7 molecules on their membrane surface. These two molecules play an important role in stimulating cell-mediated immune response and since these two molecules are readily expressed in dendritic cells, they are more potent antigen presenting cells than compared to B cell and macrophages, which need to be activated by the antigen to express these two molecules. Dendritic cells capture the antigen in the tissue by phagocytosis or endocytosis and migrate into the blood or lymph, from where they are transported to various lymphoid organs where they present the antigen to T lymphocytes. Probably the filamentous projections on the membrane of dendritic cells help them to capture the antigen in an efficient manner than the B cells and macrophages. Hence the dendritic cells play primary role in presenting the antigens. It is still not clear whether the dendritic cells have independent origin or macrophage lineage. Some evidence suggests that mature macrophages and dendritic cells may interconvert, although this has to be confirmed.

There is another category of dendritic cells, the follicular dendritic cells, appears to have a different origin, because they do not express class II MHC molecules and therefore do not act as antigen presenting cells. These cells are exclusively found in the lymph follicles, which are rich in B cells. Even though they do not express class II MHC molecules, they do express high levels of membrane receptors for antibody and complement. Circulating antigen-antibody complexes bind to the receptors on follicular dendritic cells, thereby, helping in activation of B cells in lymph nodes. The presence of antigen-antibody complexes on the membrane of follicular dendritic cells is thought to play a role in developing memory B cells within the follicles.

ORGANS OF THE IMMUNE SYSTEM

These are divided into two groups on the basis of their function, namely primary and secondary lymphoid organs. The thymus and bone marrow constitute the primary (or central) lymphoid organs where the maturation of lymphocytes takes place. The lymph nodes, spleen and various mucosal associated lymphoid tissues (MALT) compose the secondary (or peripheral) lymphoid organs. The secondary lymphoid organs help in trapping the antigen and provide site for mature lymphocytes to interact with that antigen. Once the lymphocytes mature in the primary lymphoid organ, they are released into blood and lymphatic system.

PRIMARY LYMPHOID ORGANS

In the primary lymphoid organ, maturation of lymphocytes takes place and these lymphocytes become committed to a particular antigenic specificity. Only when the lymphocytes mature in the primary lymphoid organ, they become immunocompetent cells. In mammals B cell maturation occurs in the bone marrow and T cell maturation occurs in the thymus.

THYMUS

Thymus is situated above the heart and it is bilobed structure. The thymus is internally zonated into many lobules, which are separated from each other by connective tissue strands called trabeculae. Each lobule consists of central medulla and the outer cortex. The medulla is sparsely populated by thymocytes, whereas the cortex is densely packed with immature T cells called thymocytes. It is believed that the progenitor T cells enter the thymus and start proliferating rapidly within the cortex (Fig. 4.7).

The rapid proliferation of thymocytes is coupled with apoptosis (cell death), then a small proportion of surviving T cells migrate to medulla where they continue to mature and finally leave the thymus. Some studies have shown that a small population of thymocytes mature in the cortex itself and leave the thymus without ever entering the medulla (Fig. 4.7).

Both the cortex and medulla of the thymus is composed of network of stromal cells, epithelial cells, interdigitating dendritic cells and the macrophages. These cells contribute for the maturation of thymocytes. For ex. the developing thymocytes and the stromal cells physically interact. The thymic epithelial cells act as nurse cells by having long membrane processes that surround as many as 50 thymocytes, resulting in the formation of multicellular complexes.

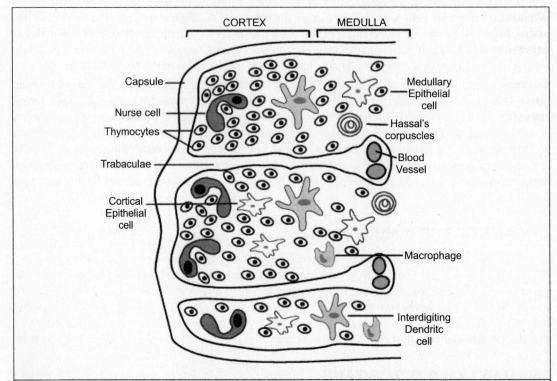

Fig. 4.7 Diagrammatic representation of cross section of the thymus showing various types of cells and the zonation of thymus lobule.

BONE MARROW

In mammals B cell maturation occurs in bone marrow, where as in birds bursa Fabricius is the primary site of B cell maturation. Immature B cells proliferate and differentiate within the bone marrow. As in the case of thymus, stromal cells interact directly with B cells and secrete certain cytokines, which help in development of B cells. As observed in thymus, during T cell maturation a selection process occurs with respect to elimination of T cells with self reactive receptors against self-antigens, similarly within the bone marrow elimination of B cells with self reactive antibody receptors occurs. Details of this process are dealt in Chapters10.

LYMPHATIC SYSTEM

The fluid portion of the blood, i.e. plasma seeps through the thin wall of the blood capillaries into tissue spaces and bathes the tissue. In the bargain it nourishes the tissue with nutrients carried by the blood. Much of this fluid returns to the blood by back pressure and the remainder of this fluid now called **lymph**, flows from the connective tissue spaces into series of large **lymphatic vessels** (Fig. 4.8). Among the lymphatic vessels, **thoracic duct** is the largest, which empties into the left subclavian vein near the heart. This is how lymphatic system restores the fluid lost from the blood by returning it into the heart. There is no separate pumping device for the circulation of lymph, it circulates in the body due to squeezing action of body muscle on the lymph ducts. A series of one way valves along the lymphatic vessels prevents backward flow of lymph.

It is the lymphatic system, which picks the foreign antigen that has entered the tissues and the antigen is carried to various lymphoid organs where the foreign antigen is trapped. As the lymph passes from the tissue to lymphatic vessels, it is enriched with lymphocytes. Thus lymphatic system not only acts as transporter of antigens but also helps in making these antigens available for the lymphocytes.

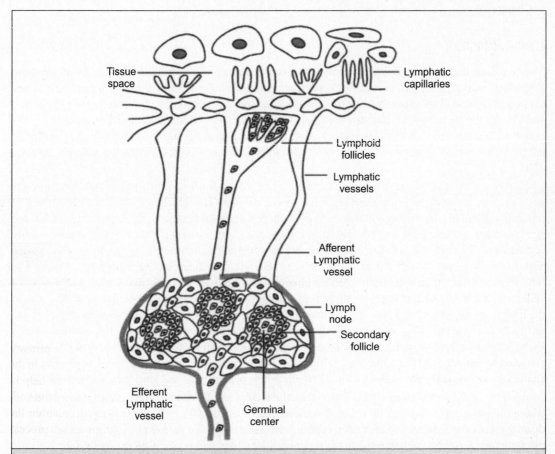

Fig. 4.8 A diagrammatic representation of lymphatic system showing lymph vessels and lymphatic capillaries and the direction of flow of lymph.

SECONDARY LYMPHOID ORGAN

Lymph nodes and the spleen are the most highly organized secondary lymphoid organs. Along the lymphatic vessels, there occurs various types of lymphoid tissues. Some of them in the lung and the lamina propria of the intestinal wall consist of diffuse collection of macrophages and lymphocytes. Such less organized lymphoid tissue is called mucosal-associated lymphoid tissue (MALT). In other lymphoid tissues, lymphoid follicles occur, which consist of aggregates of various cells surrounded by draining lymphatic capillaries. In the absence of antigenic activation, a lymphoid follicle is referred to as primary follicles, which comprises follicular dendritic cells and small resting B cells. Following antigenic challenge, the primary follicle transforms itself into secondary follicle, where a ring of concentrically arranged B-lymphocytes surrounding a germinal center, in which proliferating B cells, memory B cells and antibody producing plasma cells are interspersed with macrophages and follicular dendritic cells. The germinal center is the main center of B cell activation, consist of large population of blast cells called centroblasts. In the absence of antigenic stimulation the B cells undergo apoptosis within the germinal center. Those B cells that interact with antigen presented on the membrane of follicular dendritic cells will differentiate into plasma and memory cells. Differentiation of B-lymphocytes in germinal center is dealt in greater details in Chapter 10.

LYMPH NODE

They are bean shaped, encapsulated by connective tissue and enclose within them a reticular pattern with macrophages, lymphocytes and dendritic cells. Lymph nodes are organized lymphoid structures, first one to encounter the antigen that enters the tissue spaces and they are found at the junctions of the lymphatic vessels. As the lymph percolates thorough the lymph node, the particulate antigen brought in by the lymph will be trapped by the phagocytic cells, follicular and interdigitating dendritic cells. A lymph node internally consists of a microenvironment of its own with three zones-cortex, paracortex and medulla (Fig. 4.9).

The outer most layer of the lymph node is called cortex, which consists of B-lymphocytes, macrophages and follicular dendritic cells arranged in primary follicles. Antigenic challenge, leads to enlargement of primary follicles into secondary follicles, each containing a germinal center. In the germinal center, intense activation and differentiation of B cells occurs. Paracortex zone is beneath the cortex, which is richly populated by T lymphocytes and interdigitating dendritic cells. The interdigitating dendritic cells express high levels of class II MHC molecules, which are necessary for antigen presentation to T_H cells. The innermost zone is called medulla is sparsely populated by lymphocytes, but many of them are plasma cells, which actively secrete antibody molecules. As the antigen enters the regional lymph node through the lymph, it is processed and presented on class II MHC molecule by the interdigitating dendritic cells to the T_H cells, resulting in T_H cell activation in paracortex area. The initial activation of B cell also occurs in the T cell rich area of paracortex. Activated T and B cells form proliferating foci and the B cells are confined to the edges of the paracortex. These foci reach maximum size within 3 to 4 days of antigen challenge and some B cells in these foci differentiate into plasma cells and start secreting IgG and IgM.

After the antigen challenge, within 4 to 7 days, the B cells and T_H cells migrate to the primary follicle, where the interaction between follicular dendritic cells, B cell and T_H cells takes place, leading to the development of secondary follicle with a central germinal center. The germinal center grows in size and the follicular dendritic cells trap the antigen-antibody complex and retain it on the membrane for long period. Antigen trapped on the membrane of these cells is responsible for activation of B cells. The follicular dendritic cells on trapping the antigen on their membrane surface get self activated and start

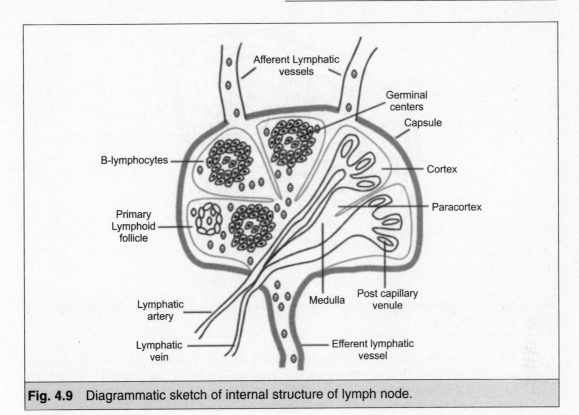

Fig. 4.9 Diagrammatic sketch of internal structure of lymph node.

producing certain growth factors, which play an important role in activation of B cells. The activated B cells in the germinal center divide rapidly and undergo differentiation to form plasma cells or memory B cells. Some self-reactive B cells go through a process of selection and undergo apoptosis. The plasma cells migrate from the germinal center into medulla and start secreting antibody.

As the lymph enters the lymphatic capsule through the afferent lymphatic vessels into the subcapsular area of the lymph node, it slowly percolates through the cortex, paracortex and medulla, giving sufficient chance for the phagocytic cells and dendritic cells to trap the antigen brought in by the lymph. The lymph leaving a node through its single efferent lymphatic vessel will carry enriched antibodies secreted by the medullary plasma cells against the antigens that entered the lymph node. Efferent lymph also carries lymphocytes, which leave the lymph node due to excessive proliferation in the lymph node on challenge with antigen. Some times visible swelling of the node occurs due to active immune response and the increased concentration of lymphocytes within the lymph nodes. Stimulation by antigen within the lymph node is also known to increase the migration of lymphocytes as an indication of active immune response.

SPLEEN

It is a secondary lymphoid organ, oval in shape, situated in the left abdominal cavity below the pancreas. Spleen responds to systemic infection, because it filters the blood and traps the blood borne antigens, unlike the lymph nodes, which trap localized antigens from the regional tissue spaces. Internally, spleen is compartmentalized by capsular connective tissue projections called trabeculae. The compartments are further subdivided into red pulp and white pulp (Fig. 4.10).

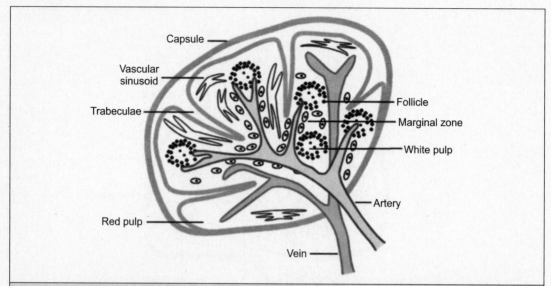

Fig. 4.10   A diagrammatic sketch of spleen showing internal zonation of red pulp and white pulp area.

The red pulp consists of network of sinusoids enriched with macrophages and RBCs. It is the site where aged and defective RBCs are destroyed and removed. The white pulp surrounds the arteries, forming periarterial lymphatic sheath (PALS) and manly consists of T lymphocytes. The marginal zone located next to the PALS is made up of B cells organized into lymphoid follicles. The initial activation and B and T cell takes place in the T cell-rich PALS. This region consists of interdigitating dendritic cells, which capture the antigen and present it to T_H cells on their class II MHC. This leads to activation of T cells, which further leads to activation of B cells. The activated T and B cells then migrate to primary follicles in the marginal zone. These ordinary follicles transform themselves into secondary follicles upon antigenic stimulation. These secondary follicles resemble the germinal centers of lymph node, where rapidly dividing B cells and dense clusters of concentrically arranged lymphocytes surround plasma cells.

The spleen is not supplied by the afferent lymphatics as found in lymph node, instead, blood passing through the spleen will carry the antigens and empties it in the marginal zone. Antigens that enter marginal zone are trapped by interdigitating dendritic cells, which carry the antigen to the periarteriolar lymphoid sheath. Lymphocytes from the blood also enter the spleen in the marginal zone and then migrate to periarteriolar lymphoid sheath.

MUCOSAL ASSOCIATED LYMPHOID TISSUE (MALT)

Mucosal surfaces of the digestive tract, respiratory, and urogenital systems are the major sites of entry of pathogens. The defense at the surface of mucosal lining is provided by a group of lymphoid tissue, collectively known as **mucosal associated lymphoid tissue** (MALT). This tissue shows remarkable variation in its structure, which may range from loosely arranged lymphoid cells, as in the lamina propria of intestinal villi to highly organized structures such as tonsils, appendix and Peyer's patches. It is observed that MALT has largest population of plasma cells as compared to spleen, lymph node and the bone marrow.

Table 4.1 Characteristics of small intestinal and colonic IEL

Characters or	Small intestinal IEL	Colonic IEL
Predominant cell type	$\gamma\delta$+ TCR and CD8$^+$	$\alpha\beta$+ TCR and CD4$^+$
$\gamma\delta$ IEL subset	CD 8$^+$	CD4$^-$/ CD 8$^-$
Receptor Association	50% with $\alpha\beta$ TCR	90% with $\alpha\beta$ TCR
Homing receptors	Small quantity of CD2 and L- selectin	Majority of them express CD2 and L-selectin
Cytolytic activity	Spontaneous	Non spontaneous
Cytokines of IL-2, IL-4, IL-5	Moderate amount	Higher levels of
Cytokines IL-1, IFN-γ and TNF-α	Similar amount	Similar amount

CD4$^+$. The ratio of CD4$^+$ to CD8$^+$ cells in the LP is similar to that found in peripheral blood (PB) (35% to 65%). As in PB, approximately 95% of the T cells bear a $\alpha\beta$ T cell receptor complex. Compared with the 10% of the human IEL that expresses the $\gamma\delta$ TCR, only 3% of CD3$^+$ LPL represses this form of TCR.

Despite the similarities described thus far between PBL (peripheral blood lymphocytes) and LPL, LPL differ in their apparent maturational state compared with PBL. Within the CD4$^+$ LP T cell subset, cell surface markers as well as functional studies demonstrate that the majority of LP T Cells are memory phenotype and helper-inducer phenotype. Majority of human LP T cells (CD4$^+$ cells) are negative for expression of L-selectin. Within the CD8$^+$ LP subset, approximately half express the CD28 molecules associated with cytolytic function. This is similar to the percentage found in PB CD8$^+$ cells. The percentage of CD8$^+$ LPL expressing the CD11 phenotype associated with suppressor effector function is the same or lower as PBL. Thus LP T cell differs from PB T cells in having predominantly the phenotypes of "helper-inducer" and cytolytic T cells, whereas the phenotype of "suppressor-inducer" cells and "suppressor-effector" cells are observed less frequently.

LP T cells are commonly thought to represent a more activated population of lymphocytes compared with PB-lymphocytes based on the expression of cell surface markers commonly found on activated cells. Both CD4$^+$ and CD8$^+$ LP T cells demonstrate increased IL-2R expression. Moreover, these IL-2R's are functions based on the increased proliferation of LP lymphocytes in response to exogenous IL-2. Unlike helper function, however, exogenous IL-2 does not enhance the CD8$^+$ suppressor function despite the increased expression of IL-2R on both CD4$^+$ and CD8$^+$ cells, suggesting that this population may be regulated in a different fashion.

FUNCTIONS OF LP T CELLS

A. Characteristics of Helper and Suppressor Functions of LP T cells

Consistent with the helper phenotype of LP T cells, T-enriched LPL have a marked helper effect for T-depleted LPL as measured by Ig production, especially for IgA. While pokeweed mitogen (PWM) has no significant effect on Ig production by colonic LPL T-depleted and T-enriched co-cultures, it is necessary for Ig production by PBL T-depleted and T-enriched co-cultures. LP T cells provided help for IgA and IgM synthesis by T-depleted PB mononuclear cells, but did not result in significant IgG production. The ability of LP T cells to provide enhanced B cell help compared with PBL's is due to the higher proportion of CD4$^+$/ L-selectin-cells in LPL compared with PBL and not an inherent difference in individual lymphocytes.

The suppressor function of CD8$^+$ LP T cells as measured by the ability of these cells to suppress Ig synthesis in B cell/CD4$^+$ cell co-culture is similar to that seen in PB-lymphocytes.

B. Cytokine Production by LP T cells

Recently, attempts have been made to categorize the patterns of cytokine secretions by LPL and IEL into T helper 1 (Th1) vs. T helper 2 (Th2). After the activation with phorbol myristyl acetate (PMA) and ionomycin, high expression of IL-2 and IFN-γ was observed. Qualitatively, both Th1 and Th2-type cytokines are produced by LPL and have the net effect of providing high helper function as measured by IgG production by PWM-stimulated PB cultures. These earlier studies demonstrating the ability of CD4$^+$ LP T cells to provide help in IgA synthesis to both PBL and LPL suggests that cytokines produced by LP T cells enhance IgA synthesis in B cells already committed to IgA secretion. The actual isotype switch to IgA synthesis occurs within the Peyer's patch. IL-5 produced by Th2 cells has been shown to enhance IgA synthesis in unstimulated PP B cell cultures as well as LPS-stimulated splenic B cell cultures.

In health therefore, Th2 cytokine secretion predominates in LP T cells and is likely responsible for supporting IgA synthesis by LP B cells as well as serving other immunoregulatory functions. In an effort to understand etiologic factors in human intestinal inflammation, several groups have analyzed LPL cytokine production in Crohn's disease and ulcerative colitis. These studies have found an increase in IL-2, IFN-γ and TNF-α production by LP mononuclear cells from patients with Crohn's disease but not patients with ulcerative colitis. On this basis, T helper cells in the lamina propria of Crohn's disease are said to have Th1 predominance compared to ulcerative colitis and control lamina propria, which have Th2 predominance.

C. Cytotoxic T cell function

Consistent with the finding that few LP mononuclear cells bear natural killer cell markers (Leu7, Leu11, and Leu15), NK cell activity is low in both health and disease in the intestinal lamina propria compared to peripheral blood. Lymphocyte activated killer (LAK) cell activity can be induced in a dose dependent manner with exogenous IL-2 but is not specific against normal or cancerous colonic epithelial cells. Cytolytic activity by LP T cells has been assessed indirectly by using antibodies to the CD3 component of the TCR and target cells bearing Fc receptors. Few granzyme positive cells were detected in lamina propria of noninflamed stomach, small intestine and colon. Phenotypic analysis showed that most of the granzyme-positive cells consisted of NK cells, not activated CTL.

COORDINATED FUNCTIONS OF THE INTESTINAL MUCOSAL IMMUNE SYSTEM

A. Antigen Presentation in the intestinal mucosa

As found in other lymphoid tissues, APCs in the intestinal mucosa include macrophages, B cells and dendritic cells but are not limited to these cell types. The growing body of evidence that mucosal T cells, IEL and LPL utilize distinct activation pathways and that the mucosal T cells recognize and respond to antigen in the context of classic and non classic restriction elements expressed by the intestinal epithelium. It is also interesting to note that the antigen sampling in the gut is not limited to specialized M cells overlying PP. Several investigators have demonstrated that murine, rat and human intestinal epithelial cells (IEL) express class II MHC molecules and can present protein antigens and elicits antigen specific T cell responses *in vitro*. Thus far, evidence of *in vivo* antigen presentation by gut epithelial cells has not been shown. The expression of class I and II MHC molecules on epithelial cells is increased by the local production of IFN-γ and TNF-α by stimulated IEL and LPL. These IEC are capable of taking up soluble antigen, processing it and presenting it to antigen primed T cells. It is interesting to note that IEC not only serve as immunoregulatory cells but also as antigen presenting cells. IEC preferentially activate the suppressor subset of PB T cells characterized by CD8$^+$/CD28$^-$ cells. This induction of antigen nonspecific suppressor function may serve to tonically downregulate mucosal immune response and facilitate the development of tolerance to ubiquitous intestinal antigens. Freshly isolated enterocytes from patients with chronic, idiopathic intestinal inflammation, Crohn's disease, of ulcerative colitis failed to induce CD8$^+$ suppressor activity and preferentially stimulated CD4$^+$ helper T cells. Thus in these human diseases characterized by a failure to downregulate the intestinal immune response, there is evidence for pathologic antigen presentation by IEC and, consequently pathologic immune regulation.

Another nonclassic, nonpolymorphic class I molecule that may be involved in antigen presentation in the gut is the **thymus leukemia (TL)** antigen, which is encoded by the T3 and T18 genes. The TL antigen is expressed primarily by IEC and thymocytes and the analysis of α1 and α2 domains of the TL antigen show homology with peptide binding site of classic class I molecules. Although antigen presentation by IEC in the context of the TL antigen has not been demonstrated, this nonpolymorphic determinant may act as an additional selection factor for CD8$^+$IEL and LPL

B. Oral Tolerance

Oral tolerance refers to the induction of specific systemic unresponsiveness to antigen by its prior feeding. The mucosal immune system has developed under dual evolutionary pressure of protecting the host from invasion of pathogens while permitting the transfer of food antigens. The phenomenon of oral tolerance has been demonstrated in humans fed keyhole limpet hemocyanin (KLH). In normal controls fed KLH, subcutaneous administration of KLH resulted in diminished delayed skin test responses and KLH-specific T cell proliferation. Although KLH ingestion alone did not result in significant anti-KLH antibody production in serum or secretions, subcutaneous administration of KLH resulted in higher titers of serum IgG and IgM and salivary IgA compared with controls not fed KLH. These data suggest that oral administration of antigen in human's results in systemic T cell tolerance but results in mucosal and systemic B cell priming. It is observed that antigen fed at low doses results in the generation of T suppressor cells within Peyers patches, antigens fed at high doses results in clonal anergy. It is proposed that this dichotomy may result from the efficient uptake of antigen fed at low doses by M cells, resulting in antigen presentation within Peyers patches compared to antigen fed at high doses that may access the systemic circulation directly. These T suppressor cells are thought to mediate their effect through release of immunosuppressive cytokines TGF-β, IL-4 and IL-10 characteristic of Th0 and/or Th2 cells. Both CD4 and CD8 cells derived from Peyers patch have been shown to secrete TGF-β. These data are consistent with the observation of diminished delayed type hypersensitivity response to orally fed antigens because DTH responses are Th1 mediated and suppressed by Th2 cytokines.

C. Regulation of Intestinal Immunoglobulin Responses

The predominant type of immunoglobulin secreted by the B-lymphocytes of the gut is IgA, accounting for 70 to 90% of all immunoglobulin present in normal intestinal mucosa. A higher percentage of B-lymphocytes from intestinal mucosa express markers of activation compared with B-lymphocytes from peripheral blood such as increased CD5 expression and spontaneous secretion of IgA. Probably this is the result of continuous exposure to antigens in the luminal environment resulting in activated T helper cells. Secretory IgA produced by B cells from mucosal lymphoid follicles is taken up by the basolateral surface of epithelial cells and released into the lumen where it prevents the invasion of epithelial cells by bacterial, protozoan and viral pathogens. In this way IgA traps potential antigens in the lumen before they elicit an amplified immune response. Unlike other types of immunoglobulins, IgA does not bind to complement and therefore, is well suited to the gastrointestinal tract to avoid cytolytic injury to epithelial cells.

The mechanism involved in B cell isotype switchover and IgA secretion is well understood at present. B cells are first exposed to environmental antigens in the B cell zone of the Peyers patch. These antigens are sampled by the specialized epithelial cells overlying the Peyers patch known as M cells, which then transport these antigens to the Peyers patch for contact with B and T cells. M cells sample luminal antigens through pinocytosis and transport these antigens to PP. M cells do not express class II MHC molecules, hence it is unlikely that they present antigens directly. Antigen specific T cells direct B cell IgA isotype switch through both direct cell to cell contact as well as cytokine secretion. T cells that reside in the PP are 95% $\alpha\beta$+TCR and 60% CD4+. Indeed, 20 to 40% of LPL are B cells and a large proportion of these, are plasma cells. The primed B cells recirculate to the lamina propria and the epithelium via mesenteric lymph nodes or thoracic ducts where they perform their effector function by differentiating into plasma cells and secreting IgA. The generation of secretory IgA response in the gut can be divided into the T helper cell-derived cytokines responsible for the isotype switch from IgM to IgA (PP) and the cytokines leading to IgA secretion by sIgA+ cells (LPL). Earlier studies using bone marrow derived pre-B cells show that these cells differentiate into IgA-secreting cells in the presence of dendritic cells and T cells from PP but differentiate into IgG-secreting cells in the presence of dendritic cells and T cells from spleen. Thus, cellular and /or soluble signals generated by the combination of dendritic cells and PP T cells drive the B cells to its tissue specific, immunoglobulin-secreting state. Multiple cytokines are known to be involved in promoting the genetic switch to the IgA isotype and the terminal differentiation of a sIgA-positive cell to an IgA secreting plasma cells. TGF-β derived from both T cells and nonlymphoid cells and IL-5, derived from Th2 cells are involved in enhancing the heavy chain isotype switch from IgM to IgA in mucosal B-lymphocytes. The finding of TGF-β acting as a critical switch factor is consistent with the observation that dendritic cells rather than T cells have to be derived from PP for IgA B cell differentiation.

IL-5 and IL-6 predominantly regulate terminal differentiation of sIgA-positive B cells to IgA-secreting plasma cells with synergistic contribution by IL-2 and IL-4. Similarly, IL-5 induces increased IgA synthesis in sIgA+ cells but not sIgA-PP derived B cells. Within the LP, there exists two separate Bcell liniage:

- A conventional B cell line capable of differentiating into antibody secreting cells of high affinity after antigen presentation in the Peyers patches.
- More primitive B cell line, B-1, with a more limited IgM secreting repertoire but that can respond quickly to bacterial invasion without the need for antigen presentation in the PP.

These B-1 cells may be stimulated to produce autoreactive antibodies in a nonspecific manner after enteric antigen stimulation. In this way, they are analogous to γ/δ IEL T cells and likely represent vestiges of a more primitive immune system in which the risk of autoimmunity in exchange for protection against invading pathogens was beneficial.

CUTANEOUS ASSOCIATED LYMPHOID TISSUE

The epidermis of the skin consists of specialized cells called keratinocytes, which secrete number of cytokines that may help in local inflammatory reaction. Skin plays an important role in innate immune response, because it acts as surface protective layer in relation to external environment. Keratinocytes on activation produce class II MHC molecules and act as antigen presenting cells. In the epidermal layer of the skin, dendritic cells are also present and they are called Langerhans cells, which internalize the antigen, by phagocytosis or endocytosis. The Langerhans cells after encountering the antigen migrate from epidermis to the nearest lymph node where they differentiate into interdigitating dendritic cells. These cells express high level of class II MHC and function as activators of naïve T_H cells. The epidermis also contains lymphocytes, which are called intraepidermal lymphocytes (IEL). These are similar to the IEL of the MALT, where they are predominantly CD8$^+$ T cells, with a larger proportion of them expressing $\gamma\delta$T-cell receptors. In the dermal layer of the skin, widely spread out CD4$^+$ and CD8$^+$ T cell and macrophages are present. All these cells help in encountering the antigen entering the body through the skin and mount an immune response against it (Fig. 4.12.).

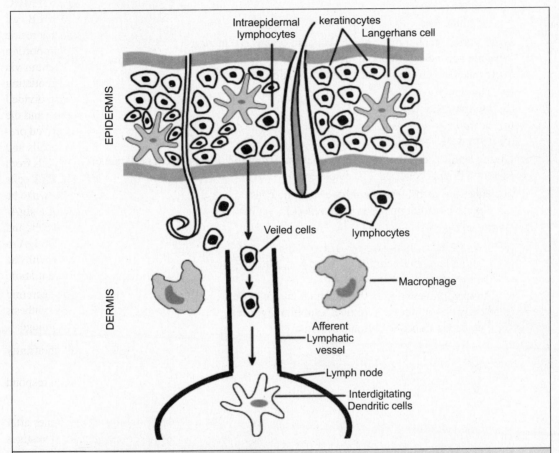

Fig. 4.12 Diagrammatic representation of section of skin showing the distribution of Langerhans cells.

Exercise

1. Write notes on any two of the following: (20 marks) or any one of the following (10 marks each)
   (a) B lymphocytes
   (b) T lymphocytes
   (c) Macrophage
   (d) Dendritic cells
   (e) Granulocytes

2. Write a brief account on primary lymphoid organs (10 marks)
3. What are secondary lymphoid organs? Write a brief account on each of them (20 marks)
4. Write notes on: (10 marks each with illustration)
   (a) Thymus
   (b) Lymph node
   (c) Spleen
   (d) Lymphatic system

5. Give a details account of mucosal associated lymphoid tissue (MALT) (20 marks)
6. Present a brief account on: (10 marks each)
   (a) Functions of IEL (intra epithelial lymphocytes)
   (b) Functions of Lamina propria T cells (LP T cells)

7. Write notes on: (5 marks each)
   (a) Intra epithelial lymphocytes (IEL)
   (b) Lamina propria T cells (LP T cells)
   (c) Oral tolerance
   (d) Antigen presentation in the intestinal mucosa
   (e) Regulation of intestinal immunoglobulin reponse
   (f) Cutaneous associated lymphoid tissue

Chapter 5

Antigens or Immunogens

- Types of Antigens
- General Properties of Antigens
- Role played by biological system in the immunogenicity
- Adjuvants
- Antigenic determinants or Epitopes
- Haptens
- Superantigens

□ □

Antigens are substances, which can induce a detectable immune response. This process is called immunogenicity, which consists of elaboration of antibody production and the development of cell-mediated immunity, or both. Antigenicity, on the other hand, is the property of a substance (antigen) that allows it to react with the products of the specific immune response. Substances that are immunogenic are always antigenic, but antigens are not necessarily immunogenic. For ex. certain low molecular weight substances, referred to as haptens, ex. penicillin, are not immunogenic unless coupled to a larger carrier molecule. Thus hapten functions as antigen but not as immunogen.

Types of Antigens

Broadly speaking, antigens are classified into two major types, namely, exogenous and endogenous antigens.

Exogenous antigens

These antigens enter the host from the exterior in the form of microorganisms, pollens, drugs, or pollutants. These antigens are responsible for a spectrum of human diseases ranging from the infectious diseases to the immunologically mediated diseases of man, such as bronchial asthma. There are also genetic mechanisms operating at the level of the exogenous antigens. Influenza virus, for ex, which is a major cause of epidemic respiratory disease in man, exist in nature in many antigenic forms recognized as A, B and C. Similarly typhoid O, H etc., these are mutated forms of the same species. Human being survives the epidemic each time when infections occur by a new strain.

Endogenous antigens

These antigens are found within the individual and include the following: Xenogenic (heterologous), autologous and idiotypic or allogenic (homologous) antigens.

(a) Xenogenic antigens   These are found within a variety of phylogenetically unrelated species. These antigens are also known as heterogenic antigens. In laboratory serological practice, cross-reactions are common source of difficulty and cross reactivity is often found between antisera to certain bacterial antigens and antigens present on cells such as erythrocytes. Antisera to these antigens will cross-react with cells or fluids of many different species of animals and with various microorganisms. The chemical determinants responsible for this cross reactivity are not known but are presumed to be similar or identical groupings possibly mucopolysaccharides and lipids present in large structural molecules. The best known of the heterophile antigens is the Forssman antigen, which is present on the red cells of many species as well as in bacteria such as pneumococci and salmonella. Cardiolipin from mammalian heart is also a heterophile antigen.

(b) Autologous antigens   Autologous body components are constituents of the host and are recognized as self-components. Under ordinary circumstances, they are non-immunogenic. It is believed that a change in these body components may cause them to become immunogenic under certain circumstances, and the host mounts an immunologic attack against its own tissues. In some instances, human tissues contain antigens that normally can be recognized by the immune system of the host but are separated from the actions of antibodies or immune cells by barriers, such as the basement membrane.

(c) Allogenic antigens   These antigens are genetically controlled by antigenic determinants that distinguish one individual of a given species from another. In human's antigenic determinants of this sort are found on RBC, WBC, platelets, serum proteins and surface cell markers, including histocompatibility antigens. These antigens are known to be polymorphic in nature. Immunization with any of these antigens can occur and progress to disease, when an individual receives an incompatible blood transfusion or a solid graft containing antigenic determinants that are absent in the recipient host. When these specificities are lacking in the recipients, they are perceived as foreign therefore lead to an immune response. In general, the intensity of the response is proportional to the degree of genetic diversity between the immunogen and the host, i.e., greater the disparity, the more intense is the response. These reactions may take the form of a transfusion reaction, as in the case of an incompatible blood transfusion, or the rejection of a solid graft, as in the case of a kidney transplant. Alternatively, immunization can occur during the course of pregnancy when fetal cells (Ex., leukocytes, erythrocytes, platelets) or proteins gain access to the maternal circulation. The maternal production and transplacental transfer of antibody into any of these paternally acquired fetal antigens can lead to severe anemia, leukopenia, thrombopenia, or aberrations in gamma globulin production by the fetus.

General Properties of Antigens

(a) Foreignness   The first and the primary requirement for any molecule to qualify as an immunogen are that the substance is genetically foreign to the host. In nature, an immune response will occur to a component that is not normally present in the body or normally exposed to the host's lymphoreticular system. On occasion, however, body constituents may be recognized as foreign, elicit an immune response, and become the adventitious targets of injury, as in the autoimmune diseases of human's. Under ordinary circumstances, the immune system discriminates between "self" and "non self". However, not all-foreign substances can induce an immune response. For ex., exposure to carbon particles will not induce antibody production; only the phagocytic response is initiated.

The recognition of a specific immunogen and the commitment to respond to the stimulation by the production of either antibody or cell mediated immunity or with tolerance also seem to depend on the physical and chemical properties of the immunogen. These responses are mediated by the specific receptors on pre-committed lymphocytes and with an influence on the type of cells recruited. For ex. Certain immunogens directly stimulate B-lymphocytes with the production of antibody without the requirement of T- cells (T-independent antigens); other types of immunogens require the interaction of T- helper cells and B - lymphocytes in the full expression of an immune response (T- dependent antigens). (For details refer to Chapter 11). Another type of cell cooperation is probably mediated by macrophages.

(b) Molecular size   For a substance to be immunogenic, it must be of certain minimum size; effective immunogens have molecular weights greater than 10,000. The best immunogen tend to have a molecular weight approximately 100,000 Daltons. Although some smaller molecules such as insulin (5000 Dalton) and glucagon (4600 Dalton), do function as immunogens, the immune response is minimal in most hosts and these substances function as haptens after combining with tissue proteins.

(c) Heterogeneity and chemical composition   In addition to foreignness and molecular size, heterogeneity and chemical composition also plays an important role in immunogenicity. For ex. A homopolymer polypeptide chain of *lysine* or *sugar* fails to be immunogenic regardless of their size. The same homopolymer when substituted with one or two different amino acids and amino sugars may become immunogenic. The addition of aromatic amino acids, such as *tyrosine* or *phenylalanine* to poly-lysine homopolymer or addition of *N-acetyl glucosamine* or *galactosamine* etc., to the homopolymer of glucose residue will have profound effect on the immunogenicity of these synthetic polymers. To know how complexity and structural heterogeneity plays a role in immunogenicity, a synthetic co-polymer of *glutamic acid* and *lysine* requires a minimum molecular weight of 30,000-40,000 to be immunogenic. To the same copolymer, addition of *tyrosine* reduces the minimum molecular weight required for immunogenicity to between 10,000 and 20,000. On addition of both *tyrosine* and *phenylalanine* to the same co-polymer, reduces the minimum molecular weight required for immunogenicity to 4000. All four levels of protein structures-primary, secondary, tertiary and quaternary contribute to the structural complexity of a protein, which affects its immunogenicity.

(d) Antigen processing and presentation is the key to immunogenicity   The development of adaptive or acquired immunity in terms of cellular and humoral immune response requires processing of antigens by antigen presenting cells. In addition to this, the antigens have to be presented on MHC molecules to the receptor of T-lymphocytes i.e. T-helper cells (T_H cells) or T-cytotoxic cells (T_C cells). Class I MHC molecule presents the antigens to the T_C cells and class II MHC molecule to the T_H cells. Any macromolecule that cannot be degraded and presented by the antigen presenting cells will lack immunogenicity. For ex. A large molecular weight polymer of D-amino acids, which is a stereo isomer of the naturally occurring L-amino acids will not be immunogenic because the cellular system does not have the enzyme to degrade D-amino acid polymer unlike in the case of L-amino acids polymer.

It is observed that large insoluble macromolecules are strongly immunogenic than the small soluble molecules because, macromolecules are more readily phagocytized and processed by the antigen presenting cells.

(e) Complexity and Conformation   The factors that determine the complexity of an immunogen include both physical and chemical properties of the molecule. For ex, the state of aggregation of a molecule influences immunogenicity. A solution of monomeric proteins may actually induce a refractory state or tolerance when present in monomeric form but is highly immunogenic in its polymeric or aggregated state. Several antigens that do not induce an immune response when isolated in pure form do so when they are part of a larger particle or substance.

There is no one molecular configuration that is immunogenic. Linear or branched polypeptides or carbohydrates, as well as globular proteins are all capable of inducing an immune response. Nonetheless, antibody that is formed to these different conformational structures is highly specific and can readily discriminate between these differences. When the conformation of the antigen is changed, the antibody induced by the original form no longer combines with it. When a determinant group consists of a sequence of amino acids derived from different portions of a folded polypeptide chain, an antibody directed to it cannot recognize the extended chain when denaturation and unfolding takes place.

(f) Charge   Immunogenicity is not restricted to any particular molecular charge; positive, negative and neutral substances can be immunogenic. However, the net charge of the immunogen does appear to influence the net charge of the resultant antibody. It has been shown that immunization with some positively charged antigens results in the production of negatively charged antibodies. These data suggests that the production of antibody may be influenced by the overall charge of an immunogen.

(g) Accessibility   The accessibility of the determinant groups to the recognition system will determine the outcome of an immune response. Recent developments leading to preparation of synthetic polypeptide that contain limited number of amino acids in which chemical structure can be defined are used to confirm this fact.

In the Fig. 5.1 three types of multichain, branched synthetic polypeptides are shown. In the first ex., alanine side chains are attached to the amino groups of polylysine backbone, and on the outside the immunodominant tyrosine and glutamic acid groups are added.

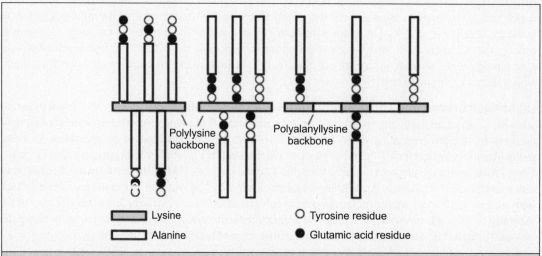

| | Lysine | ○ Tyrosine residue |
| | Alanine | ● Glutamic acid residue |

Fig. 5.1   Three types of multichain-branched synthetic polypeptides used for immunization. (After Sela, M.: Studies with synthetic polypeptides. Adv. Immunol., 5: 29, 1966).

An immune response will occur to these immunodominant groupings when this polymer is injected into a rabbit. In the center diagram, the immunodominant tyrosine and glutamic acid determinants are placed next to the polylysine backbone and the alanine side chains or "whiskers" protrude into outside milieu. No immune response occurs to this configuration. In the third ex., however, alternating alanine with lysine residues forming a polylysine-polyalanine backbone structure has modified the spatial configuration of the side chains. Since the side chains can be inserted only at the location of the lysine groupings, the space between them is greatly lengthened. When injected into an experimental animal, this polymer will induce an immune response. Thus the accessibility of determinant groupings on an immunogen will influence whether an immune response will occur.

Role Played by Biological System in the Immunogenicity

Even though a macromolecule qualifies to be an antigen by having all the basic properties explained earlier, its ability to induce an immune response depends on certain properties of the biological system that antigen encounters.

(a) Genetic constitution of the individual   The degree of immune response or the type of immune response shown by an individual will depend on the genetic constitution of the individual. For ex. When two different inbred strains of mice are immunized with a strong immunogen, one strain will produce high titer antibodies, whereas other strain produces low titer antibody. If the two strains are crossed and the F1 hybrid is immunized with same immunogen, it will produce intermediate level of antibody. From the back cross data the gene responsible for antibody production was mapped to a sub-region of the major histocompatibility complex (MHC). From several experiments conducted with different immunogens with varying immunogenicity, it is evident that MHC gene products, which function as antigen presenters to T cells play a central role in determining the degree of immune response to an antigen.

The genes encoding B cell and T cell receptors and the genes encoding various types of proteins of immune regulatory mechanisms also play an important role in determining the immunogenicity of given macromolecule in different individuals.

(b) Dosage and route of administration of immunogens   Each immunogen has a characteristic dose response curve like a fingerprint, which is determined by measuring the immune response produced by an immunogen at various doses and route of administration. For some immunogens, certain combination of optimal dosage and route of administration will produce a peak immune response in a given individual.

Non-responsiveness for a potent immunogen can be induced in an individual by an insufficient dose, because it fails to activate sufficient number of lymphocytes. Similarly, an excess dose of antigen also fails to induce an immune response because it causes lymphocytes to enter into a non-responsive state. For ex. In mice, 0.5 mg dose of *Pneumococcal* capsular polysaccharide as antigen fails to induce an immune response. This phenomenon is called immunological unresponsiveness or tolerance (For details refer to chapter 21) whereas a thousand fold lower dose of same antigen (5×10^{-4} mg) induces humoral immune response. For most antigens, single dose of administration will not induce a strong immune response; hence, repeated administration after a gap of 1 week or 2 weeks interval is required to induce a strong response. Such repeated administration of immunogens is called **booster** dose, which is a general practice followed in normal immunization schedules. Booster increases the clonal expansion of T and B cells.

Immunogens are generally administered parenterally (other than gut). Commonly, following routes of administration are used:

Intravenous (into a vein), intradermal (into the skin), subcutaneous (beneath the skin), intramuscular (into muscle) and intraperitoneal (into the abdominal cavity).

The route of administration of an immunogen determines which immune organ and cell population will be involved in the immune response. An immunogen administered intravenously is carried first to the spleen, whereas subcutaneously administered antigen first moves to the local lymph node. Each of these lymphatic organs differs in lymphoid cells within them, accordingly difference in quality of the subsequent immune response occurs.

ADJUVANTS

Adjuvants are defined as a group of structurally heterogenous compounds, which evoke or increase an immune response to an antigen (Latin-adjuvare-to help). Classically recognized examples include oil emulsions, saponins, aluminium or calcium salts, non-ionic block polymers surfactants, derivatives lipopolysaccharides (LPS), mycobacteria and many others. Freund's demonstrated Immunopotentiation by adjuvants, hence the adjuvants are called Freund's complete and incomplete adjuvants.

Freund's complete adjuvant: It is a water-in-oil emulsion-containing antigen in the aqueous phase and a suspension of killed bacteria (tubercle bacilli) in the oily phase.

Freund's incomplete adjuvant: It is similar to the previous one except that the oily phase (liquid paraffin) does not contain tubercle bacilli.

In addition to these two adjuvants aluminum compounds such as phosphates and hydroxides are also used as adjuvants.

The mechanism of action of adjuvants fall under 4 categories:

1. Depot effect, 2. Macrophage activation, 3. Effect on lymphocytes, 4. Anti-tumor action.

1. Depot Effect Free antigen usually disperses rapidly from the site of entry (injection) draining the injection site. An important function of repository adjuvants is to counteract this effect by providing long-lived reservoir of antigen, either at an extracellular location or within the macrophages. In addition to this immune-stimulatory activity of repository adjuvants has been ascribed to prolonged delivery of antigens to lymphoid organs, which constitutes signal 1. Preferentially the antigen should trigger T cells in the lymph nodes for a sufficient period of time. In particular, antigen retention on follicular DCs (dendritic cells) within the draining lymph node is responsible for stimulating continued antibody production. Antigen maintenance at the injection site is effectively established by oil-based adjuvants that form a deposit of antigens

Adjuvants of emulsion type produce higher and far more sustained antibody levels with a broadening of the response to include more of the antigenic determiners (epitopes) in the antigen preparation.

2. Macrophage Activation Repository adjuvants influence the macrophages to form granulomata, which provide the sites for interaction with antibody forming cells. The maintenance of consistent antigen concentration by depot, particularly on the macrophage surface, ensures that as antigen sensitive cells divide within the granuloma, their progeny are highly likely to be stimulated by antigens.

All adjuvants stimulate macrophages, majority of them through direct interaction, but complete Freund's adjuvants appear to act on macrophage through T cells. The activated macrophages are thought to act by improving immunogenicity through an increase in their efficiency of antigen presenting activity on their surface and presentation to lymphocytes and by the enhanced secretion of soluble stimulation factors (ex. Interleukin-1), which influences the proliferation of lymphocytes.

3. Effects on lymphocytes The immunopotentiating effect of mycobacterium component in complete Freund's adjuvant are so striking that, their use in immunization of human beings is not in practice. In humans, BCG is a potent stimulator of T and B cells and macrophages. Bacterial lipopolysaccharides and polyanions such as dextran sulfate are B cell mitogens and are said to be good adjuvants. Polylysine stabilized poly I:C that produces good interferon levels in primates is said to be an effective adjuvant for immunization to influenza virus.

4. Anti-tumor action   Major effect of adjuvants in this case is mediated through cytotoxic and cytostatic actions of activated macrophages on tumors, with the stimulation of T cell specific immunity to the tumor antigens.

Antigenic Determinants or Epitopes

These are recognition sites of an immunogen molecule, which interact with lymphocyte through their receptors and stimulate them. Antigenic determinants are immunologically active sites of an immunogen that bind to secreted antibodies or to antigen specific membrane receptors. An antigen can have many different epitopes, which are recognized by B and T cells. It is observed that, when mouse is immunized with glucagon a small peptide hormone of 29 amino acids, antibodies are produced corresponding to epitopes of amino terminal portion and the T cells respond only to epitopes of carboxyl terminal portion. In the case of complex protein antigens, an epitope may involve component of the primary, secondary, tertiary and even quaternary structures of the protein. In the case of heteropolysaccharide antigens, extensive side chain branching via glycosidic linkage affects the overall three-dimensional conformation of individual epitopes.

There is fundamental difference in recognition of antigen by the T cells and B cells. B cells are know to recognize soluble antigens, where the epitopes recognized by the B cells tend to be highly accessible sites on the exposed sites of the immunogen. As mentioned earlier T cells recognize only processed antigenic peptides by MHC molecules on the surface of APCs and altered self-cells.

HAPTENS

Landsteiner and Pauling defined hapten as a small molecule, which by it self cannot stimulate antibody production but will combine with antibody once formed. Haptens are also called as partial antigens. Many low molecular weight chemical compounds have the ability to be haptens. One-way in which, antibodies can be elicited to haptens is by coupling such haptens to either a carrier molecule or a carrier particle and then introduce into an appropriate host. When a soluble macromolecule is used as a carrier, it is essential that the macromolecule be immunogenic in the host in question. When insoluble particles (such as latex or polystyrene particles or polymethylmethacrylate) are used as carriers for the introduction of the hapten into the animal, it is not essential that the particles be antigenic to the animals. Antibodies elicited to hapten in the above desired fashion will once formed specifically react with the single haptens even in the absence of carrier molecules or particles.

Antibodies produced against the haptens could be against the charged or uncharged hapten molecule. When the antibodies are against the charged haptens, the charge appears to play an important role in the combination of hapten with antibodies. Haptens can induce a strong immune response if coupled to an active carrier protein of appropriate size greater than 10,000 Dalton. It should be noted that the response to hapten protein complex would be directed to (1) the hapten, (2) the carrier, and (3) an area of overlapping specificity involving the hapten and the adjacent carrier constituents.

Karl Landsteiner in the early part of this century carried out very extensive studies on the antigenic specificity of such hapten chemical determinants resulting in a new appreciation of how critical and precise was the fit between antibody and antigenic determinants.

Landsteiner studied in detail hapten carrier system by immunizing rabbits with hapten carrier conjugate and tested the reactivity of the rabbit serum with minor modifications coupled to different carrier protein. From this study, he could measure specifically the reaction of the antihapten antibodies in the serum, whether they bind to other haptens having slightly different chemical structure. Whenever closely resembling haptens reacted with some anti-hapten antibodies it is called as cross-reactivity. Landsteiner, by observing, which hapten modifications prevented or permitted cross-reactions was able to explain the specificity of antigen antibody interactions.

Landsteiner used various derivatives of aminobenzenes as haptens to understand what role does overall configuration of hapten play in determining the specificity of antibody reaction. For. ex. Antiserum specific for o-aminobenzoic acid, m-aminobenzoic acid and p-aminobenzoic acid reacted only with the original immunizing hapten and did not show any cross-reactivity with other haptens (Table 5.1)

Table 5.1   Antisera showing highly specific reactivity depending on *o-, m-,* or *p-* position substitution.

Antiserum against	Reactivity with			
	Aminobenzene (Aniline)	o - Aminobenzoic acid	m - Aminobenzoic acid	p - Aminobenzoic acid
Aminobenzene	+ + +	0	0	0
*o-*Aminobenzoic acid	0	+ + +	0	0
m- Aminobenzoic acid	0	0	+ + + +	0
p- Aminobenzoic acid	0	0	0	+ + + ±

Key: 0 indicates no reactivity; + + + and + + + + indicate strong activity; + ± and + + indicate lesser degrees of reactivity

On the other hand, when the overall configuration of the hapten was kept the same and the hapten was modified in the para position, into various non-ionic derivatives, then the anti-sera showed varying degree of cross-reactivity (Table 5.2)

Table 5.2   Antisera showing varying degree of cross-reactivity with hapten due to change in substitution at paraposition.

Antiserum against	Reactivity with			
	Aminobenzene (Aniline)	p- Chloroamino-benzene	p- Toluidine	p- Nitroamino - benzene
Aminobenzene	+ + +	+	+ ±	+
p- chloroamino-benzene	+ + +	+ +	+ +	+ ±
p- toluidine	+ ±	+ +	+ +	+
p- nitroamino-benzene	+	+ +	+ ±	+

Key: 0 indicates no reactivity; + + + and + + + + indicate strong activity; + ± and + + indicate lesser degrees of reactivity

It was concluded from this study that:

- acidic and basic groups are very important in regulating the specificity of an antigenic determinant,
- spatial configuration of the haptens is important,

- terminal groups in an antigen are often important determinants of specificity and
- Interchange of non-ionic groups of similar size had little effect on specificity of a determinant.

Many drugs, peptide hormones and steroid hormones can act as haptens.

Superantigens

Superantigens are bacterial or viral proteins that bind simultaneously to Vβ region of the TCR and α chain of class II MHC molecule. There are two categories of superantigens: exogenous and endogenous, which are capable of cross-linking TCR and class II MHC provide an activating signal resulting in activation of T cells and proliferation (Fig. 5.2).

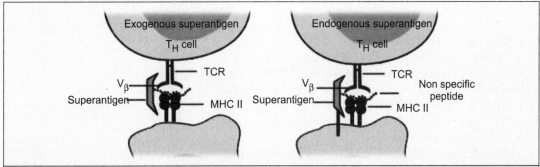

Fig. 5.2   Cross-linkage of T-cell receptor and class II MHC molecules mediated through superantigen. Note Exogenous superantigens are soluble bacterial proteins. Endogenous superantigens are membrane embedded proteins.

Exogenous antigens are soluble antigens secreted by bacteria and they belong to variety of exotoxins of gram-positive bacteria, ex. exfoliative dermatitis toxin, staphylococcal enterotoxin, streptococaal pyrogenic toxin, toxic-shock syndrome toxin.

On the other hand endogenous superantigens are cell-membrane proteins encoded by certain mammalian viruses. Mouse mammary tumor virus produces 4 different types of superantigens called minor lymphocyte stimulating determinants.

Certain superantigens can not only bring about T cell activation but also maturation of T cells in the thymus. These superantigens bind to TCR Vβdomain of the thymocytes and when these thymocytes interact with thymic stromal cells, it leads to deletion of these thymocytes. Sometimes, such deletions by superantigens may reach a massive proportion, which is called "holes in the repertoire" characterized by absence of T cells with Vβ domain.

Exercise

1. Define antigens and antigenicity. Write briefly on classification of antigens. (10 marks)
2. Give a descriptive account of general properties of antigens (20 marks)
3. Write an account on role played by the biological system in immunogenicity (10 marks)
4. What are adjuvants? Write a brief account on adjuvants and their properties (10 marks)
5. Define haptens? Write a note on molecules that qualify as haptens and role played by haptens (10 marks)
6. Write a brief account on superantigens (10 marks)

Chapter 6

Major and Minor
Histocompatibility Complex

- Structure of MHC Molecules
- Peptide Interaction with MHC Molecule
- Genetic Polymorphism of Class I, II and III MHC Molecules
- Cellular Distribution and Regulation of MHC Expression
- MHC and Immune Responsiveness
- MHC and Susceptibility to Infectious Diseases
- Minor Histocompatibility (H) Antigens
- Identification of Minor H Antigens and their Genes

Investigators working on tissue transplantation originally identified major histocompatibility complex (MHC) molecules. In 1930s George D. Snell of Jackson Laboratories in Bar Harbor, USA, and Peter A. Gorer of the Lister Institute of Preventive Medicine in Middlesex, England, described a locus on chromosome 17 of mice and later investigation revealed that in humans it is situated on chromosome 6. The locus has collection of genes hence it is called **HLA (Human leukocyte antigens) complex** in humans, but MHC is now accepted as general label.

Viruses and many other bacteria and protozoan parasites, such as those that cause malaria, sleeping sickness and leishmaniasis, are not so easily thwarted. They establish their infections inside the host's cells, where antibodies cannot reach them. To rebuff these organisms, another arm of the immune system comes into play. The host's cells carry MHC molecules on their surface, which are associated with self/nonself recognition. In infected cells, these MHC molecules bind to and display small peptides, or fragments of proteins, that come from the parasites. The peptides of parasite and host MHC molecules from the complex, which acts as an antigens that can be recognized by antigen receptors on cytotoxic (killer) T lymphocytes or T_C cells. In this way, the killer cells can identify and kill infected cells selectively, sparing healthy cells. One function of the MHC peptide complexes is therefore to signal that a cell is infected.

MHC peptide complexes are also important in the regulation of immune responses. Some specialized cells, such as macrophages, roam the body, ingesting extracellular materials they find, degrading them to produce peptides and presenting the peptides as antigens. These antigen presenting cells travel from sites of infection to the lymph nodes, where they recruit lymphocytes for the immune response. When helper T cells or T_H cells recognize a MHC-peptide complex on these antigen-presenting cells, they secrete cytokines that promote the differentiation of immune system cells.

Thus the recognition of a MHC-peptide complex on the surface of a cell is a critical event in the initiation of cellular and humoral immune responses. During the past 25 years, immunologists around the world have sought to discover how the complex between a MHC molecule and a peptide forms. These studies have led to an understanding of how the structure of MHC molecules enables them to bind to many different peptides from the extraordinary variety of infectious agents and foreign tissue origin that an organism encounters. Therefore, MHC has been implicated in the susceptibility to disease and in the development of autoimmunity.

Inheritance of HLA system, location and functions

The major histocompatibility complex is a collection of genes arrayed within a long continuous stretch of DNA on chromosome 6 in humans and these genes are organized in to regions encoding three classes of molecules (Fig. 6.1)

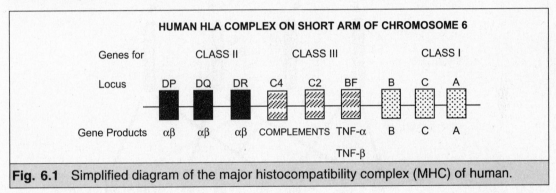

Fig. 6.1 Simplified diagram of the major histocompatibility complex (MHC) of human.

- Class I MHC genes encode glycoproteins that are expressed on the surface of all nucleated cells and they present peptide antigens of altered self-cells or the antigens of intracellular parasite. Class I MHC molecule is necessary the antigen presentation to T_C cells.
- Class II MHC genes encode glycoproteins primarily expressed on antigen presenting cells (macrophages, dendritic cells and B cells) and they are responsible for presentation of processed antigens to T_H cells for recognition and discrimination.
- Class III MHC genes encode proteins of complement system, soluble serum proteins and tumor necrosis factors.

As shown in the diagram (Fig. 6.1), in humans, class I MHC molecules are encoded by A, B, and C region. C4, C2 and BF encode class III MHC molecules, and DP, DQ, and DR regions encode class II MHC molecules.

MHC haplotypes

The loci D-B-C-A are situated very close to each other on chromosome 6, and therefore the alleles at each of these four loci on the maternal chromosome will nearly always be inherited together and likewise with four alleles that happen to be on the paternal chromosome. The alleles are therefore codominantly expressed as in the case of AB blood group. Thus one need to consider while working out the inheritance of the tissue type is the group of specificities carried on each of the homologous chromosomes. The particular combination of specificities on the same chromosome is called the **haplotype.** The haplotype of one chromosome need not necessarily be the same as the other chromosome, and in fact about 90% of people are heterozygous with two different alleles at each locus. For our convenience, let us consider loci A and B only for the inheritance pattern. Fig. 6.2, using the usual chromosome diagram, shows the parental haplotypes being inherited unchanged. This is by far the commonest pattern of inheritance, occurring about 99%. The unusual occurrence of chromosomal crossing over between loci A and B results in the production of recombinant haplotype (Fig. 6.3).

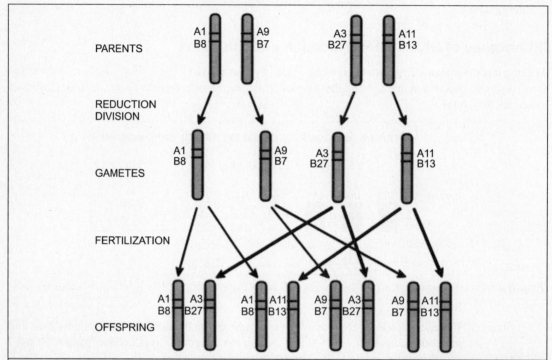

Fig. 6.2 Chromosome diagram showing the usual mechanism of transmission of the parental HLA haplotypes. Source: KISSMEYER-NIELSON, F. (ED). 1975. Histocomaptibility testing. Report of the 4th international histocompatibility workshop and conference, Copenhagen.

In the example illustrated in Fig. 6.2, both parents are heterozygous and have no alleles in common; and in this mating it is obvious that any child cannot have the same two haplotypes as his mother or his father. In this case any search for a matching donor for a child would best be started amongst the sibling who have a 1 in 4 chance of carrying the same two haplotypes. It is not rare for parents to have one haplotype in common, particularly a haplotype such as A1, B8, which occurs frequently in the population. In this situation 1 in 4 of the children will carry the same two haplotypes as the mother, and 1 in 4 the same haplotype as the father. A cross over between A and B loci can occur occasionally. The family pedigree shown in Fig. 6.3 contains single instance of crossing over and illustrates how a recombinant haplotype arise. The father has passed on one or other of his haplotype to each children unaltered, and the same is true of the mother where the first four children are concerned. However, II_5 has received the haplotype A2, B8 from her mother, which means that during the reduction division that led to the ovum fertilized in this pregnancy, there was a crossover between the mother's two No.6 chromosomes at a site between loci A and B.

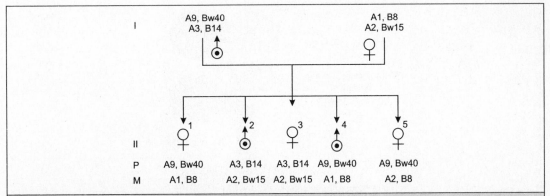

Fig. 6.3 A pedigree illustrating linkage between HLA-A and HLA-B loci. Generally a particular combination of A and B alleles, or haplotypes on one chromosome is transmitted unchanged. In II_5 a crossover has occurred during gamete formation in I_2 to produce the recombinant haplotype A2, B8. P=paternal, M=maternal, numbers 1, 2, 3, and 8, 14, w15 etc., to the alleles represent corresponding tissue antigens at the two loci. The letter w before a number indicates that his antigenic specificity if provisional. Source: CUDWORTH, A. G. AND WOODROW, J. C. (1975). *Brit. Med. J.* **iii**, 133.

STRUCTURE OF MHC MOLECULES

Structure of class I MHC molecule

Class I MHC molecule consists of a large α chain noncovalently associated with a small β_2-microglobulin molecule (Fig. 6.4). The α genes within the A, B, C regions of human HLA complex encode the chain and it is a polymorphic transmembrane glycoprotein of 45 kD. β_2-microblogulin is coded by gene located on different chromosome and it is invariant protein of 12kD. For the expression of class I MHC molecule on the cell surface, association of α and β_2 microglobulin is required. The α chain is anchored in the plasma membrane by inserting its hydrophobic transmembrane segment and hydrophilic cytoplasmic tail. The α chain of the class I MHC molecules is organized into three external domains of $\alpha 1$, $\alpha 2$, and $\alpha 3$, each containing approximately 90 amino acids. The transmembrane domain has 40 amino acids and the cytoplasmic anchor segment has 30 amino acids. Amino acid sequence analysis has shown that, there exist a considerable homology between the $\alpha 3$ domain $\beta 2$-microglobulin and the constant region domain of immunoglobulin. Therefore, it is called as immunoglobulin superfamily. In size and organization $\beta 2$-microglobulin is similar to $\alpha 3$ domain.

Peptides that bind to **peptide-binding cleft** of class I MHC molecules are usually 8 to10 amino acid residues long. The peptide-binding cleft is situated on top of the MHC molecule and is made up of $\alpha 1$ and $\alpha 2$ domains, which interact to form a platform of eight antiparallel β strands spanned by two long α-helical regions. The long α-helices form the sides and the β strands of the β sheet form the bottom of the cleft (Fig. 6.4).

The $\alpha 3$ domain appears to be highly conserved among class I MHC molecules and contain sequence that is recognized by the CD8 membrane receptor of T_C cells.

Structure of class II MHC molecule

Class II MHC molecule is a heterodimer consisting of two different polypeptide chains, a α chain of 33kD and a β chain of 28kD, which associate with each other noncovalently. Class II MHC molecules are also

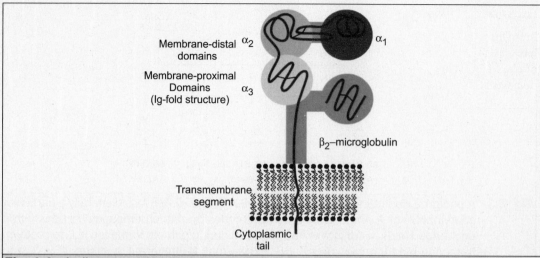

Fig. 6.4 A diagrammatic representation of class I MHC molecule showing the external domains, transmembrane segment and cytoplasmic tail.

membrane bound glycoprotein molecules like class I MHC. Class II MHC also contains an external domain, a transmembrane segment and a cytoplasmic tail or anchor segment. The external domain contains $\alpha 1$ and $\alpha 2$ domains and $\beta 1$ and $\beta 2$ domains and bear sequence homology to the immunoglobulin-fold domain structure, hence class II MHC molecules are classified as immunoglobulin superfamily. The top of the class II MHC molecule is composed of the $\alpha 1$ and $\beta 1$ domains and forms the antigen-binding cleft for processed antigen (Fig. 6.5).

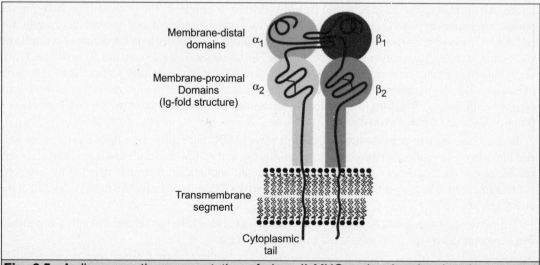

Fig. 6.5 A diagrammatic representation of class II MHC molecule, showing the external domains, transmembrane segment and cytoplasmic tail.

Organization of class I and class II MHC genes

From the cloning experiments and the amino acid sequence study of class I and class II MHC molecules have revealed that separate exons encode each domain. Figs. 6.6 and 6.7 represent a diagrammatic sketch of class I and class II MHC genes and molecules showing the correspondence between exons and the domains in the gene products.

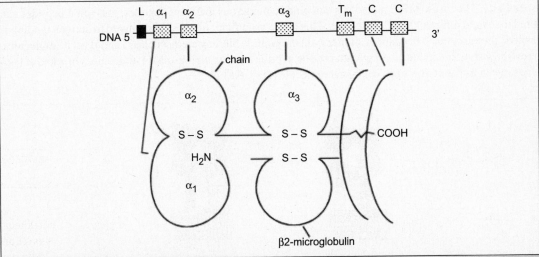

Fig. 6.6 A schematic diagram showing the class I MHC genes and the association of exon with corresponding product.

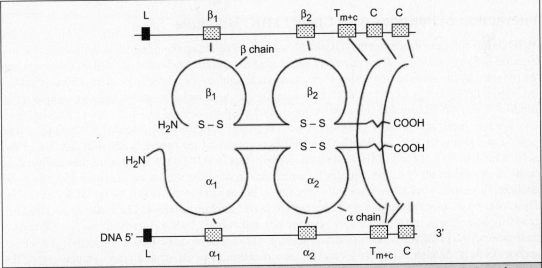

Fig. 6.7 A schematic diagram showing the class II MHC genes and the association of exon with corresponding product.

PEPTIDE INTERACTION WITH MHC MOLECULE

In humans several different allelic variants of class I and class II MHC molecules have been identified. At any given time, an individual is suppose to express up to 6 different class I molecules and up to 12 different class II molecules. Yet these limited numbers of molecules are capable of presenting antigens to the T cells and induce cellular and humoral immune responses against variety of antigens. It is observed that unlike the specificity of immunoglobulin molecule corresponding to antigen, MHC molecules do not show specificity. Therefore, MHC molecules can bind to numerous different peptides, and some peptides can bind to several different MHC molecules. This broad specificity of MHC with regard to antigen binding is called "promiscuous". Because of similarity in the peptide binding clefts of class I and II MHC molecules, they show similar peptide binding features. The peptide binding cleft in class I molecule is blocked at both ends, whereas the cleft is open in class II molecules (Fig. 6.8).

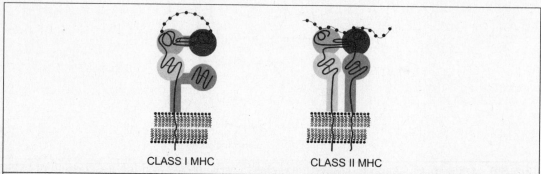

CLASS I MHC   CLASS II MHC

Fig. 6.8   A diagrammatic representation of class I and class II MHC molecules showing their interaction with peptides.

Interaction of Peptides with Class I MHC Molecule

MHC class I molecules display on the cell surface, samples of cellular protein composition thereby allowing monitoring by cytotoxic T cells for microbial infection or malignant transformation. Most of these peptides are provided by intracellular processing of proteins synthesized by the presenting cell in a pathway shown in Chapter 12. Each type of class I MHC molecule, for ex. A, B, and C in humans binds a unique set of peptides. The peptides bound to class I MHC molecule have been isolated and studied, which reveals that they are nonamers with specific amino acid sequences that appears to be essential for binding of the peptide to a particular MHC molecule. The nonameric nature of the peptide aptly suits the size of the peptide binding cleft of class I MHC. All those peptides that bind to class I MHC molecules analyzed so far have shown that all of them share similar amino acid residues at several defined positions along the peptide. These amino acids are responsible for fitting the peptide in the groove of the MHC molecule. Therefore, these conserved amino acid residues are called **anchor residues.** These anchor residues are generally hydrophobic residues (leucine, isoleucine) and contain carboxyl-terminal anchor. Of course there are few exception, where charged amino acids also have been reported. Besides the carboxyl terminus anchor residues, another anchor at second or second and third positions at amino terminal end of the peptide have also been found. Majority of contacts between class I MHC molecules and peptides involve residue 2 at the amino terminal end and residue 9 at the carboxyl terminus of the nonameric peptide. The class I MHC bound peptide arches away from the middle of the cleft but interacts with MHC at both ends

(Fig. 6.8). It is because of this feature, peptides that are slightly longer or those that have different middle residues but the correct anchor residues at each end can be bound to the same MHC molecule. Arching away of peptide bound to class I MHC gives an additional advantage to MHC molecule for antigen presentation to T cells, because arched regions are better exposed than the bound regions, hence arched regions can directly interact with T cell receptors.

Interaction of Peptides with Class II MHC Molecule

Peptides bound to class II MHC molecules are presented to $CD4^+$ T cells. Similar to class I MHC, class II MHC can also bind to variety of peptides. Generally these peptides are derived from the exogenous proteins, i.e. of pathogens, which are degraded within the endocytic pathway as explained in Chapter 13. It is observed that the peptides bound to class II MHC are membrane bound proteins are proteins associated with endocytic vesicles. Digestion of invariant chain, which is involved in the intracellular vesicular transport of class II MHC molecules also bind to class II MHC. Almost all class II MHCs analyzed so far have been shown to bind to same invariant chain peptide. The peptides isolated from the class II MHC peptide binding cleft have been found to contain 13 to 18 amino acid residues. The peptide-binding cleft of class II MHC is open at both ends, thus allowing peptides to extend beyond the ends (Fig. 6.8). The peptides bound to class II MHC are known to have roughly constant elevations on the floor of the binding cleft and also have conserved motifs, but unlike the class I binding peptides, they do not have conserved anchor residues at the ends of the peptides. Class II binding peptides have hydrogen bonds distributed throughout the binding site rather than clustered predominantly at the ends as observed in class I binding peptides. Generally, the peptides that bind to class II MHC molecule contain core sequence of 7 to 10 amino acids, mainly aromatic or hydrophobic residue at the amino terminus and three additional hydrophobic anchors in the middle portion and carboxyl terminal end of the peptide. Nearly 30% of the peptides bound to class II MHC contain proline residue at position 2 and another cluster of proline at the carboxyl terminal end.

GENETIC POLYMORPHISM OF CLASS I, II AND III MHC MOLECULES

There is enormous diversity in MHC molecules expressed within a species. This diversity results from polymorphism due to the presence of multiple alleles at a given genetic locus within a given species. MHC molecule expressed by one individual may significantly differ from the one expressed by another individual of the same species. The number of amino acid differences between MHC alleles can be quite significant, up to 20 amino acid residues contributing to the uniqueness of each allele. Analysis of human class I molecule has revealed 59 A alleles, 111 B alleles and 37 C alleles. This enormous polymorphism creates a major hurdle when it comes to matching MHC molecules for successful organ transplants. A sequence divergence of 5 to 10% has been observed in amino acid residues of several allelic MHC molecules encoded by the single locus. Another unusual feature is that the sequence variation among MHC molecules is not randomly distributed along the entire length of polypeptide, instead it is clustered in short stretches, mainly within the α1 and α2 domains of class I molecule and α1 and β1 domains of class II molecules.

Class III MHC molecules are functionally diverse proteins, which includes complement components C2, C4a, C4b and factor B, two steroid 21 hydroxylase enzymes (21-OHA, 21-OHB), tumor necrosis factor α and β and two heat shock proteins. Class II MHC molecules are free proteins that play some role in immune response but have no role to play in antigen presentation unlike that of class I and II MHC molecules. Certain genetic disorders of humans show strong association with class III locus. For ex.

Ankylosing spondylitis is associated with B locus of the HLA complex, where HLA-B27 allele is involved. TNF-α and TNF-β genes are found in this B locus and these cytokines may be involved in cartilage destruction, which is the characteristic feature of this disease. Systemic lupus erythematosus is another disease associated with MHC alleles and is associated with the regulatory defects in the expression of class III complement components may contribute to the severity of the disease.

Recent evidences suggest that heat-shock proteins may be linked to certain autoimmune diseases is discussed in detail in Chapter 21. They are a group of conserved proteins that are produced by cells in response to various types of stress such as, lack of oxygen and nutrients, viral infection of a cell, and heat itself.

CELLULAR DISTRIBUTION AND REGULATION OF MHC EXPRESSION

The level of class I MHC expression varies among different nucleated cell types. The highest level of class I MHC expression is found in lymphocytes, i.e. 5×10^5 molecules per cell, which constitute approximately 1% of the total plasma membrane proteins. On the other hand, liver cells, fibroblasts, muscle cells and neural cells express very low levels of class I MHC. Since a single nucleated cell expresses many class I MHC molecules, as noted earlier, any particular MHC molecule can bind many different peptides. Therefore, each cell will display a large array of MHC molecules with peptides bound to their groove. If a cell is normal one, its class I molecules will display self-peptides of cell origin like histones, ribonucleoproteins and cytochrome c. On the other hand, if a cell is transformed or virally infected, class I MHC molecule will display viral peptides or altered self-peptides. Since a cell expresses different class I molecules belonging to different allelic sets, each class I MHC will display different viral peptides depending on the binding ability of different peptides with different class I MHC molecules. A heterozygous individual will express A, B and C alleles from each parent that involves six different class I MHC molecules on the membrane of each nucleated cell.

Class II MHC molecules are expressed only by the antigen presenting cells that include macrophages, dendritic cells, B cells and thymic epithelial cells. Expression of class II MHC molecules by these cells differs at different stages of development. For ex. Pre B cells do not express class II MHC but mature B cells constitutively express class II MHC. Naive macrophages and monocytes express only low levels of class II MHC, but on encountering an antigen their expression significantly increases. Since the human class II MHC gene contains three loci, DP, DQ and DR, a heterozygous individual expresses six parental class II molecules and six molecules containing α and β chain combination from either parent.

Regulation of MHC expression

Since the level of expression of class I and II MHC varies among different cells types, there is indication that differential gene expression occurs under regulated manner in different cells. Exact mechanism involved in the differential expression of class I and II MHC is still under investigation. The transcriptional regulation of MHC is mediated by both positive and negative elements. For ex. MHC II transactivator, called **CIITA,** and **RFX,** both have been found to bind promoter region of class II MHC genes. Defects in this transcription factor is associated with **bare lymphocyte syndrome**, where patients with this disorder lack class II MHC molecules on their cells, as a result suffer from severe immunodeficiency due to lack of T cell stimulation.

The expression of MHC molecules is also regulated by various types of cytokines like interferons-α, β, and γ and tumor necrosis factor, all have been implicated in enhanced expression of class I MHC molecules. IFN-γ induces the formation of specific transcription factor that binds to the promoter sequence flanking class I MHC genes, results in up-regulation of transcription of the genes encoding the class I α chain, β2-microglobulin, the proteasome subunits (LMP), and the transporter subunits (TAP). IL-4 increases the expression of class II MHC by resting B cells. IFN-γ down regulates class II MHC expression by B cells. In addition to this corticosteroids and prostaglandins also decrease the expression of class II molecules.

MHC expression is also affected by variety of viruses, in greater number of cases, it is decreased as in the case of human cytomegalovirus (CMV), hepatitis B virus (HBV) and adenovirus 12 (Ad12). The mechanism by which these viruses cause decreased expression of class I MHC molecule has been explained in Chapter 18 with recent evidences.

MHC AND IMMUNE RESPONSIVENESS

It is well established now that the class II MHC plays a central role in immune responsiveness because it is involved in presenting the antigen to T_H cells. There is variability in immune responsiveness among the different haplotypes, for which, two models have been proposed-**determinant selection model** and **holes in the repertoire model.**

Determinant-selection model

According to this model, the structure of a particular MHC molecule determines the strength of its association with any given antigen. The MHC polymorphism within a species will generate different patterns of responsiveness and nonresponsiveness to different antigens. The haplotype of the class II molecule showing the highest affinity binding for a particular peptide is generally is the same as the haplotype of responder strain or individual for that peptide. The non-responder status of some individuals has been linked to deletion of a class II MHC gene.

Holes-in-the-repertoire model

T cells bearing receptors that recognize foreign antigens closely resembling the self-antigens may be eliminated during thymic processing. The T cell response to an antigen involves trimolecular association-T cell receptor, antigenic peptide and the MHC molecule of APC. Any alteration in this association will lead to lack of immune responsiveness. That is the absence of an MHC molecule that can present an antigenic peptide to T cell or the absence of T cell receptor that can recognize antigenic peptide on MHC could result in the absence of immune responsiveness.

MHC AND SUSCEPTIBILITY TO INFECTIOUS DISEASES

There are number of diseases associated with particular MHC alleles like autoimmune diseases, certain viral diseases, bacterial diseases, disorders of the complement system, certain neurological disorders and some types of allergies. Susceptibility to a given pathogen is related to the expression of particular type of MHC alleles expressed by an individual. Variation in antigen presentation by different MHC alleles also determines the effectiveness of the immune response to a given pathogen. Some times, major epitopes of pathogens mimic certain self-MHC peptides, which results in lack of functional T cells specific for those epitopes. Various MHC alleles also code for binding site for specific viruses, bacteria or their products, resulting in immune nonresponsiveness. Some naturally occurring evidences suggests that, a reduction in MHC polymorphism within a species may predispose that species to disease. For. ex. Inbreeding population of animals restricted to a ecological niche are predisposed to pathogenic infections. One of the best examples is that of Cheetas, whose population is confined to narrow belt in Africa are highly susceptible to various viral diseases due to inbreeding in natural population. MHC polymorphism ensures that at least some members of species will be able to respond to any one of a very large number of potential pathogens. Infection with *Mycobacterium tuberculosis* appears to be more frequent in individuals with HLA-DR2. Among unrelated infectious agents, the human MHC class II allele DRB1*1302 is associated with protection against *Plasmodium falciparum* malaria and persistent hepatitis B infection in Gambia. Protection against one disease in one population can be associated with susceptibility to another infectious agent. The human MHC class II allele DQB1*0501 is protective against cerebral malaria in Gambia but confers susceptibility to river blindness caused by the nematode *Onchocerca volvulus*. Overall, the epidemiological data show that specific MHC haplotypes are associated with resistance or susceptibility to specific infectious diseases.

MINOR HISTOCOMPATIBILITY (H) ANTIGENS

Minor histocompatibility (H) antigens were originally defined in mice by *in vivo* rejection response against skin graft and tumors exchanged between mice of different inbred strains. The existence human counterpart of non-MHC transplantation antigens was established by two clinical findings, one relating to the host-versus-graft (HVG) response, which causes skin graft rejection between HLA-identical siblings, and the other to the graft-versus-host disease (GVHD) manifest in recipients of bone marrow grafts from HLA-identical siblings. It has recently been appreciated that the minor H antigens may also cause the insidious clinical complication of chronic rejection of MHC matched solid tissue grafts.

Minor H antigens are peptides

The peptide nature of minor H antigens was implicit from the work of Townsend et al on the MHC-restricted T cell recognition of influenza nucleoproteins derived peptides. Many investigators have subsequently confirmed this, thus indicating that short, MHC-bound peptides derived from endogenous proteins are the basic biochemical elements responsible for minor H antigens.

Graft Rejection due to Minor H Antigen is a Complex Genetic Trait

Classical genetic analysis required that a locus exhibits a phenotypic trait that can be monitored in genetic crosses. The trait originally used to map the minor H loci was very complex, that of graft rejection. Most minor H loci were selected on this basis and used to construct congenic strains of mice that differed from their partner strains at the selected trait. *Hya,* the Y chromosome locus responsible for male-specific histocompatibility (H-Y) antigens represents an extreme example of genetic complexity. The Y chromosome does not undergo meiotic recombination except for a small segment referred to as the pseudoautosomal region; thus, almost all Y chromosome genes cosegregate in genetic crosses, as if they were a single locus.

Generation of *in vitro* T cell response to minor H antigens requires *in vivo* immunization before *in vitro* secondary mixed lymphocyte culture (MLC). Both CD4$^+$ helper T cells and CD8$^+$ cytotoxic T cells can be elicited in this way, and both recognize their specific minor H antigens in an MHC-restricted manner. This cooperation was implicit from the earlier studies on response to H-Y antigens in which permissive and nonpermissive MHC class I and class II alleles could be identified that affected CTL generation and skin graft rejection. The same type of cooperation is responsible for CTL generation and allograft rejection against autosomally-encoded minor antigens isolated in congenic strains of mice.

CD4$^+$ and CD8$^+$ T cell cooperation has genetic implications because genes distinct from those encoding epitopes that stimulate CD8$^+$ CTLs frequently encode minor H epitopes that stimulate CD4$^+$ T cells.

When these two gene types cosegregate, as is the case for at least three classically-defined mouse minor H loci, H3, H4 and Hya, they form a functional unit that confers the trait of CTL generated and allograft rejection. Thus these classically-defined minor H loci are haplotypes rather than single loci. There are circumstances in which the requirement for T cell cooperation can be overridden. One example is of skin graft differing by minor H genes encoding epitopes capable of stimulating only CD8$^+$ T cells sometimes being chronically rejected. In addition, CD4$^+$ T cells alone can mediate rejection of syngeneic male cells in a mouse strain that cannot generate CD8$^+$ H - Y specific T cells but has high responder H-2 class II allele.

Immunodominance

When grafts are exchanged between MHC-matched but genetically disparate individuals, there are multiple minor H differences presented but surprisingly the T cell response is limited to a small number of immunodominant peptide epitopes. This hierarchy is observed when T cells are given the opportunity to respond to minor H antigens presented by different H-2 antigens on the same cell. Several explanations have been put forward to explain why certain minor H peptides are immunodominant over other. Firstly, the frequency of T cells responding to the dominant peptides may be higher than those responding to dominated peptides. Secondly, dominant minor H peptides may occupy more restricting MHC molecules than are occupied by dominated peptides. Thirdly, dominant peptides may more efficiently stabilize the interaction between the MHC-peptide complex with the TCR. Evidence to date is suggestive of the dominant peptides binding MHC molecules more avidly, thus augmenting the TCR-peptide-MHC molecular interaction.

Identification of Minor H Antigens and their Genes

Genetic variation underlies all phenotypic differences among individuals of a species. An indirect consequence of this variation can be the generation of self-peptides that act as alloantigens (minor H antigens). There are currently examples of alloantigens encoded by genes located on the mitochondrial genome, the Y chromosome and the autosome.

Minor H peptides encoded by the mitochondrial genome

Maternally transmitted mouse minor H antigens were the first minor H antigens to be identified. They are encoded by the mitochondrial genes ND1 and COI and are generally presented by the MHC class Ib molecules H2-M3 that selectively binds N-formylated peptides. A non-N-formylated minor H peptide derived from the mitochondrial ATPase6 protein has also been identified that binds classical MHC class Ia RT1.A^a molecule in rats. In every case, the alloantigens arise from single amino acid changes within the peptide. These observations set the paradigm that minor H antigens arise from allelic variation within peptide sequence presented by the restricting class molecule.

Minor H peptides encoded by the Y chromosome

Some of the genes of this chromosome control expression of the H – Y antigens, the most studied of all the minor antigens. Identifying the genes encoding the H – Y antigens required coupling of different tools including the following: mice and human carrying deletions that affect sex differentiation, cell lines selected to carry deletions in gene encoding H – Y antigens, physical mapping of the Y chromosome, cosmid and cDNA testing by transfection for candidate H – Y antigen genes and testing of synthetic peptides for H – Y antigens. At the moment it is unclear how many more H – Y encoding genes on the Y chromosome, autosome or the X chromosome are there in humans and rodents.

Minor H antigens encoded by autosomal chromosomes

First minor H peptide to be sequenced was HA-2, a GVHD-associated minor H antigen recognized in association with HLA-A2.1 and homologous to myosin heavy chain proteins, although the gene encoding this peptide has not yet been established. A second minor H peptide (AAPDNRETF; in single letter amino acid code) was recently discovered. It is the immunodominant peptide detected with CTLs from MLCs of C3H.SW mice immunized with C57BL/6 cells. Interestingly, donor T cells from mice immunized with this peptide appeared capable of inducing the dermal lesions characteristic of GVHD in irradiated recipient mice.

Minor H peptides isolated biochemically lack information about the genes that encode them, the two cases in which autosomal minor H genes have been identified lack information about their peptides. The interferon-inducible nuclear myxovirus resistance gene, Mx1, appears to be a minor H gene. Natural allelic variation results in some strains carrying a functional Mx1 allele, while other strains carry an inactive allele. Mx⁻ mice reject skin graft from Mx⁺ congenic mice, and CTLs can be raised that lyse interferon-γ target cells transfected with a functional Mx1 gene. Mx1 is thus an example of a minor H barrier conferred by the absence/presence of an intact gene. The minor H peptide determined by this gene has not been identified. The most unusual example of a putative mouse minor H gene is β2-microglobulin, which lies within the H3 minor H complex and encodes the light chain of the MHC class I molecule heterodimer. An amino acid substitution at position 85 is responsible for the two most common variants, α and β of β2-microglobulin. It has been hypothesized that the amino acid change subtly influences the shape of the MHC class I molecules, thus enabling novel peptides to bind and stimulate CTLs when immune responses are elicited in H3 congenic strain combinations that differ at alleles of β2-microglobulin.

Exercise

1. Describe the gene clusters that are responsible for inheritance of HLA system and explain how MHC haplotypes are inherited (20 marks).
2. Give a detailed account of structure of MHC molecules (20 marks).
3. Write a note on (10 marks each)
   (a) Organization of class I and II MHC genes.
   (b) Cellular distribution and regulation of MHC expression
   (c) Minor histocompatibility antigens encoded by sex chromosomal and autosomal genes
4. Explain the mechanism of interaction of peptides with MHC molecules (15 marks).
5. Write notes on (5 marks each):
   (a) Genetic polymorphism of MHC molecules
   (b) MHC and immune responsiveness
   (c) MHC and susceptibility to infectious diseases
   (d) Graft rejection due to minor H antigen

Chapter 7

Antibodies (Immunoglobulins)

- ■ Immunoglobulin Structure and Function
- ■ Antigenic Determinants on Immunoglobulins
- ■ Immunoglobulin Classes
- ■ Immunoglobulin G (γ-globulin G or IgG)
- ■ Immunoglobulin M (γ-globulin M or IgM)
- ■ Immunoglobulin A (γ-globulin A or IgA)
- ■ Immunoglobulin E (γ-Globulin E or IgE)
- ■ Immunoglobulin D (γ-Globulin D or IgD)

❏ ❏

Immunoglobulin Structure and Function

Circulating antibodies produced by plasmablast cells of lymphoid tissue develops this. Humoral immunity does not last longer like cellular immunity and it does not act on smaller quantity of antigens. Since these proteins secreted by plasma blast cells are globular in nature they are called as globulins. These proteins are involved in immunological reactions by reacting with invading antigens they are also called as immunoglobulins. Immunoglobulins function as antibodies and they are classified into five major categories, based on their physicochemical and biochemical properties. They are IgG (γ globulin G or immunoglobulin G), IgM (γ globulin M or immunoglobulin M), IgA (γ globulin A or immunoglobulin A), IgD (γ globulin D or immunoglobulin D), and IgE (γ globulin E or immunoglobulin E). Despite their diversity the family of immunoglobulins have common properties. They all cross react with same antigen indicating that common structure exists between molecules and all appear to be associated with antibody activity.

Immunoglobulins are also present on B cell membrane and serve as membrane bound antibodies, which confer antigenic specificity on B cells. Antigen specific proliferation of B cells is dependent on membrane bound antibody interaction with antigen. The serum antibodies produced by the plasmablast cells in response to a particular antigen belong to heterogeneous category because of multiple B cell epitopes. Therefore, circulating antibodies produced are of polyclonal type.

Basic structure of Immunoglobulin

In the 1950s experiments by Porter and Edelman revealed the basic structure of the immunoglobulin (Ig) molecule. The chain structure of immunoglobulin was first suggested by Edelman and was later confirmed by Porter. IgG was subjected to papain, pepsin and mercaptoethanol digestion in various aliquots and various fraction produced were analyzed by separating them through column chromatography. This experiment revealed that 150,000-MW IgG molecule was composed of two 50,000-MW polypeptide chains designated as heavy (H) chains and two 25,000-MW chains, designated as light (L) chains (see Fig. 7.1).

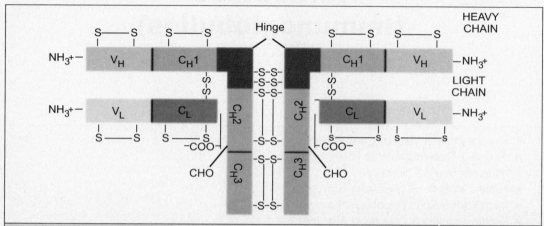

Fig. 7.1   A diagrammatic representation of immunoglobulin structure. Each heavy and light chain in an immunoglobulin molecule consist of an amino-terminal variable (V) region made up of 100-110 amino acids and differ from one antibody to other. The remainder of the immunoglobulin molecule is made up of constant region, which exhibits limited variation and consist of carboxyl terminal. The hinge region is present only in IgG, IgD and IgA molecules.

For each immunoglobulin molecule there are two Fab sites, because they bind to antigen and one Fc site that crystallizes under freezing conditions. Porter raised antisera to these two portions and found that antibody to Fab fragment could react with both the H and L chains, whereas antibody to the Fc fragment reacted only with the heavy chain. These observations led to the conclusion that Fab consists of portions of a heavy and light chain and the Fc contains only heavy chain component. On the basis of these results, Porter and Edelman proposed a model of IgG (Fig.7.1). According to this model, the IgG consists of two identical H chains and two identical L chains, which are linked by disulfide bonds.

Light chain sequencing

The amino acid sequencing of different light chains derived from different immunoglobulins revealed that the amino-terminal half of the light chain consist of 100-110 amino acids and showed lots of variation among different immunoglobulins. This region was called the **variable (VL) region**. The carboxyl terminal half the light chain is called, **constant (CL) region**, has two different types of protein chains among different immunoglobulins. They are designated as *kappa (κ) and lambda (λ)*. In humans 60% light chain constant regions are kappa and 40% are lambda. In humans, four IgG subtypes are present and they differ from one another by interchange of two or three amino acid positions in the kappa or lambda chain. A single antibody molecule contains either kappa chain or lambda chains but never both.

Heavy chain sequencing

The amino acid sequences of several heavy chains obtained from different antibodies were compared and it was found that a similar pattern existed here also like that of light chain. The amino terminals, consisting of 100-110 amino acids showed remarkable variation among different antibodies, therefore called as **variable region of heavy chain (V_H)**. The remainder of the heavy chain region terminating with carboxyl end revealed several different types of proteins among different classes of antibodies called μ, δ, ε, α, and γ corresponding to **constant region of the heavy chain (CH)**. Each of the different constant regions of the heavy chain is called isotype. The length of the constant region is approximately 330 amino acids for γ, δ, and α and 440 for μ and ε. The heavy chain of a particular antibody molecule determines the class of the antibody i.e. IgM, IgG, IgD, IgA, and IgE respectively. A single antibody molecule has two identical heavy chains and two identical light chains.

Immunoglobulin Domains

On careful analysis of the amino acid sequence of the heavy and light chain, it was observed that both the chains contain several homologous units of 110 amino acid residues. Within each unit called as **domain**, an intrachain disulfide bond results in formation of a loop of about 60 amino acids in each loop. The heavy chain contains one variable domain (V_H), and three or four constant region domains (C_H1, C_H2, C_H3 and C_H4) depending on the class of antibody. The light chain contains one variable domain (V_L) and one constant domain (C_L). X-ray crystallographic analysis of the immunoglobulin revealed that each domain is thrown in to characteristic folds called immunoglobulin fold (Fig. 7.2). The structure consists of two β pleated sheets, each containing antiparallel β strands on amino acids, which are connected by loops of various lengths. The β strands are characterized by alternating hydrophobic and hydrophilic amino acids whose side chains are arranged perpendicular to the plane of the sheet; the hydrophobic amino acids

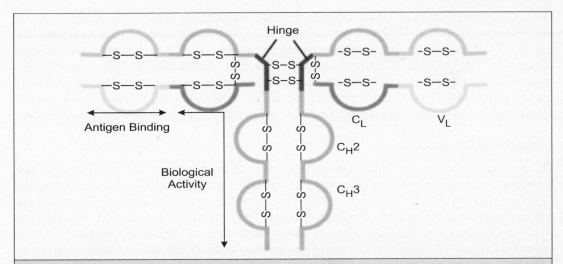

Fig. 7.2   Diagrammatic representation of immunoglobulin structure showing different domains of heavy and light chains with intrachain disulfide bonds positions. The IgM and IgE immunoglobulins will not possess hinge region, hence contain an additional domain in the central portion of the heavy chain.

are oriented toward the interior and the hydrophilic amino acids free outward. It is observed that the V domain is slightly longer than the C domain and contains an extra pair of β strands within the β-sheet and an extra loop sequence connecting this pair of β strands (Fig. 7.3).

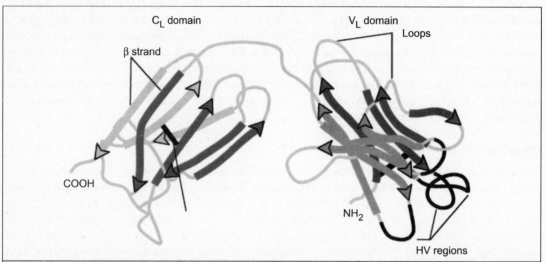

Fig. 7.3   A diagram representing the variable and constant region of the immunoglobulin fold representing the β pleated sheet.

Variable region domains

Detailed analysis of amino acid sequence of the light and heavy chain variable region domain revealed that, it has several hypervariable (HV) regions within it. These are also called complementarity-determining regions (CDRs). Three such hypervariable regions are present in human and mouse variable region domains of heavy and light chains and it constitutes about 15-20% of the variable domain. The remainder of the variable region of heavy and light chain shows very less variation and these stretches are referred as frame work regions (FRs). The wide range of specificities exhibited by the antibodies lies in the six hypervariable loops in Fab fragment. The framework region acts as supporting region of these six loops.

Constant region domains

The amino acid sequence of this domain shows slight variation among different classes of antibodies and is associated with various biological functions of the antibody. The Fab region of the antibody is extended by the presence of CH1 and CL domains, thereby facilitating interaction with antigen by increasing the maximum rotation of the Fab arms. The constant region of the light chain is linked to CH1 by a disulfide bond between them. It is presumed that more random association of VH and VL domains with their respective CH1 and CL domains may contribute to antibody diversity and this association is driven by VH and VL interaction alone. Recent experiments conducted in this regard have contributed some information. For ex. when VH and VL domains from two different antibodies having different specificities a and b were prepared separately and mixed. Each domain reassociated exclusively with its original partner to form homogeneous VLa/VHa or VLb/VHb complexes.

Hinge region

The heavy chains of γ, δ, and α contain an extended peptide link between CH1 and CH2 domains and it has no homology with the other domains (refer to Fig. 7.1 & 7.2). This region is called **hinge region**, which is made up of proline rich residues and gives flexibility to Fab arms movement. As a result, the Fab arms can assume various angles relative to each other. The hinge region contains two prominent amino acids, namely proline and cystein. Presence of large number of proline residues in the hinge region has resulted in making this region more vulnerable to papain or pepsin digestion. The cystein residues in this region helps in establishing the disulfide bond with the opposite heavy chain. The number of interchain disulfide bonds in the hinge region varies considerably among different classes of immunoglobulins and between types. μ and ε chains lack hinge region, instead they have an additional 110 amino acids domain that has hinge like features. In other words, heavy chain of IgE and IgM contain four constant region domains, where as the heavy chains of IgA, IgD and IgG contain three constant region domains and a hinge region. The sequence of constant region domains in different antibodies can be shown as follows:

IgG, IgD, and IgA	IgM and IgE
C_H1/C_H1	C_H1/C_H1
Hinge region	C_H2/C_H2
C_H2/C_H2	C_H3/C_H3
C_H3/C_H3	C_H4/C_H4

In IgG, IgA, and IgD the two CH2 domains and CH3 in IgM and IgE are separated by oligosaccharide chains, which makes them more accessible for aqueous environment and complement components. The CH3 domain in IgG, IgA, and IgD and CH4 domain in IgM and IgE is designated as carboxyl-terminal of the immunoglobulin. In membrane bound immunoglobulins (mIg) the carboxyl-terminal domain differs in both structure and function from the corresponding domain in secreted immunoglobulins (sIg). The characteristics of carboxyl terminal domain of mIg is as follows:

- A hydrophilic extracellular spacer sequence of 26 amino acid residues
- A transmembrane hydrophobic sequence
- A short tail directed into cytoplasm

Among all immunoglobulin isotypes, the length of the transmembrane sequence is constant but the lengths of the extracellular spacer sequence and cytoplasmic tail varies remarkably. B cell is known to express different classes of mIg at different stages of development. Each of the subclasses of immunoglobulins and the five types are capable of binding to membrane and can be expressed membrane bound antibodies. The immature pre-B cell expresses only mIgM in the beginning and later in the mature B cell mIgD is also expressed together with mIgM. Memory B cell is known to express different classes of immunoglobulins in various permutations and combinations of mIgM, mIgG, mIgA and mIgE. The antigenic specificity of all membrane bound antibody molecules is identical, so that each antibody molecule binds to the same antigenic determiner or epitope, when different classes of antibody molecules are expressed on a single cell. The genetic mechanism involved in the expression of different types of antibody molecule by the single B cell is discussed in Chapter 10.

Antigenic Determinants on Immunoglobulins

The antigenic determinants or epitopes on immunoglobulin molecules fall into three major categories: isotypic, allotypic and idiotypic determinants, which are located in characteristic position of antibody molecule.

Isotypic Determinants

These are constant region determinants, which define heavy chain class and subclass and each light chain type and subtype within a given type of immunoglobulin molecule. The constant region is encoded by separate gene, and all members of a species carry the same constant region gene. Therefore, antibody of one type injected into another individual of the same species will never be immunogenic to the same species but in another species it will be certainly immunogenic and induce antibody production against the constant region epitope. Within a species, each normal individual will express all isotypes in their serum. Different species inherit different constant region genes and therefore express different isotypes (Fig. 7.4.).

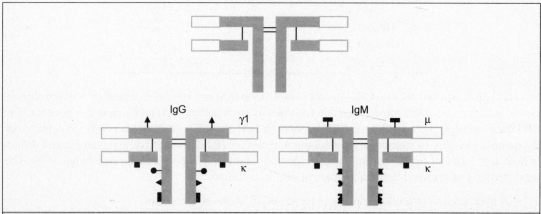

Fig. 7.4   Isotypic variants of the constant region of different classes and types of immunoglobulins.

Allotypic Determinants

In somewhat the same way as the RBCs in genetically different individuals can differ in terms of blood group antigen systems, so the immunoglobulins heavy chains differ in the expression of their allotypes. All the members of a species inherit the same set of isotype genes, but multiple alleles exist for some of the genes. These genes encode subtle amino acid differences, called the allotypic determinants that occur in some, but not in all the members of the species. In humans all four IgG subclasses and one IgA subclass and for κ light chain allotypes have been characterized. The γ chain allotypes are called as Gm markers and to date 25 of them have been identified. They are designated by the class and subclass followed by the allele number. For ex. G1m(1), G2m(23), G3m(11), G4m(4a). An individual with G1m(a) locus on IgG1 would have a peptide sequence: Asp-Glu-Leu-Thr-Lys on each of the IgG1 molecule. Another person whose IgG1 if negative would have the sequence Glu-Glu-Met-Thr-Lys, i.e. It differs by two amino acids from the previous one. Of the two subclasses of IgA, only IgA2 subclass has allotypes, designated as A2m(1) and A2m(2). The κ light chain has three allotypic determinants, designated as κm(1), κm(2), and κm(3).

Antibodies to allotypic determinants may arise following blood transfusion or may be produced by the pregnant mother in response to paternal allotypic determinants on the fetal immunoglobulins (Fig. 7.5)

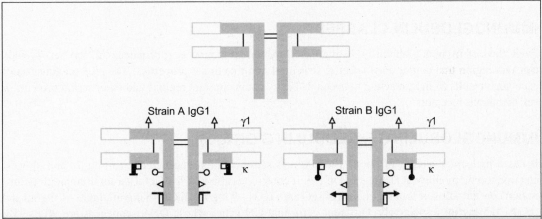

Fig. 7.5 A diagrammatic representation showing the positions of allotypic determinants of an antibody.

Idiotypic Determinants

Each individual antigenic determinant of the variable region is referred to as an idiotype (See Fig. 7.6).

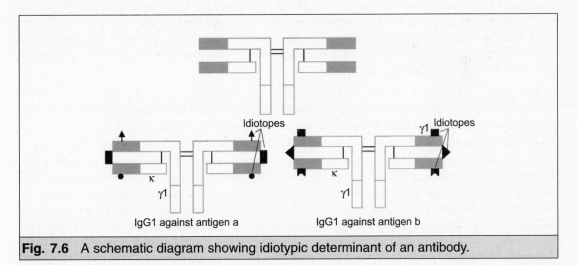

Fig. 7.6 A schematic diagram showing idiotypic determinant of an antibody.

The unique amino acid sequences of the VH and VL region of a given antibody can function as antigenic determiner but also as an antigen-binding site. Idiotypic determinants are generated by the conformation of the heavy and light chain variable region. In some cases the idiotypic determinant may be the actual antigen-binding site and in some cases it may comprise variable region sequences outside of the antigen-binding site. Each antibody will present multiple idiotypes and sum of the individual idiotypes is called the idiotype of the antibody. In an individual the antibodies produced by the same B cell clone are known to have identical variable region sequences and they all have the same idiotype. One theory states that, anti-idiotypic antibody produced naturally during the course of immune response plays an important role in regulating the immune response.

IMMUNOGLOBULIN CLASSES

Each class of immunoglobulin is distinguished by unique amino acid sequences in the heavy chain constant region that confer class specific structural and functional properties. The effector function of each class results from interaction between its heavy chain constant regions and other serum proteins or cell membrane receptors.

IMMUNOGLOBULIN G (γ GLOBULIN G OR IgG)

It has a molecular weight of about 150,000 and sedimentation coefficient of 6s to 7s and slowest electrophoretic mobility at alkaline pH of 8.6. It constitutes about 75% of total serum immunoglobulins. Serum concentration of four subclasses of IgG are : IgG1 - 9 mg/ml, IgG2 - 3 mg/ml, IgG3 - 1 mg/ml and IgG4 - 0.5 mg/ml respectively. Different germ-line CH genes whose DNA sequences are 90 to 95% homologous encode the four IgG subclasses. The structural characteristics that distinguish these subclasses from one another are the interchain disulfide linkage between the heavy chains and the length of the hinge region. Besides this there are subtle amino acid difference between subclasses of IgG, which affects the biological activity of the molecule (Fig. 7.7.).

- IgG1, IgG3, and IgG4 can readily cross the placental barrier and is thus found in fetal circulation, hence plays an important role in protecting the developing fetus.
- IgG3 is the most effective complement activator, followed by IgG1; IgG2 is relatively poor in complement activation and IgG4 is not able to activate complement at all.
- IgG1 and IgG3 bind to Fc receptor on phagocytes with high efficiency; IgG4 has intermediate affinity to Fc receptors and IgG2 has extremely low affinity. Binding to Fc receptors permits the IgG to function as major opsonin.

Functionally this class of immunoglobulin is bacteriolytic, viricidal and precipitating antibody but is a poor agglutinating and complement-fixing antibody compared to other immunoglobulins. In an immune response it appears late and persists for longer duration. The half-life of IgG in the body is 18-23 days. IgG monomer has one carbohydrate moiety on the Fc fragment and the carbohydrate content is 3%.

IgG diffuses more readily into extravascular spaces than other immunoglobulins. It carries the major burden of neutralizing bacterial toxins and of binding to microorganisms to enhance their phagocytosis. The complexes of the IgG antibody with bacteria enhances the complement reaction chemotactically by attracting polymorphonuclear phagocytes, which adhere to bacteria through surface receptors for complements and the Fc portion of the IgG. The interaction of IgG complexes with platelet Fc receptor presumably leads to aggregation and release of vasoactive amines. Transplacental passage, complement fixation and binding to various cell types is mediated by Fc part of the IgG molecule. With respect to overall regulation of IgG levels in the body the catabolic rate appears to depend directly upon the total IgG concentration. Whereas, synthesis is largely governed by antigen stimulation, so that in germ free animals IgG levels are extremely low but rise rapidly on transfer to a normal environment.

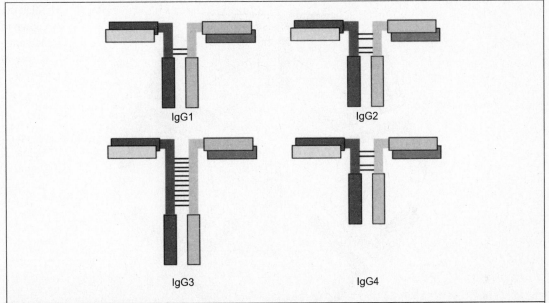

Fig. 7.7 A diagrammatic representation of different classes of IgG molecules, showing positions of the disulfide bond and the length of the hinge region.

IMMUNOGLOBULIN M (γ-GLOBULIN M OR IgM)

It is often referred to as macroglobulin, because of its higher molecular weight. IgM exists as pentamer with a molecular weight of 900,000and a monomer with a molecular weight of 180,000. IgM accounts for 5-10% of the total immunoglobulin with an average serum concentration of 1.5 mg/ml. IgM has a half-life of 5 days. Monomeric IgM is expressed as membrane bound antibody on B cells and it is used as an antigenic receptor by the B cells. Pentamer of IgM is secreted by plasmablast cells, in which 5 monomeric units are held together by disulfide bonds linking their carboxyl terminal (Cμ4/Cμ4) domains and (Cμ3/Cμ3) domains (Fig. 7.8). The Fc regions of the monomer are directed toward center of the pentamer and 10 antigens binding sites (Fab) directed to the periphery of the molecule.

Each pentamer has an additional peptide chain linked to Fc region called the J (Joining) chain. It is disulfide bonded via cystein to 2 of the Cμ4 domains of two monomers. The J chain is added, just before the formation of pentamer, hence it is believed that J chain is required for the formation of pentamer. The presence of J chain also helps IgM to bind to receptors on secretory cells, which transport it across epithelial linings to the external secretions that bathe mucosal surface. Although IgA is the major antibody found in the secretory fluids, IgM plays an important accessory role as secretory immunoglobulin. It cannot cross the placental barrier and it is the first one to appear in a primary response to an antigen and also the first one to disappear from the serum. It is the first immunoglobulin to be synthesized by the neonates. It is a better agglutinating, complement fixing and bacteriolytic antibody. IgM is intravascular, hence largely confined to bloodstream. Natural antibodies like Anti A and Anti B, and antibodies against microorganisms are usually IgM.

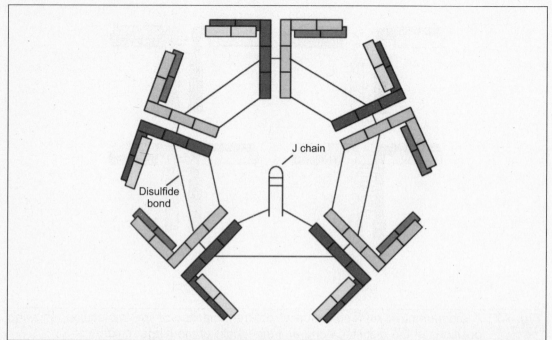

Fig. 7.8 A diagrammatic representation of structure of IgM pentamer showing the disulfide bonds and J chain link with the pentamer.

An IgM molecule can bind to 10 small haptens at a time, but can only bind to 5 large antigens because of steric hindrance. Serum IgM has a higher valency than the other isotypes, therefore pentameric IgM is more efficient than other isotypes in binding such multidimensional antigens as viral particles and RBCs. For ex. The corresponding antibodies when react with RBCs, they clump together and aggregate and the process is called agglutination. It is observed that, it takes 100 to 1000 times more molecules of IgG than of IgM to achieve the same level of agglutination. IgM facilitates complement activation much easily than IgG, because complement needs two adjacent Fc regions for activation, and the pentameric molecule of IgM can easily do this.

As shown in the Fig. 7.9. the IgM molecule has five carbohydrate residues on each monomer whereas the IgG molecule has one carbohydrate residue attached to the constant region of the heavy chain. The C_1, C_2, C_3, carbohydrate residues of the IgM molecule are complex and contain Fucose, Mannose, Galactose, N-acetylglucosamine and possibly sialic acid arranged in a highly branched structure. C_4, and C_5, are simple and contain only Mannose and N-acetylglucosamine in an unbranched linear array. The carbohydrate moieties affect the conformation and general properties of the IgM antibodies.

IMMUNOGLOBULIN A (γ-GLOBULIN A OR IgA)

IgA appears selectively in the sero-mucous secretions such as: saliva, nasal fluid, sweat, colostrum and secretions of the lung, genito-urinary tract and GI tracts where it defends against attack by microorganisms. IgA constitutes only 10 to 15% of the total immunoglobulin in serum. IgA has a half-life of 6 days. IgA primarily exists as a monomer in the serum but polymeric forms are more common in secretory fluids.

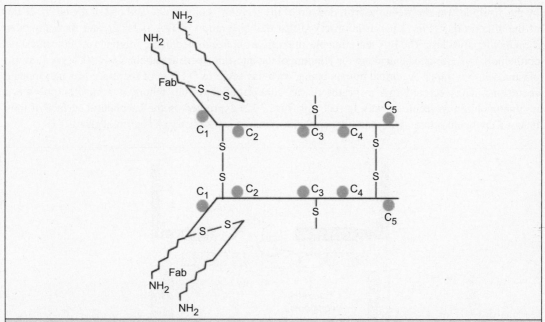

Fig. 7.9 A diagrammatic representation of monomer of IgM showing positioning of carbohydrate residues.

IgA found in secretory fluids is called secretory IgA (sIgA). IgA monomer has a molecular weight of 150,000 and a dimer 600,000. The dimeric IgA has a J-chain polypeptide, which is identical to the J-chain of IgM molecule with a molecular weight of 15,000 and a polypeptide chain called secretory component (Fig. 7.10.). The J-chain component facilitates polymerization of both serum IgA and secretory IgA.

The secretory component is the intestinal epithelial cells and the hepatocytes secrete polypeptide of 70,000 MW. It is made up of 5 immunoglobulin like domains and is found attached to the plasmamembrane of the epithelial cells or hepatocytes. It binds to Fc region of IgA dimer and this interaction is stabilized

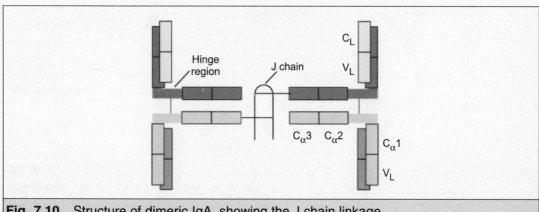

Fig. 7.10   Structure of dimeric IgA, showing the J chain linkage.

by the disulfide bond between the fifth domain of the secretory component, and one of the heavy chains of the dimeric IgA (Fig. 7.11). It is observed that daily secretion of IgA is far greater than any other immunoglobulin class. The IgA secreting plasma cells are concentrated in the submucosa of the intestinal epithelium. It is estimated that along the jejunum of the intestine, there are about 2.6×10^{10} IgA secreting plasma cells are found. A normal human being, each day secretes 5-15gm of secretory IgA into mucous secretions. The secreted IgA migrates to the subepithelial tissue, where it binds for polymeric immunoglobulin molecule or poly Ig receptor (Fig. 7.12) expressed on the basolateral surface of most mucosal epithelial cells and the glandular epithelia of mammary, salivary and lacrimal glands.

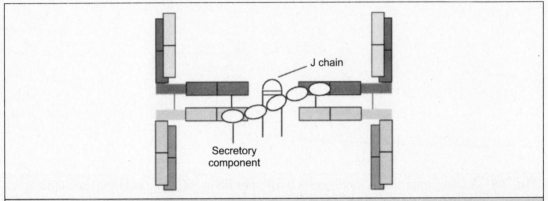

Fig. 7.11   Structure of dimeric IgA molecule showing association with secretory component to form secretory IgA (sIgA).

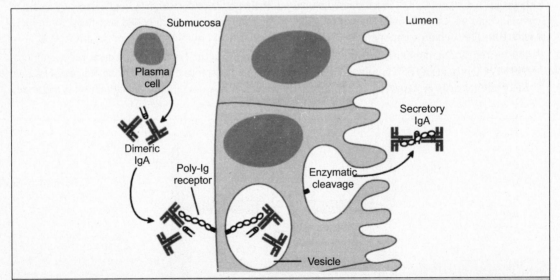

Fig. 7.12   Schematic diagram showing formation of secretory IgA during a passage through mucous epithelial cells. Note the poly Ig receptor is found on the basolateral membrane of the epithelial cells to which the polymeric IgA binds and transported across to the luminal membrane through the cytoplasm of the epithelial cells.

When the polymeric IgA binds to poly Ig receptor, the receptor IgA complex is endocytosed in to coated pits and directed across the cytoplasm of the epithelial cell toward the luminal membrane, where the vesicle fuses with the plasma membrane. At this juncture the poly Ig receptor is cleaved from the plasma membrane and becomes the secretory component. The secretory component is bound to polymeric IgA and together with IgA released in to the mucosal secretion. The secretory component protects the hinge region from proteolytic digestion in the protease rich mucosal environment. Since secretory IgA is polymeric, it can bind to large antigens with multiple epitopes, hence secretory IgA serves as an important antibody at the mucous membrane surfaces, which are main entry sites of most pathogens. Binding of secretory IgA to bacterial and viral surface antigens prevents them from binding to mucosal surfaces. This inhibits colonization by bacteria and viruses. The mucous helps in entrapping the complexes of IgA and antigens and eliminates them by peristalsis of gut or ciliated epithelium of respiratory tract. Secretory IgA has been known to provide protection against bacteria such as *Salmonella, Neisseria gonorrhoea, Vibrio cholera* and viruses such as *polio, influenza and reoviruses*. IgA activates complement only through alternative pathway.

Because IgA transported across the intestinal epithelial cells, it can act at three different levels of the intestinal lining. It can bind to viral or bacterial antigen in the submucosa region, within epithelial cells and within the mucosal secretion. This is a unique example of antibody acting in an intracellular location. The second function of intracellular IgA is to excrete foreign antigens trapped in the intracellular location.

In some animals like rats, rabbits and chickens 30 to 75% the IgA produced in the intestinal wall, enters into enterohepatic circulation through the portal vein. In these species hepatocytes make poly Ig receptor. From the hepatocytes, the IgA is excreted in bile, therefore in these animals bile the major route of elimination of IgA-antigen complexes. However, in ruminants, mice, dogs and humans, less than 1% of IgA produced in the intestinal lining enters the bile. More than 90% of IgA enters the intestinal lumen.

IMMUNOGLOBULIN E (IgE OR γ-GLOBULIN E)

It is largely cell bound, especially to mast cells. It mediates immediate hypersensitivity reactions that are responsible for the symptoms of hay fever, asthma, hives, and anaphylactic shock. These symptoms would occur when an antigen complexes with IgE, which is bound to mast cells. Average concentration of IgE in the serum is 0.3 µg/ml. It has a half-life of 2.5 days and molecular weight of 190,000. Its carbohydrate content is 12% linked to constant region of the heavy chain. The main physiological role of IgE would appear to be protection of the external mucosal surface of the body by the local recruitment of plasma factors and effector cells through triggering an acute inflammatory reaction. IgE binds to Fc receptor on the mast cells of basophils and complexes with infectious agents or antigens (allergens) and triggers the release of vasoactive agents and granulocyte chemotactic factor, leading to an influx of plasma IgG, complement, polymorphs and eosinophils. In such a context, the ability of eosinophils to damage IgG coated helminths and the IgE response to such parasites would constitute an effective defense. IgE does not cross the placental barrier and it activates alternative pathway of complement. See Fig. 7.13 and 7.14 also Fig. 17.3 in helminth infection).

IMMUNOGLOBULIN D (IgD OR γ-GLOBULIN D)

It is a membrane bound antibody, found attached to B cell membrane together with mIgM, but appears later and is considered to be an indicator of the mature or 'virgin' resting B cell. On a give B cell membrane IgD has the same antigen binding specificity as IgM. It has a molecular weight of 150,000 and a half-life of 3 days. Serum concentration of IgD is about 0.03 mg /ml and it represents about 0.25% of total serum

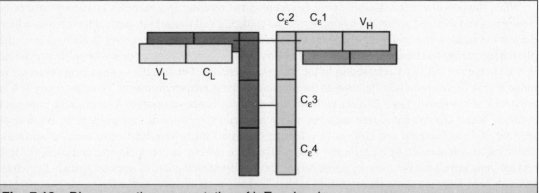

Fig. 7.13   Diagrammatic representation of IgE molecule.

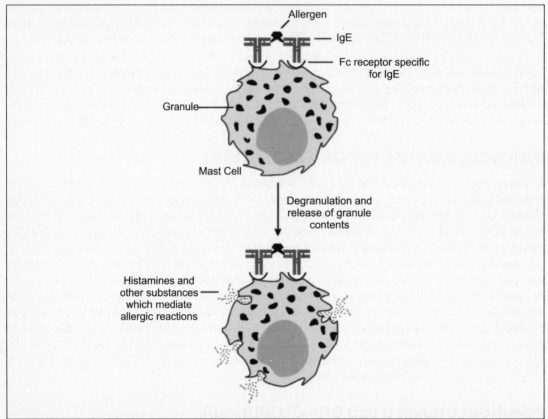

Fig. 7.14   A schematic diagram to show allergen cross-linkage to receptor bound IgE on the mast cells induces degranulation and release of vasoactive substances.

immunoglobulin and 1% of immunoglobulins synthesized daily, therefore it is unlikely that it has an important direct role in the neutralization of antigens (Fig. 7.15). On the other hand, it can function as a receptor, for when heterologous antibodies against the μ and δ constant regions are used to mimic stimulating 'antigen', both stimulate replication. When the cell is stimulated either in this way or with mitogens or T cell factors, IgM is synthesized and secreted whereas IgD production is shut off. This is consistent with low level of IgD. Its carbohydrate content is 13%. Antibodies to certain antigens such as insulin, penicillin, milk protein and diphtheria toxoid and thyroid antigen is found to stimulate IgD production. Since it is found on B cells together with mIgM it seems likely that they may function as mutually interacting antigen receptors for the control of the lymphocyte activation and suppression.

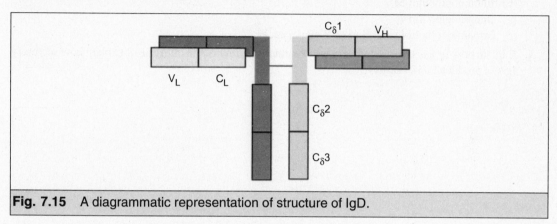

Fig. 7.15 A diagrammatic representation of structure of IgD.

A controversial issue is the role of IgD in memory. Some hold that the majority of cells giving rise to the secondary response have lost IgD from their surface, whereas others argue that IgD loss is not a necessary stage in memory cell maturation.

Ablation of population of B cells that carries IgD on their surface (IgD+) by administration of heterologous anti-δ antibodies to the animal continuously from birth does not abolish the immune response. This contrasts with the profound immunodeficiency engendered by suppression of IgM cells with anti-μ antibodies. This difference may simply be due to the fact that IgM+ B cells are produced early in ontogeny and are precursors of most or all of the other cells involved in producing antibody, whereas IgD expression occurs after the B cell is competent to respond. IgD suppression *in vivo* and anti-δ antibodies administered *in vitro* do give rise to subtle shifts in the quantitative responsiveness of B cells to T-dependent antigens. This may indicate that IgD is involved in interactions between T and B cells and in the regulation of B-cell populations. Since IgD appears on the mature virgin B cell and decreases when the B cell is stimulated by antigen, the virgin cell would be the one in whose regulation IgD would be likely to participate.

It is more difficult to account for the secreted form of IgD (sIgD). However, secreted form of IgD could complete a feed back loop by supplying afferent signals representative of all the idiotypes present in the B-cell repertoire to the T –cell population. The low stability of serum IgD would also serve a function, since an intercellular messenger molecule should not have an excessive half life it is to function properly in that role. There, is in fact, some evidence that a factor emitted by B cells is needed for the development of a class of isotype-specific TH cells. This factor might be the secretory form of IgD.

Exercise

1. Give a detailed account of Porter and Edelman model of immunoglobulin or Explain the general structure of immunoglobulin (20 marks)
2. What are antigenic determinants on immunoglobulins? Give an account of each type (15 marks) or (5 marks each if individual type is asked-isotype, allotype and idiotype)
3. Write notes on any one of the following: (10 marks each)
   (a) Immunoglobulin G
   (b) Immunoglobulin M
   (c) Immunoglobulin A
   (d) Immunoglobulin D and E (5 or 8 marks each)
4. Explain how IgA is transported across the epithelial lining of the intestine or explain how secretory IgA is produced. (10 marks)

Chapter 8

Antigen-Antibody Interactions

- Precipitin Reactions
- Radial Immunodiffusion (Mancini Method)
- Two Dimensional Immunoelectrophoresis
- Immunoelectrophoresis
- Radioimmunoassay (RIA)
- Immunofluorescence
- Experimental Assessment of Humoral Immunity
- Elispot Assay
- Immunodiffusion (Ouchterlony Technique)
- Rocket Immunoelctrophoresis
- Counter Current Immunoelectrophoresis
- Agglutination Reaction
- Enzyme Linked Immunosorbent Assay (ELISA)
- Western Blotting
- Direct Hemolytic Plaque Assay

The antigen antibody interaction is similar to that of enzyme substrate interaction except that this interaction does not lead to irreversible alteration either in antibody or antigen and therefore reversible. The reaction between an antigen and antibody is of noncovalent type, where the antigenic determinants or epitopes interact with V_H/V_L domain of the antibody molecule, particularly hypervariable region or CDRs (complementarity determining regions). The noncovalent interaction between antigen and antibody is brought about by hydrogen bonds, vander Waals interactions, ionic bonds and hydrophobic interactions. All these interactions are week type when compared to covalent interactions. Therefore, a strong affinity interaction should occur between antigen and antibody to form a stable complex. Mostly these interactions are highly specific, hence they are always strong, but some times due to nonspecific interactions weak and unstable complexes is formed (Fig. 8.1).

Antibody avidity

The strength of multiple interactions between a multivalent antibody and antigen is called avidity. This can be proved by mixing antigens with multiple, repeating antigenic determinants with antibodies containing multiple binding sites, the interaction of antigen with antibody will increase the probability of binding at second site. The avidity of an antibody is its binding capacity than its affinity of individual binding sites. Affinity at one binding site does not always reflect the true strength of the antibody-antigen interaction. It is observed that high avidity compensates for low affinity. For ex. Pentameric IgM molecule has low affinity but has high avidity when compared to IgG, because of its multivalent antigen binding ability.

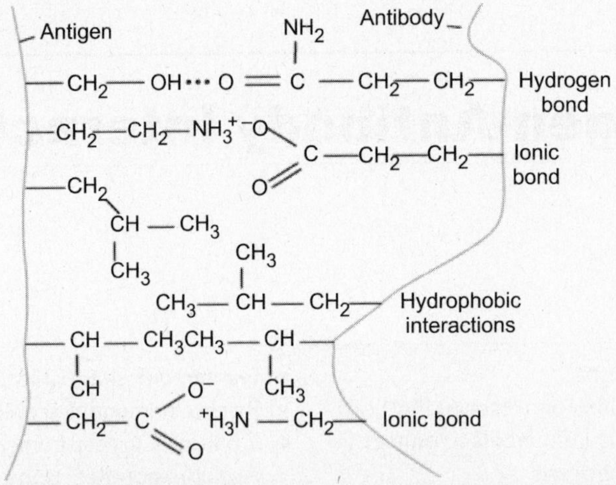

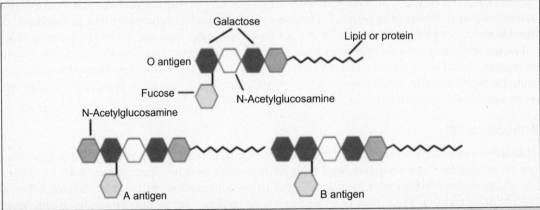

Fig. 8.1 Schematic representation of different types of antigen antibody interactions showing involvement of different types of bonds.

Antigen-antibody cross reactivity

Most of the antigen antibody reactions are highly specific type, but once in a while certain antigens show cross reactivity with unrelated antibodies. Such cross reactivities are possible only when two different antigens share similar epitope or antibodies specific for one epitope also bind to an unrelated epitope possessing similar chemical properties. Cross reactivity is generally observed with ABO blood group antigens, because they are made up of polysaccharide antigens having similar oligosaccharide residues. Only difference in AB antigens is subtle differences in terminal sugar residues (Fig. 8.2).

Fig. 8.2 Structure of A, B and O antigen showing differences in terminal sugar residue in the side chain. Shaded and un-shaded components in the structure represents the same chemical constituent as labeled in O antigen or in A antigen.

In an individual cross reactivity to blood group antigens may be induced by exposure to cross reacting microbial antigens present in the intestinal flora. Individuals lacking these blood group antigens develop antibodies against the microbial antigens. The blood group antibodies elicited by the microbial antigens will react with antigens with similar oligosaccharides found on the red blood corpuscles.

Different types of viruses and bacteria are known to possess antigenic determiners that resemble normal host cell antigens. It is observed that in some cases these antigens of viral or bacterial origin induce antibody production in the host, which cross-reacts with host cell antigens leading to tissue damaging adverse autoimmune reactions. For ex. Following streptococcus pyogenes infection, some individuals suffer from heart and kidney damage due to development of antibodies against streptococcal cell wall protein antigen M. This antigen has similar determiners like that of myocardial and skeletal muscle proteins. Therefore, antibodies formed against M antigen will cross reacts with host tissue antigens specifically with heart and skeletal muscle leading to autoimmune disease.

Jenner's invention of small pox vaccine using vaccinia virus is due to cross reacting epitopes found between these two viruses.

PRECIPITIN REACTIONS

The reaction between soluble antigen and antibody leads to visible precipitate formation, which is called precipitin reaction. Antibodies that bring about precipitate formation on reacting with antigens are called as precipitins. To form the visible precipitate, the antibody should be bivalent, i.e. more than one Fab site should be available for reacting with antigen. Similarly antigen should be bivalent or polyvalent, i.e. it must have at least two similar epitopes or different epitopes reacting with different antibodies. To form a visible precipitate of antigen-antibody complex, the concentration of both antigen and antibody plays an important role. The concentration of Ag and Ab should be equal otherwise if the concentration of one exceeds the other, it results in soluble complex and precipitate will not form. When the antigen-antibody ratio is optimal, maximum precipitate will be formed, which is called **equivalence zone** (Fig. 8.3).

From the curve it is evident that when the antibody is in excess, unreacted antibody will be found in the supernatant with small soluble complex of antigen consisting of one molecule of antigen bound by multiple molecules of antibodies. In the antigen excess region, unreacted antigen will be found in the supernatant with one or two molecules of antigen bound to a single molecule of antibody.

Precipitins may be produced against most of the proteins, some carbohydrates and carbohydrate-lipid conjugates. Precipitin reactions can be demonstrated in agarose gel by various techniques, such as Immunodiffusion (Ouchterlony method), radial Immunodiffusion (Mancini method), countercurrent immunoelectrophoresis (CIEP), immunoelectrophoresis, rocket immunoelectrophoresis (Laurel method), two-dimensional immunoelectrophoresis and centrifugation.

IMMUNODIFFUSION (Ouchterlony Technique)

Molten agarose prepared in suitable buffer of pH 8.4 – 8.6 is poured on a microscope slide and allowed to solidify. Each microscope slide would need about 3.5 ml of agarose, which on solidifying forms a gel layer on the slide of 3mm thickness. Using a punching device (Fig. 8.4) wells are punched on the gel (Fig. 8.5). Generally 7 well pattern is punched, which will enable six unknown samples (antigens) could be tested for precipitin reaction against an antibody in the middle well.

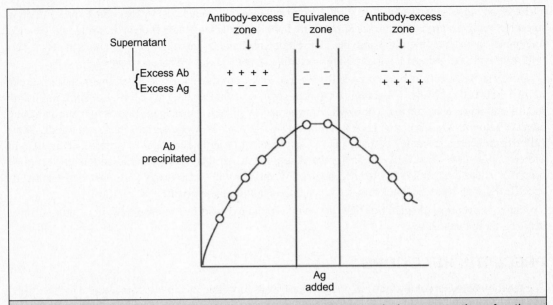

Fig. 8.3 Precipitation curve for antigen-antibody reaction at varied concentration of antigen and antibody to show equivalence zone for maximum precipitation.

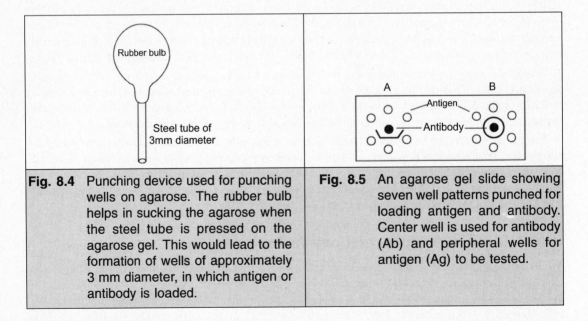

Fig. 8.4 Punching device used for punching wells on agarose. The rubber bulb helps in sucking the agarose when the steel tube is pressed on the agarose gel. This would lead to the formation of wells of approximately 3 mm diameter, in which antigen or antibody is loaded.

Fig. 8.5 An agarose gel slide showing seven well patterns punched for loading antigen and antibody. Center well is used for antibody (Ab) and peripheral wells for antigen (Ag) to be tested.

Ouchterlony method works on the principle of diffusion of antigen and antibody radially from wells toward each other through a concentration gradient. As the equivalence is reached a white precipitin band appears at the junction of antigen-antibody complex. Precipitin bands formed in this reaction can be classified into three types, which indicate whether or not they share epitopes (Fig. 8.6).

Line of identity: this type of precipitin band like a smooth curve will be formed when the antigens share identical epitopes against single antibody, giving a single curved line of identity (Fig. 8.6A).

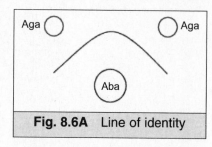

Fig. 8.6A Line of identity

Line of partial identity: This type of precipitin band is observed when the antigens share some epitopes but one of them has unique epitope(s). The antibody will form line of identity with the common epitope(s) and a curved spur with unique epitope(s). Here one should note that the concentration of unique as well as shared epitopes should be equal than only the precipitin band will be overlapping otherwise two precipitin bands may be formed with a spur as shown in the diagram. In this case antibodies to the unique epitope(s) diffuse past the common precipitin line to form a precipitin line (spur) with the unique epitopes of the more complex antigen (Fig. 8.6B).

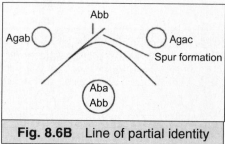

Fig. 8.6B Line of partial identity

Line of nonidentity: This type of precipitin band would occur when two antigens are unrelated and do not share any epitopes. Therefore, two independent precipitin lines are formed which cross each other and do not form a smooth curve. In this case, precipitin lines cross because the unrelated antigen and antibody do not precipitate and therefore are free to diffuse past the precipitin lines; as a result, the precipitin line of each related antibody-antigen system extends beyond that of the other (Fig. 8.6C).

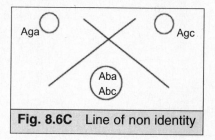

Fig. 8.6C Line of non identity

RADIAL IMMUNODIFFUSION (Mancini method)

In this case, the antigen or antibody is readily incorporated in the gel and the wells are punched as shown in the Fig. 8.7. If the gel contains the suitable dilution of antibody, antigen is added to the wells and allowed to diffuse through the agarose overnight. As the antigen diffuses into the agarose, the region of equivalence is established and a ring of precipitate is formed around the well (Fig. 8.7). The diameter of the precipitin ring is proportional to the concentration of antigen. By preparing a standard curve by measuring the diameter of rings formed against known concentration of antigen against a known dilution of antibody, it is possible to find out the concentration of unknown antigen. (Fig. 8.8). This method has its own limitations. It cannot detect antigens at concentrations lower than 5 μg/ml. Mancini method is used for quantitation of serum levels of IgM, IgG and IgA by incorporating specific anti-isotypic antibodies in the agarose gel.

ROCKET IMMUNOELECTROPHORESIS

The gel readily contains the antibody of known concentration and the negatively charged antigen is loaded in the wells punched on one corner of the gel plate as shown in the Fig. 8.9A. Antigen well side is connected to negative pole and the opposite end to the positive pole. Electrophoresis is carried out. Since the gel readily contains antibody, as the antigen starts travelling in the gel toward the positive pole,

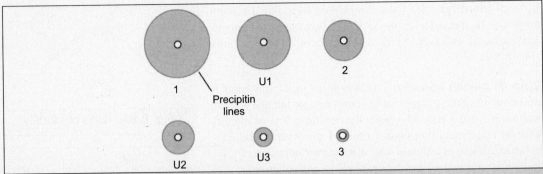

Fig. 8.7 A diagrammatic sketch of radial immunodiffusion depicted in the form of rings around the well. Note the difference in size of the rings, which is proportional to concentration of antigen.

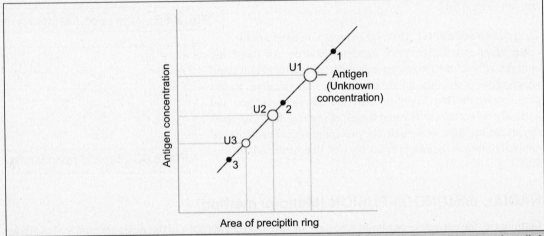

Fig. 8.8 A standard curve is prepared by measuring the diameter of the rings of radial immunodiffusion of known concentration of antigen against a known dilution of antibody (wells 1, 2 and 3). From the standard curve, the unknown antigen concentration can be determined (wells U1, U2 and U3).

precipitin band appears in the form a rocket. The height of the rocket is proportional to the concentration of antigen in the well (Fig. 8.9B). Some limitations of rocket immunoelectrophoresis are, only negatively charged antigen will be able to move in the agarose matrix, it is not possible to quantitate several antigens in a mixture at the same time, some antibodies, which are not sufficiently charged can not be quantitated by this method.

TWO-DIMENSIONAL IMMUNOELECTROPHORESIS

This is slightly modified version of rocket immunoelectrophoresis. By this method several antigens in a complex mixture can be quantitated simultaneously. In this method, first the antigen is separated into

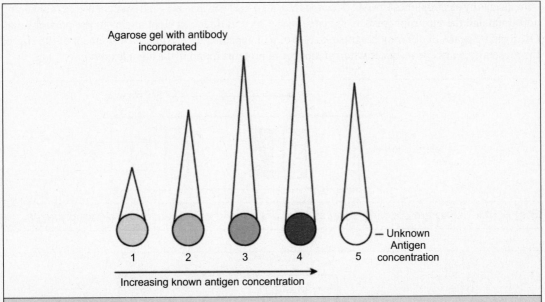

Fig. 8.9A   Demonstration of rocket immunoelectrophoresis on a gel plate, showing precipitin reaction in the form of rocket formation.

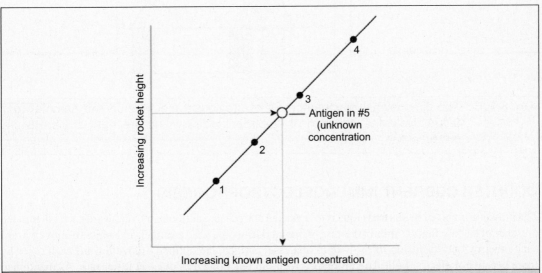

Fig. 8.9B   A Standard Curve prepared by measuring the height of the rocket for known concentration of antigen against a known concentration of antibody, height of the rocket of unknown antigen can be compared with standard curve to determine the concentration of unknown antigen.

components by electrophoresis in one direction (Fig. 8.10A). Then the gel is laid over another gel containing antiserum and the electrophoresis is repeated in the second direction right angles to the previous one. Overlapping peaks of different heights like rocket will appear (Fig. 8.10B). Measurement of the size of the rockets or peaks allows quantitation of number of proteins found in the complex mixture.

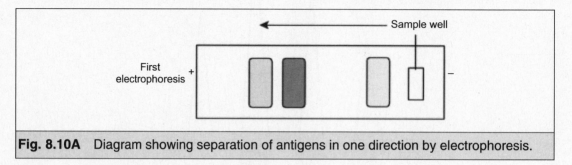

Fig. 8.10A   Diagram showing separation of antigens in one direction by electrophoresis.

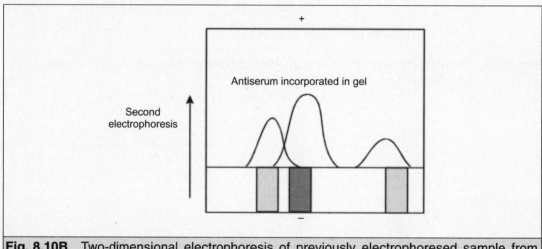

Fig. 8.10B   Two-dimensional electrophoresis of previously electrophoresed sample from 8.10A. Note the direction of electrophoresis, which are right angles to the previous one.

COUNTER CURRENT IMMUNOELECTROPHORESIS

The principle involved in this technique is to make the antigen and antibody move toward each other in the presence of electric field. Unlike in the case of immunodiffusion, where antigen and antibody move toward each other by only diffusion force, here in this case, antigen and antibody move toward each other by force because of electric field. Therefore the precipitin reaction takes place at faster rate. As mentioned earlier agarose slide is prepared and rows of wells are punched, it is called two well patterns. The distance between each pair of well is about 4mm and the distance between each paired row is maintained at 1 cm. A single well is punched at right-hand top corner of the slide to indicate that side of the slide is to be connected to positive pole. In the paired row all the left-hand side wells are loaded with unknown serum sample to be analyzed for antigens and the right hand side wells are loaded with antibody (Fig. 8.11). Antibody side is to be connected to the positive pole, provided the antibody is positively charged. Electrophoresis is run for one hour and at the end of electrophoresis if the precipitin band appears between the paired wells in any row, it indicates the presence of antigen corresponding to the antibody. In this way many samples of unknown serum can be analyzed for the presence of antigens. Only the limitation of this technique is that, the antibody and the antigen should be oppositely charged at a given pH. This technique is routinely used for testing the blood samples in the blood bank for hepatitis antigen.

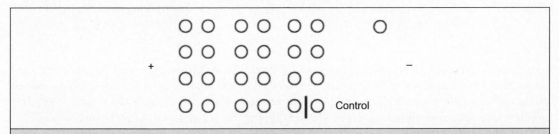

Fig. 8.11   Two well pattern of punching the wells for counter current immunoelectrophoresis. Note the wells of the left-hand side are used for loading antigen and the right hand side for antibody. A single well is punched at right-hand top corner to indicate that this side of the slide is to be connected to the positive pole.

IMMUNOELECTROPHORESIS

This technique involves combination of two different methods, first, electrophoresis of sample followed by immunodiffusion to identify the precipitin bands. An antigen mixture is loaded in the well punched at one-fourth corner of a gel plate. Antigen loaded side is connected to negative pole and electrophoresed (Fig. 8.12A). After the completion of electrophoresis (1 hr later), a trough is cut in the middle of the slide (Fig. 8.12B) with the help of a fine blade. Antiserum is loaded in the trough and the gel is kept for immunodiffusion in a moist chamber over night.

The antiserum diffuses from the trough toward antigen components and forms precipitin bands with different antigen component if the antiserum is polyvalent. If the antiserum is specific for a particular component of antigen only one precipitin band will form (Fig. 8.12B). Immunoelectrophoresis is used for checking the purity of isolated serum components like antigens or antibodies, which are used for

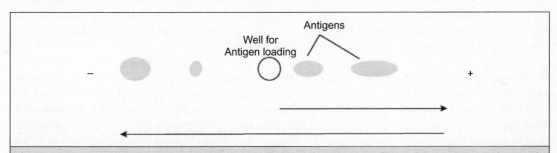

Fig. 8.12A   Immunoelectrophoresis of an antigen mixture. First the antigen mixture is electrophoresed. Antigen components get separated on the basis of charges.

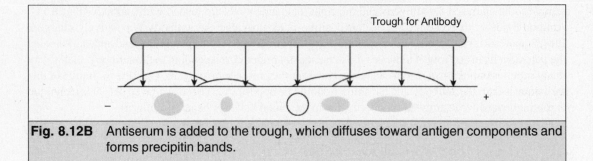

Fig. 8.12B   Antiserum is added to the trough, which diffuses toward antigen components and forms precipitin bands.

immunization schedule. Moreover, it is also used for identification of plasma or serum components for the presence or the absence of certain proteins. This technique also helps in determining whether a patient produces abnormal amounts of serum proteins. Immunoelectrophoresis is a qualitative technique and is useful in quantitation of antigen levels as low as 0.2µg/ml and it can detect antibody concentrations of 3-20µg/ml.

AGGLUTINATION REACTION

Whenever a particulate antigen interacts with its antibody, it would result in clumping or agglutination of the particulate antigen, which is called agglutination reaction. The antibody involved in bringing about agglutination reaction is called **agglutinin**. As observed in precipitin reactions, just as excess of antibody inhibits precipitin reactions, an excess of antibody also inhibits agglutination reaction. This mechanism of inhibition is called prozone effect. High concentration of antibodies that bind to the antigen but may fail to induce agglutination; such antibodies are called incomplete antibodies. IgG antibodies may act as incomplete antibodies and at high concentration may occupy all of the antigenic sites, thereby blocking the access to IgM. Certain particulate antigen may possess antigenic determiners in deep pockets of the plasma membrane and may not be easily available for antibodies. Therefore, in such cases agglutination reaction fails.

Hemagglutination

Typing of ABO blood group is hemagglutination reaction. For which, a drop of blood is taken on a slide and mixed with a drop of antiserum to A and B antigens. If the blood corpuscles possess any of these antigens they will form visible clumps on reacting with antiserum. Agglutination with an antiserum of A or B would indicate to which blood group the person belongs. Many bacteria can be identified by agglutination reaction. Similarly molecular antigens antigens can be also identified by agglutination reaction by specially coating the antigens over an inert particle surface.

(a) Bacterial agglutination (Tube agglutination)   Routinely in the clinical laboratories, bacterial agglutination reactions are carried out to identify the bacterial species as well as to know the intensity of infection. Bacterial infections induce production of serum antibodies specific for surface antigens of the bacterial cell wall. Such antibodies can be identified by bacterial agglutination reaction. Generally, the serum obtained from a patient, suspected to have been infected with bacteria is serially diluted (1:2, 1:4, 1:8, etc.) and to these serial dilutions suspected bacteria is added. The last tube showing visible agglutination reaction will indicate the antibody titer of the patient. Patients suffering from typhoid fever will show significantly elevated agglutination titer to *Salmonella typhi*. Agglutination reaction also helps in identifying the type and species of bacteria, for which typing sera is used. Important clinical application of this technique are the *Widal* test for the diagnosis of typhoid fever, *Brucella* agglutination test for *Brucellosis* and the *Weil Felix* test for *Rickettsiosis*.

(b) Passive agglutination   This technique is used for demonstration of agglutination reaction of particulate antigens by adsorbing them on the inert particulate surface. Particulate surface used here may consist of tanned and killed RBCs of O blood group, or sheep or chicken RBCs. Many antigens will spontaneously couple with red cells and form stable reagents for antibody detection. These include antigens of *E.coli, Yersinia*, lipopolysaccharide of *N. meningitides, toxoplasma, mycoplasma* species and purified protein derivatives of *Mycobacterium* species. Particles of latex or polystyrene, mineral colloid-bentonite are used to coat them with suitable antigens. To coat the red blood corpuscles with soluble antigen, RBCs are tanned by treating them with tannic acid or chromium chloride; both of these are known to enhance the adsorption of the antigen to the surface of the RBCs. Serum from the patient is serially diluted and added to the micrometer plate wells containing antigen coated RBCs. Agglutination reaction is assessed by the spread pattern of the RBCs. If the RBCs settle down as solid buttons, it indicates no agglutination. If a mat like appearance is seen, then it indicates agglutination. Size of the mat would indicate the titer of the antibody, greater the antibody concentration; larger will be the mat. Passive hemagglutination reaction is much more sensitive than precipitin reaction. It detects antibody concentration as low as 0.001mg/ml.

(c) Reverse Passive hemagglutination test   When red blood cells are coated with antibody instead of antigen and used for detection of antigen in the patients serum or from the blood of a professional donor it is called reverse passive hemagglutination test. It is commonly used for the detection of hepatitis B surface antigens (HbsAg) in patients serum or in donors blood in the blood bank.

Agglutination inhibition reaction

It is used in the pregnancy test kits, where latex particles are coated with human chorionic gonadotropin. Anti-HCG is added to the test urine sample on a slide. After thorough mixing latex particles coated with human HCG are added. If there is agglutination and clumping of latex particles, it would indicate that the sample is negative. If the agglutination does not take place then the sample is positive for pregnancy. Agglutination inhibition reaction is also used for clinical diagnosis of certain viral infections. For ex. Premarital determination of immune status of a women to rubella virus. A titer greater than 10 is considered to be good and the women is immune to rubella, whereas a titer of less than 10 is indicative of a lack of immunity and the need for immunization. Certain types of viruses are capable of causing agglutination of red blood corpuscles. If an individual infected with such a virus contains antiviral antibodies in the serum, then the antibodies will bind to the virus and interfere with hemagglutination by virus.

Coomb's Test

Some times certain antibody molecules directed against deeply embedded membrane antigenic determinant can not cause agglutination even after binding to antigenic determinant. Such antibody molecules are considered to be short, because their Fab arms cannot bridge antigenic determinants on two different cells. Therefore agglutination fails to occur even after the antibody molecule binds to the antigenic determinants on the membrane. For. ex. Rh antibodies are of this category. They are called as incomplete antibodies because they fail to bring about strong agglutination of RBCs even after the binding of antibody molecules to the red blood cells carrying Rh antigen. These red cells already bound to Rh+ve red cell membranes can be reacted upon by anti-human immunoglobulin produced against Rh antibody. Anti-human immunoglobulins are produced in sheep, rabbits etc. Addition of anti-human antibodies to the sample containing blood corpuscles reacted upon by Rh antibodies will result in strong agglutination reaction (Fig. 8.13). This is called Coomb's test. It is performed in two ways: direct and indirect test.

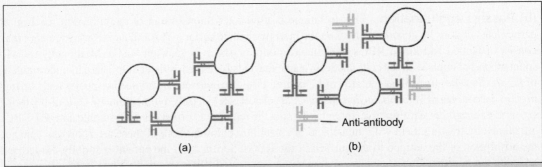

Anti-antibody

(a)   (b)

Fig. 8.13 The Coomb's test, **(a)** RBCs sensitized by anti-Rh or incomplete antibodies, **(b)** Antiglobulin (anti-anti Rh) reacts with Rh antibodies bound to RBCs and bring about agglutination.

(a) Direct Coomb's test   This test detects immunoglobulin already bound to the red blood corpuscles by addition of antiglobulin. For ex. Rh+ve child, born to Rh-ve mother. The Rh+ve antigen of the infant would have already sensitized Mother and Rh antibodies, which have diffused passively through the placenta into child's blood, bind them. To this blood sample, when antiglobulin (anti-anti Rh) is added, immediate agglutination reaction takes place indicating the presence of sensitized RBCs.

(b) Indirect Coomb's test   It is a two step reaction used for detection of circulating incomplete antibodies against Rh antigens, which is usually present in the mothers serum after the birth of Rh+ve infant. Patient's (mother's) serum is incubated with Rh+ve RBCs. Rh antibodies in the mothers serum react with Rh determinants on Rh+ve RBC membrane. After some time, to this antiglobulin (anti-anti Rh) is added and the appearance of agglutination indicates the presence of anti Rh antibodies in maternal blood.

Complement Fixation Test

Generally, as soon as the antigen-antibody complex is formed, the complements are activated and it binds to Fc arm of IgG or IgM antibodies. Complements facilitate destruction of antigen-antibody complexes. Attachment of complement to Fc arm of the antibody molecule, when antigen-antibody complex is formed is called complement fixation test. It can be demonstrated in vitro and the test depends on use of hemolytic indicator system, which consists of sheep RBCs (SRBCs) bound by antibodies to sheep RBCs (anti-SRBC) and a complement. Antibodies to sheep RBCs are raised in rabbit or guinea pig. When SRBCs + anti-SRBC + complement is mixed together, the complement binds to Fc arm of the anti-SRBC and initiates cytolytic reaction, thereby causing hemolysis of SRBCs (Fig. 8.14A). The actual complement fixation test is done in two steps:

- In the first step patient's serum to be tested for antibody or antigen is added to the serum containing known antigen or antibody and the mixture is incubated for promoting antigen-antibody reaction. After some time, to this mixture known complement is added (Fig. 8.14A).

• In the second step to the above mixture sensitized SRBCs (SRBCs bound by anti-SRBC) are added (Fig. 8.14B).

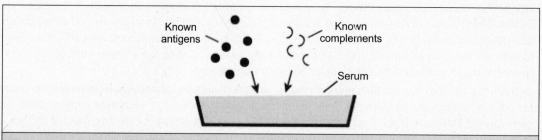

Fig. 8.14A   Step 1 of complement fixation test. Patient's serum, known antigen and known complements are added.

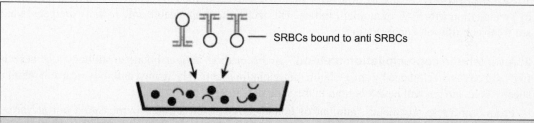

Fig. 8.14B   Step 2 of complement fixation test. To the above mixture (Fig. 8.14A), sensitized SRBCs are added (SRBCs bound by anti-SRBC).

The results are interpreted like this:

In the first step, if the antigen and the antibody have formed the complex, then the complement will be bound to this complex. Therefore, the complement will not be available for hemolysis of sensitized SRBCs when added to the mixture (Fig. 8.14C). If, in the first step, antigen-antibody complex did not occur then the complement will be freely available for the sensitized SRBCs to undergo hemolysis (Fig. 8.14C).

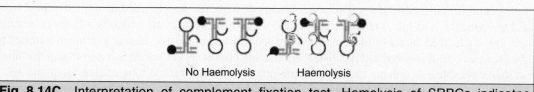

No Haemolysis   Haemolysis

Fig. 8.14C   Interpretation of complement fixation test. Hemolysis of SRBCs indicates absence of antigen antibody reaction in the test serum. No hemolysis of SRBCs indicates non-availability of complement (complement is fixed) and presence of antigen antibody reaction in test serum.

RADIOIMMUNOASSAY (RIA)

It is one of the most sensitive test for detecting the antigen or antibody, which is radioactively labeled. Hence it is called radioimmunoassay. It is used for quantitation of hormones such as thyroxine and insulin. The principle of RIA involves competitive binding of radiolabeled antigen and unlabeled antigen to high affinity antibody. The labeled antigen is mixed with antibody at a concentration sufficient enough to saturate the antigen binding sites of the antibody molecule, then the sample containing known concentration of unlabeled antigen is added in increasing amounts.

Since the antibody can not distinguish between unlabeled and labeled antigen, both antigens compete for antigen binding site on antibody. With the increasing concentration of unlabeled antigen, more and more labeled antigen will get displaced from the binding site. By measuring the free-labeled antigen in the solution, it is possible to determine the concentration of unlabelled antigen. There are two methods, by which, antigen-binding capacity can be found out (1) Farr technique, (2) Antiglobulin coprecipitation technique.

1. Farr technique   In this method, the complexed antigen-antibody is separated out from the solution by precipitation with 50% ammonium sulfate. This technique is applicable only to those antigens, which are soluble at this salt concentration.

2. Antiglobulin coprecipitation method   In this method, antigen bound to antibody together with free antibody is precipitated by antiglobulin (antiglobulin is antibody against antibody raised in rabbit or sheep). Free antigen will be left behind in the supernatant.

From both these techniques, amount of bound radiolabeled antigen is measured out at various concentrations of unlabeled antigen and a curve is prepared (Fig. 8.15). The curve is linear over a limited range; therefore unknown sample needs to be diluted such that the readings fall within the linear range of the curve. Once the standardization is achieved, the experiment is carried out with unknown sample of patient's serum. Percentage of labeled antigen bound to antibody is estimated in the presence of unknown patient's serum. Using the standard graph (Fig. 8.15), the concentration of the hormone or unlabeled antigen in the patient's serum is found out.

Radio immunosorbent test or RIST

The antibody content of a patient's serum can be assessed by the ability of antibody to bind to antiglobulin, which has been immobilized on a solid surface by adsorption. The solid surface could be polycarbonate tube or nitrocellulose paper discs. This test is usually done for the detection of IgE antibodies in severely allergic patients. Anti-IgE is raised in rabbits and used in labelled as well as unlabeled form. Unlabeled anti-IgE is adsorbed on to a solid surface (polycarbonate tube) and to this, patient's serum to be tested for the presence of IgE is added and incubated. After some time excess of serum is removed and the tube is washed with saline to remove excess of serum proteins. To the washed tube, radiolabeled anti-IgE is added. Radiolabeled anti-IgE will bind to IgE, which has already complexed with adsorbed anti-IgE (Fig. 8.16). Geiger counter measures radioactivity in the tube and the bound antibody quantity is detected.

Radioallergosorbent test (RAST)

It is used for measuring the amount of IgE to specific allergen in the patient's serum. Specific allergen is adsorbed on to a solid surface and treated with patient's serum. The mixture is incubated for some time, and later the excess of serum is washed by saline. Specific IgE from the patient's serum will bind to

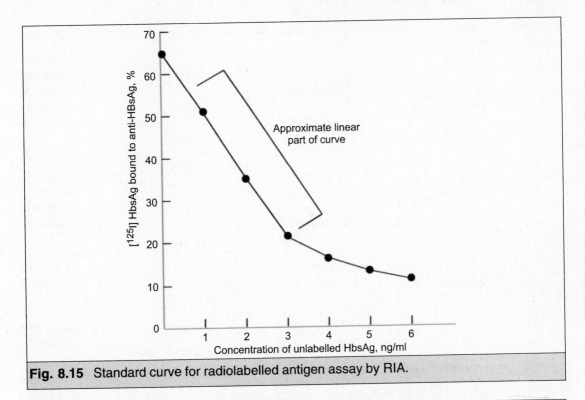

Fig. 8.15 Standard curve for radiolabelled antigen assay by RIA.

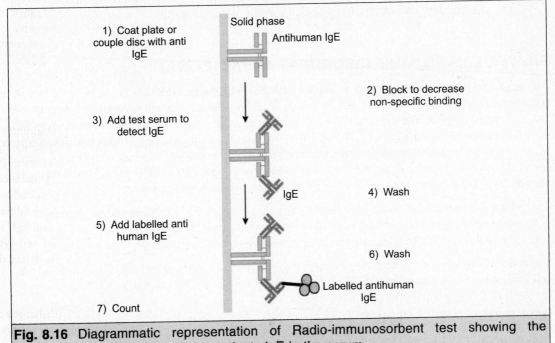

Fig. 8.16 Diagrammatic representation of Radio-immunosorbent test showing the methodology to detect patients IgE in the serum.

specific allergen, which is immobilized (Fig. 8.17). Bound IgE is detected by adding radio labeled anti-IgE as explained in RIST.

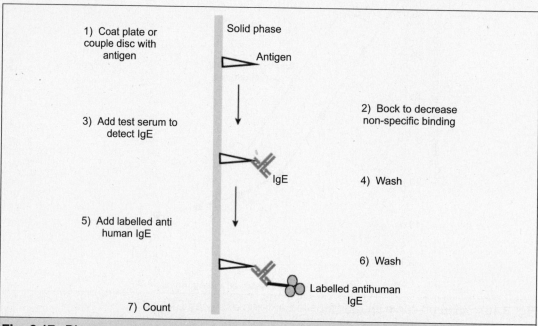

1) Coat plate or couple disc with antigen

Solid phase

Antigen

2) Bock to decrease non-specific binding

3) Add test serum to detect IgE

IgE

4) Wash

5) Add labelled anti human IgE

6) Wash

Labelled antihuman IgE

7) Count

Fig. 8.17 Diagrammatic representation of Radio allegosorbent test showing the methodology involved in detection of specific IgE in the patients serum.

ENZYME LINKED IMMUNOSORBENT ASSAY (ELISA)

All the laboratories are not equipped to handle radiolabeled substances. There is always a danger of contamination of human subjects, if proper measures and procedures are not used while handling the radioisotopes. Therefore, the technique of using enzyme linked immunosorbent assay comes handy and it is cheaper than radioimmunoassay. ELISA relies on the principle of enzyme substrate reaction, where a known enzyme is coupled to an antibody, which when exposed to colored substrate complexes releases color. The intensity of color is measured by taking the optical density on a colorimeter. Most commonly used enzymes for coupling with antibodies and their color substrate complexes are:

1. Horse radish peroxidase (enzyme)- substrate: hydrogen peroxide + orthophenylene diamine.
2. Alkaline phosphatase (enzyme)- substrate: p-nitrophenyl phosphate.
3. β-galactosidase (enzyme)- substrate: o-nitrophenyl-β-d-galactopyranoside.

The methodology involved in ELISA to detect antibody binding capacity or indirect ELISA (Fig. 8.18A) and antigen binding capacity (sandwich ELISA) is diagrammatically shown in (Fig. 8.18B).

IMMUNOFLUORESCENCE

Fluorescent dyes such as **fluorescein** and **rhodamine** can be coupled with antibody without destroying their specificity. Both dyes can be conjugated to Fc region of an antibody molecule. These dyes absorb

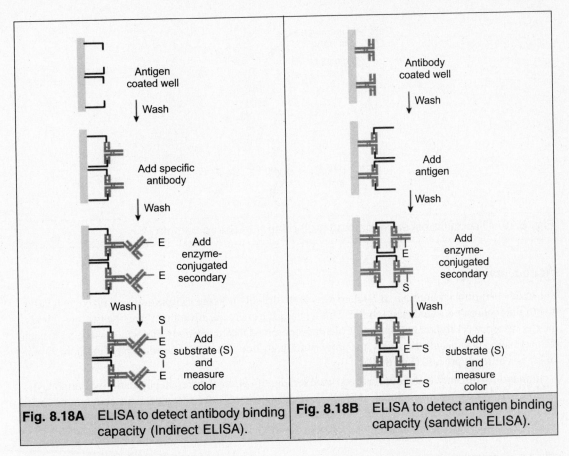

| **Fig. 8.18A** ELISA to detect antibody binding capacity (Indirect ELISA). | **Fig. 8.18B** ELISA to detect antigen binding capacity (sandwich ELISA). |

light at one wavelength and emit light at a longer wavelength. Fluorescein absorbs blue light at 490 nm and emits an intense yellowish green fluorescence at 517 nm. Rhodamine absorbs light in the yellow green range at 515 nm and emits a deep red fluorescence at 546 nm. The emitted light is viewed through a fluorescent microscope, which is fitted with UV light source and excitation filter. Differential staining of cells with two fluorescent substances can achieved by tagging one antibody with fluorescein and the other antibody with rhodamine and simultaneously two different antigens of the cell preparation can be identified.

Staining of cell membrane molecules or tissue sections by fluorescent antibody molecules can be carried out in two ways: Direct and indirect.

Direct staining

In this method, the primary antibody is conjugated to fluorescent substance and applied directly to the cell or tissue preparation. For ex. Gastric auto-antigens reacting with autoantibodies present in the serum of a patient suffering from *pernicious anemia*. From the serum of the patient IgG autoantibodies are isolated and tagged with fluorescein and applied to the gastric mucosa cell preparation. The cytoplasm of parietal cells will fluoresce brightly indicating the presence of antibodies (Fig. 8.19).

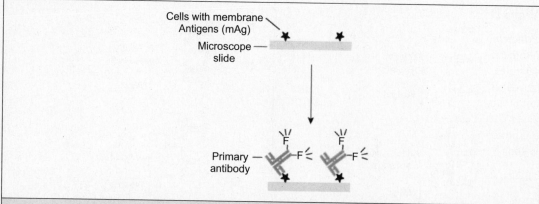

Fig. 8.19 Direct fluorescence staining method for the tissue sample.

Indirect staining

The unlabelled primary antibody is applied directly to the cell or tissue sample and visualized by treating it with fluorochrome-labeled antiglobulin. This technique has several advantages over the first one. Firstly, the fluorescence is brighter because multiple fluorochrome labeled antibody molecules will bind to each primary antibody molecule. Secondly, the primary antibody does not need to be conjugated to fluorochrome and it is a difficult process (Fig. 8.20).

Immunofluorescence technique has been used for identification of different population of lymphocytes by specially preparing monoclonal antibodies against their specific receptors and conjugating these antibodies with fluorochrome. The technique is suitable for identifying bacterial species, complement components in tissues, hormones and hormonal receptors.

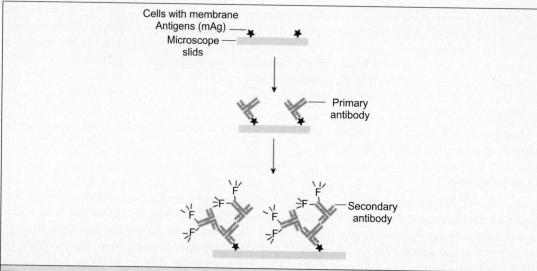

Fig. 8.20 Indirect fluorescence staining method for tissue sample.

WESTERN BLOTTING

Principle involved in this technique is similar to Southern blotting, which detects DNA fragments and Northern blotting, which detects RNAs. Western blotting is a jargon used for detection of protein in a complex mixture by applying similar principle used for DNA or RNA. The protein mixture is electrophoretically separated by SDS polyacrylamide gel electrophoresis. The separated bands of protein are blotted on to nitrocellulose paper and the protein bands are identified by treating the nitrocellulose paper with radiolabeled monoclonal antibodies or by enzyme-linked monoclonal antibodies specific for the protein of interest. The protein band is visualized by autoradiography or by addition of substrate leading to color complex formation (Fig. 8.21).

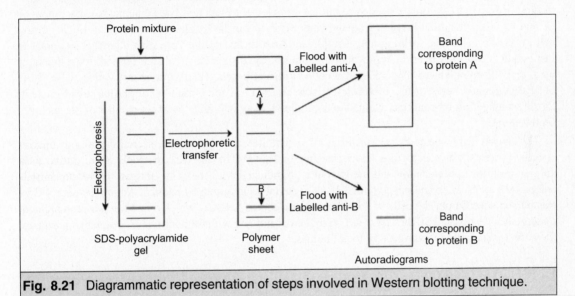

Fig. 8.21 Diagrammatic representation of steps involved in Western blotting technique.

Western blotting technique can be also used for detecting the antibody bands against various antigenic determiners. For which, labeled antigens visualize antibodies separated by polyacrylamide gel electrophoresis. For ex. Antibodies to HIV core proteins in the serum of HIV infected individual are identified by this method.

EXPERIMENTAL ASSESSMENT OF HUMORAL IMMUNITY

N. K. Jerney, A. A Nordin and C. Henry developed an hemolytic plaque assay for the determination of plasma cells producing antibodies to quantify humoral immune response, which is later modified by many researchers has been currently used for the study of humoral response.

DIRECT HEMOLYTIC PLAQUE ASSAY

Principle involved in this assay is similar to the one used for viral plaque assay. This assay is used to measure the number of plasma cells in mice primed with SRBCs. Spleen cells from the sensitized mice are mixed in warm melted agar with an excess of SRBCs. This mixture is poured in a Petre dish, which already contains hardened agar. Newly poured agar containing cell suspension is allowed to cool and solidify. Solidified agar contains immobilized splenic lymphocytes surrounded by large number of SRBCs.

The Petre dish is incubated for 1 hr at 37°C, during which time, stimulated plasma cells secrete antibodies, which diffuse into the agar matrix and bind to SRBCs in the vicinity of plasma cells. A serum containing active complement is added. The complement binds to antibody molecule, which is already bound to SRBCs and mediated lysis. The lysis of SRBCs surrounding the plasma cells will cause clear plaque formation, which is devoid of SRBCs. The number of plaques counted is equal to the number of antibody producing plasma cells specific for SRBC antigen. This assay primarily identifies IgM producing plasma cells, and it is also called as **direct plaque-forming cells (PFC)** assay.

The hemolytic plaque assay can not only determine the number of IgM secreting plasma cells, but also it can be used for determining IgG secreting plasma cells with slight modification. Since, single IgG molecule can not initiate complement-mediated cytolysis and two molecules of IgG or Fc regions of IgG located within 30 to 40 nm are needed to initiate complement-mediated lysis. Such close attachment of Fc regions does not normally occur from the random binding of IgG molecules secreted by single plasma cell to SRBC membrane. Adding anti-isotypic antibody to IgG to the Petri dish after the first hour of incubation does a modification in procedure. After this, the dishes are incubated for additional one hour by adding the complement. This method is called **indirect hemolytic plaque assay,** which causes lysis of SRBCs bound by IgM or IgG molecules. In this case, subtraction of number of plasma cells formed in the direct assay from the number formed in the indirect assay will give the exact number of plasma cells secreting IgG.

The hemolytic plaque assay can be also used to quantitate the plasma cells secreting antibody against specific proteins, polysaccharides, glycoproteins, or haptens. In this case the SRBCs are coated with antigen used for immunization and the animal is immunized with the same antigen. From the animals spleen cells are isolated and mixed with SRBCs coated with immunizing antigen. Antibodies secreted by the antigen specific plasma cells will bind to antigen coated SRBCs, which on addition of complement undergo lysis. Uncoated SRBCs serve as control and do not lyse with the addition of complement, because they are neither bound to antigens or to antibodies.

ELISPOT ASSAY

It is the modification Jerney hemolytic plaque assay. In this method, plasma cells are quantitated without using SRBCs. The antigen -primed lymphocytes are incubated in a Petri dish, which is coated with antigen. As the plasma cells secrete antibody, it binds to the antigen in the immediate vicinity of the plasma cell. Excess of lymphocytes is removed after some time and the Petri dish is washed with saline and ELISA visualizes the bound antibody. Enzyme substrate reaction leads to colored spot formation, which are counted for enumeration of plasma cells.

Exercise

1. Explain different methods involved in demonstration of precipitin reaction. (20 marks).
2. Give detailed account of different method involved in demonstration of agglutination reaction (20 marks)
3. Write notes on: (10 marks each)
   (a) Radio immuno assay (RIA)
   (b) Enzyme linked immunosorbent assay (ELISA)
4. Write briefly on: (5 to 8 marks each)
   (a) Coomb's test
   (b) Complement fixation test
   (c) Precipitin reaction
   (d) Immunoflurescence
   (e) Western blotting
   (f) Direct haemolytic plaque assay
   (g) Radio immunosorbent test (RIST)
   (h) Radio allergosorbent test (RAST)
   (i) Immunodiffusion (Ouchterlony technique)
   (j) Radial immunodiffusion
   (k) Rocket immunoelectrophoresis
   (l) Two dimensional immunoelectrophoresis
   (m) Counter current immunoelectrophoresis
   (n) Immunoelectrophoresis
   (o) Haemagglutination test
   (p) Mechnism of antigen antibody interaction
   (q) Antigen antibody cross reactivity

Chapter 9

Immunoglobulin Genes—Organization and Expression

- Genetic Model for Immunoglobulin Structure
- Organization of Immunoglobulin (Ig) Genes
- Gene Rearrangements in Variable Region
- Mechanism of Variable Region DNA Rearrangements
- Allelic Exclusion
- Generation of Antibody Diversity
- Expression of Ig Genes
- Regulation of Ig Gene Transcription

❏ ❏

The organization of immunoglobulin gene is highly complex, which is apparent from the fact that each antibody produced against limitless array of foreign antigens displays unique amino acid sequence in its variable region but only one of a limited number of invariant sequence in its constant region. The most remarkable feature of the vertebrate immune system is its ability to respond to an apparently limitless number of antigens by the same gene. There are several segments in the immunoglobulin gene involved in the production of a single immunoglobulin heavy and light chain. These gene segments are present in the germ cell DNA but cannot be transcribed and translated until they are arranged in a proper sequence. Rearrangement of genetic sequences of immunoglobulin gene occurs during B cell maturation in the bone marrow. The rearrangement of immunoglobulin genes is a well-regulated process and is capable of generating more than 10^8 specificities at a time. After the completion of rearrangement of the genes a mature B cell will be committed to an antigenic determiners or epitope and starts producing a variable-region heavy chain and a variable region light chain. When the peripheral mature B cells encounter an antigen it undergoes stimulation and shows further rearrangement of constant region gene segments leading to change in the associated biological effector functions and different isotypes are expressed. Thus mature B cells contain chromosomal DNA that is no longer identical to germ line DNA. The whole array of different types of immunoglobulins produced by B cells rests on the principle of organization and rearrangement of immunoglobulins genes, the mechanism of class switching, differential RNA processing in the expression of immunoglobulin genes and the regulation of Ig-gene transcription.

Genetic Model for Immunoglobulin Structure

From the amino acid sequencing and antibody specificities studies it was apparent that an immunoglobulin molecule is highly specific for an antigen yet it is of different types, which cannot be explained by conventional genetic models. All most all immunoglobulins show following properties:

- Both light and heavy chain of immunoglobulin have variable region at the amino terminus and a constant region at the carboxy terminus.
- Each class of antibody shows vast diversity of antibody specificities.
- Association of a variable region with different heavy-chain constant region results in isotype formation with same antigenic specificity.

At present two models exists to explain the genetic variability in immunoglobulin structure and function namely, Germ-line and somatic-variation models and Dryer and Bennett Two-gene model.

Germ line and somatic variation models

At any time in a well-nourished and healthy individual, the germ line cells of antibody production can generate more than 10^8 different antibody specificities, which is essential for encountering wide variety of potential antigens. It is possible to achieve this only if a genetic system capable of generating diversity exists. Immunologists put forward two different theories to explain such diversities. The germ line theory maintains that the genome contains a large repertoire of immunoglobulin genes that are sufficient to produce more than 10^8 different antibody specificities. According to this model no special genetic mechanism was thought of to account for antibody diversity. The model proposer's argued that the 15% of the genome dedicated to the production of antibodies are sufficient for the survival of the immune system. On the contrary, somatic variation theories maintained that from relatively small number of the immunoglobulin genes large numbers of antibodies are produced with varied specificities by localized mutations and recombinations.

Proponents of germ line theory had the difficulty in explaining the mechanism that could generate diversity in the variable part of the each gene while preserving the constant region unchanged. Proponents of somatic variation theory found it difficult to conceive the idea of diversity of the variable region of a single gene in the somatic cell without allowing a single alteration in the amino acid sequence of constant region. Another interesting feature of the immunoglobulin gene is the production of different classes or isotypes of antibody i.e. IgG, IgM etc., can be expressed with identical variable region sequences but with different constant regions.

Dryer and Bennett two gene model

In 1965, W. Dryer and J. Bennett proposed that two separate genes encode a single immunoglobulin heavy or light chain, one gene encoding the V region and one gene encoding the C region. It was only a theoretical proposition on the basis of assumptions and suggested that some how the two different fragments of proteins produced by V and C genes come together at DNA level to transcribe a continuous message, which is later translated into a single Ig heavy or light chain. They also proposed that 100 to 1000 copies of V region genes exists in the germ line and only one copy of C region will be sufficient to produce different classes of immunoglobulins with different specificities. This hypothesis contradicted the existing concept of one gene-one polypeptide principle, because it involved two genes coding for a single polypeptide. Therefore, initially the hypothesis met with resistance and skepticism because it was a theoretical model and no experimental proof was available. Even then the model could account for those immunoglobulins in which a single V region was combined with various C regions. By postulating single constant region gene for each immunoglobulin class and subclass, the model also could account for the conservation of necessary biological effector functions while allowing for evolutionary diversity of variable region.

With the availability of newer techniques in molecular biology and with the availability of genetic probes it has been possible to prove now that Dryer and Bennett hypothesis is essentially correct, which made the opponents to eat humble pie. Indeed, it is now proved that, there exists a more complex mechanism than could have been imagined at the Dryer and Bennett came out with their idea.

S. Tonegawa and N. Hozumi in 1976 provided the first evidence of existence of separate genes encoding V and C regions of immunoglobulins and these genes are rearranged during the course of B cell differentiation and maturation. This work revolutionized the approach in biological science with newer idea, hence in 1987 Tonegawa was awarded Nobel Prize for this work.

Organization of Immunoglobulin (Ig) genes

There are two families of immunoglobulin light chains, κ and λ, and one family of heavy chains (H). Each family consists of its own set of both V genes and C genes. Each family resides on a different chromosome. In the pattern inherited by any animal, the V genes and C genes for each family is a considerable distance apart. This is called germ-line pattern, and it is found in the germ line and in somatic cells of all lineages other than the immune system. But in a cell expressing an antibody, each of its chains - one light type (either κ or λ) and one heavy type-is coded by a single intact gene. The recombination event that brings V gene to partner a C gene coding sequences called gene segments creates an active gene consisting of exons that correspond precisely with the functional domains of the protein. The non-coding sequences or introns are removed in the usual way by RNA splicing. The number of V genes and C genes in a family varies with the species Table 9.1 describes the components of each immunoglobulin family in human and mouse.

Table 9.1 Chromosomal location of cluster of immunoglobulin genes in human and mouse.

Family	Location on chromosome		Number of V genes		Number of C genes	
	Human	Mouse	Human	Mouse	Human	Mouse
Lambda	2	16	<300	3	>6	4
Kappa	22	6	<300	300	1	1
Heavy	14	12	~300	>1000	9	8

Each V gene segment at the 5' end is preceded by a **signal** or **leader** (L) separated by a single intron from the variable (V) segment. The signal peptide is cleaved from the nascent light and heavy chains before assembly of the final immunoglobulin molecule. Therefore, the immunoglobulins coded by the leader sequence do not appear in the immunoglobulin molecule. The κ and λ light chain families contain **V, J, (J for joining) and C** gene segments, which after rearrangement encode variable region of the light chain. The heavy chain family consists of **V, D, J and C** gene segments which, after rearrangements encode the variable region of the heavy chain.

κ-Chain genes

The κ-chain gene family in the mouse consists of approximately 300Vκ gene segments, each with an adjacent leader sequence. There are five Jκ gene segments and a single Cκ gene segment. The Vκ and Jκ gene segments encode the variable region of the κ light chain, and the Cκ gene segment encodes the constant region. Since there is only one Cκ gene segment, there are no subclasses of κ light chains. The κ -chain gene family in humans is similar to that of mouse and contains approximately 100 Vκ segments, 5 Jκ segments and a single Cκ segment (Fig. 9.1a).

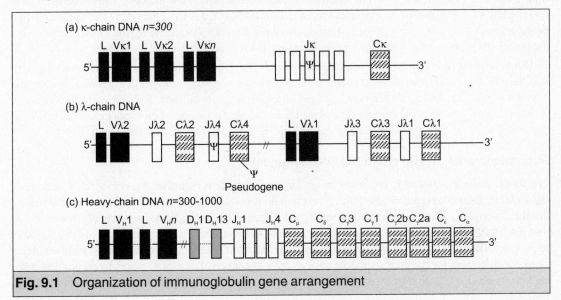

Fig. 9.1   Organization of immunoglobulin gene arrangement

λ-Chain genes

The functional λ variable region gene contains two coding segments-a 5' V segment and a 3' J segment-which are separated by a non-coding DNA sequence in un-rearranged germ line DNA. In humans there are an estimated 100 Vλ gene segments, 6Jλ segments and 6Cλ segments (Fig. 9.1b).

Heavy-chain genes

The heavy chain gene family is situated on chromosome 12 in the mouse and on 14 in humans. In mouse it has an estimated 300 to 1000 V_H gene segments, located upstream from a cluster of about 13 D_H gene segments. As with the light chain genes, each V_H gene segment has a leader sequence a short distance upstream from it. Down stream from the D_H gene segments are four J_H gene segments, followed by a series of C_H gene segments.

Each C_H gene segment encodes the constant region of an immunoglobulin heavy-chain isotype. The C_H gene segments are organized into a series of coding exons and non-coding introns. Each exon encodes a separate domain of the heavy chain constant region. A similar heavy chain gene organization is found in humans with an estimated 100 V_H gene segments, 30 D_H segments and 6 functional J_H segments followed by a series of C_H segments. In the mouse or in humans the C_H gene segments are arranged in a sequential order Cμ-Cδ-Cγ-Cε-Cα (Fig. 9.1c). This sequential arrangement is generally related to the developmental appearance of the immunoglobulin classes in the course of immune response. During B cell differentiation there occur sequential changes in the classes of the immunoglobulins expressed, while the antibody specificity remains the same. This phenomenon of sequential change in immunoglobulin class is called class switching, which is discussed in the later section.

Gene Rearrangements in Variable Region

Variable region gene rearrangements occur in an orderly fashion during B cell maturation in the bone marrow. As discussed in the earlier section, the assembly of functional genes encoding immunoglobulin light chain and heavy chain involves recombinational events, which are the only known form of site-specific DNA rearrangement in vertebrates recorded so far. First the heavy chain gene rearrange and then the light chain genes, resulting in the formation of single, functional variable region DNA sequence for the heavy chain and single, functional variable region DNA sequence for the light chain.

Ultimately, variable region gene rearrangement leads to the generation of mature, immunocompetent B cells, which is committed to a single antigenic determiner or epitope and starts expressing membrane bound antigenic receptors or antibodies (mIgM and mIgD) on its surface. Subsequently, heavy-chain constant region gene also shows rearrangements leading to the formation of different classes (isotype) of immunoglobulin without changing the antigenic specificity of the variable region.

Rearrangements in light chain V-J DNA segment

The name of the **J segment** is an abbreviation for joining since it identifies the region to which the V segment becomes connected. So the joining reaction does not directly involve V and C genes, but occurs via the J segment; when we say joining of V and C genes for light chains, we actually mean V-J-C joining. The J segment is short and actually codes for the last few, i.e. 13 amino acids of the variable region, as defined by amino acid sequences. In the intact gene, the V-J segment therefore constitutes a single exon coding for the entire variable region. Vλ gene has a choice of C genes to recombine with; each has same J – C despartite structure. The λ light chain is assembled from two parts as illustrated in Fig. 9.2.

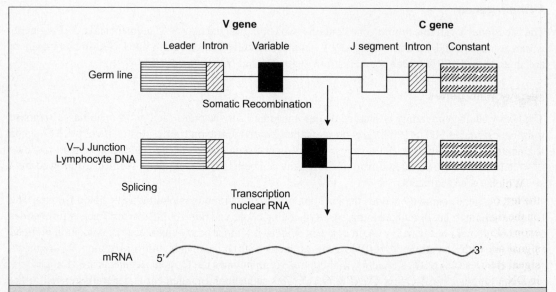

Fig. 9.2 Schematic representation of sequential arrangements of λ chain gene. C gene is preceded by a J segment so that V – J recombination generates a functional λ light chain.

A κ light chain is also assembled from two parts, but there is a difference in the structure of the C gene. A group of five J segments is spread over a region of 500-700 bp, separated by a intron of 2 – 3 kb from the single Cκ exon. In the mouse, the central J segment is nonfunctional (ψJ3). A Vκ segment may be joined to any one of the J segments. The consequences of the kappa joining reaction are illustrated in Fig. 9.3.

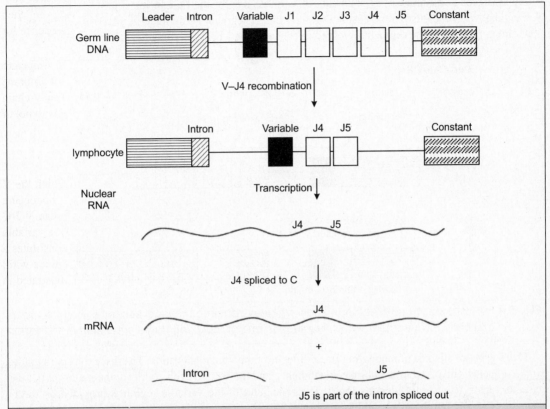

Fig. 9.3 A schematic representation of sequential arrangement of κ light chain genes. The κ C gene is preceded by multiple J segments in the germ line; V – J joining may recognize any one of the J segments, which is then spliced to the C region during RNA processing.

Whichever J segment used becomes the terminal part of the intact variable exon. Any J segments on the left of the recombining J segments are lost (J1 and J2 have been lost in the fig. 9.3). Any J segment on the right of the recombining J segment is treated as part of the intron between the variable and constant exons (J5 is included in the region that is spliced out in the fig. 9.3). All functional J segments possess a signal at the left boundary that makes it possible to recombine with the V segment; and they possess a signal at the tight boundary that can be used for splicing to the C exon. Whichever J segment is recognized in DNA joining uses its splicing signal in the RNA processing.

Rearrangements in Heavy chain V – D – J DNA segment

V – D – J joining takes place in two stages. The **D** (diversity) segment was discovered by the presence of 2 to 13 amino acids between the sequences coded by the v segment and the J segment. An array of > 10 D segments lies on the chromosome between the V_H segments and the $4J_H$ segments (which carry in length between 4 and 6 codons). First one of the D segments recombines with J_H segment; then a V_H segment recombines with DJ_H combined segment. The reconstruction leads to expression of the adjacent C_H segment (which consists of several exons). The d segments are organized in tandem array. The mouse heavy chain locus contains 12 D segments of variable length; the human locus has ~30 D segments. Some unknown mechanism must ensure that the same D segment is involved in the D – J joining and V – D joining reactions. The segment involved in constructing a heavy chain gene is illustrated in Fig. 9.4.

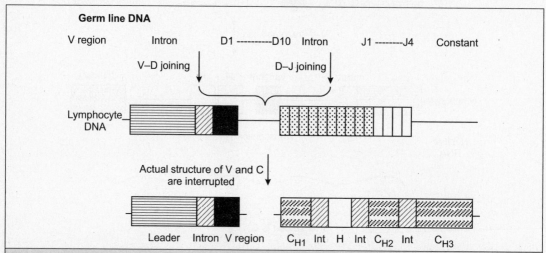

Fig. 9.4   A schematic representation showing Heavy chain genes are assembled by joining V gene to a D segment, which is joined to one of the J segments preceding the C gene.

The V genes of all three immunoglobulin families are similar in organization. The first exon codes for the signal sequence (involved in membrane attachment), and the second exon codes for the major part of the variable region itself (<100 codons long). The remainder of the variable region is provided by the D segment (in the H family only) and by a J segment (in all three families).

The structure of the constant region depends on the type of chain. For both κ and λ light chains, the constant region is encoded by a single exon (which becomes the third exon of the reconstructed active gene). For H chains, the constant region is coded by several exons corresponding to antibody protein chain. Separate exons code for the regions C_{H1}, hinge, C_{H2}, and C_{H3}. Each C_H exon is shorter. Than its ~100 codons long; the hinge is shorter. The introns usually are relatively small (~300 bp).

MECHANISM OF VARIABLE REGION DNA REARRANGEMENTS

Assembly of both light and heavy chain genes involves the same mechanism is indicated by the presence of the same consensus or conserved sequences at the boundaries of all germ line segments that participate in joining reactions. Each conserved sequence consist of a palindromic (both way reads the same) heptamer separated by either 12 or 23 bp from a conserved AT rich nonamer. These are called **recombination signal sequences (RSSs)** flanking each germ line V, D, and J gene segments. One RSS is located 3' to each V gene segment, 5' to each J gene segment, and on both sides of each D gene segment. These sequences act as facilitators of recombination process. These conserved sequences correspond to one and two turns of the DNA helix; accordingly the sequences are referred to as **one-turn signal sequence** and **two turn signal sequences.**

Fig. 9.5 illustrates the relationship between the conserved sequences at the mouse Ig loci. At the kappa locus, each Vκ gene is followed by conserved sequence of one turn spacer with a 12 bp spacing and is preceded by two-turn spacer with 23 bp precedes κ segment. The V and J conserved sequences are inverted in orientation. The reverse arrangement is found at the lambda locus each Vλ gene is followed by a conserved sequence with 23 bp two-turn spacer and Jλ gene is preceded by a one-turn signal sequence of 12 bp type

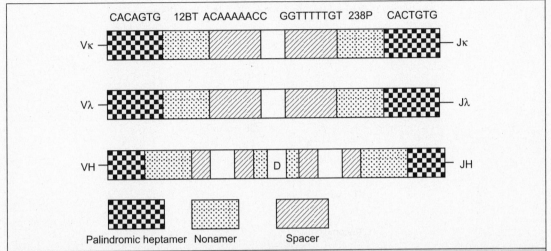

Fig. 9.5 A diagrammatic representation of conserved sequences. Conserved sequences are present in inverted orientation at each pair of recombining site. One member of each pair has a spacing of 12 bp between its components; the other has 23 bp spacing.

In the heavy chain DNA, a two-turn spacer occurs in the signal sequences of the V_H and J_H gene segments and a one-turn spacer occurs in the signals on either side of the D_H gene segment. The joining of these signal sequences follows a rule, the so-called **one-turn/two-turn joining rule**, where signal sequence having one-turn spacer can only join with sequences having two-turn spacer. This rule ensures that a V_L segment joins to a J_L segment and not to another V_L segment. Similarly the rule ensures that V_H, D_H and J_H segments join in proper order and that segments of the same type do not join each other.

The recombination event that occurs while joining the components of the immunoglobulin genes is quite different from the conventional reciprocal recombination between homologous sequences. The recombination of immunoglobulin genes represents a physical rearrangement of sequences, involving breakage and reunion. The recombination of RSSs and coding sequences is catalyzed by **V(D)J recombinase.** On the basis of transcriptional orientation of the gene segments to be joined determines the fate of the signal joint and the intervening DNA. When the two gene segments are in the same transcriptional orientation, joining results in **deletion** of the signal joint and the intervening DNA as a circular excision product.

It is observed that when the two gene segments are oppositely oriented, the joining occurs by **inversion** of DNA resulting in the retention of both coding joint and the signal joint on the chromosome. Human κ locus is found to be of this character, with half of the Vκ, gene segments are inverted with respect to Jκ. Therefore joining in this segment of human chromosome occurs by inversion.

In 1990, David Schatz, Marjorie Oettinger and David Baltimore identified two V(D)J recombination-activating genes. They designated them as RAG-1 and RAG-2 as a short form for recombination-activating gene and both act synergistically to mediate V(D)J joining. The protein products of RAG-1 and RAG-2 as well as the enzyme terminal deoxynucleotidyl transferase (Tdt) are found to be the key requirements for V(D)J rearrangement. Fig. 9.6 illustrates the deletion model of recombination and Fig. 9.7 illustrates the inversion model of V(D)J recombination.

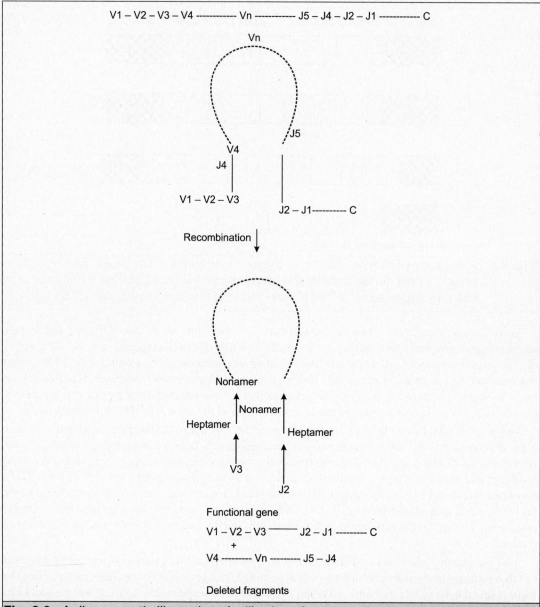

Fig. 9.6   A diagrammatic illustration of utilization of conserved sequences to bring V and J regions into juxtaposition of that a breakage and reunion excises the material between them.

Allelic Exclusion

Each B cell is known to express a unique combination of immunoglobulin chains, where each V – J and V – D – J recombination is different. A single productive rearrangement of each type occurs in a given lymphocyte to produce one light and one heavy chain gene. Because each event involves the expression of genes of only one homologous chromosome, the alleles on the other homologous chromosome are not expressed in the same cell. This phenomenon is called **allelic exclusion**.

This process ensures that the functional B cells never contain more than one $V_H D_H J_H$ and one $V_L J_L$ unit. But the expression of both alleles occurs in the development of B cells with multispecificity. With the process of allelic exclusion completed and once a productive $V_H – D_H – J_H$ and a productive $V_L – J_L$ rearrangements have occurred, the recombination machinery is turned off so as to prevent the expression of heavy and light chain genes on the homologous chromosomes.

Yancopoulos and Alt proposed a model to explain allelic exclusion. According to them, once a **productive rearrangement** is attained, the particular B cell expresses its encoded protein, and the presence of this acts as a signal to prevent further gene rearrangement. According to their model, the presence of μ heavy chain signals the maturing B cells to turn off rearrangement of the other heavy chain allele and turn on rearrangement of the κ light chain genes. If a productive κ light chains are produced and then pair with μ heavy chain to form a complete unit of IgM antibody molecule on the membrane of the B cells. The presence of IgM antibody molecule on the B cell turns off further light chain rearrangement. If κ rearrangement is **non- productive** for both alleles, rearrangement of the λ chain genes begins. If neither λ allele rearranges productively, the B cell undergoes apoptosis.

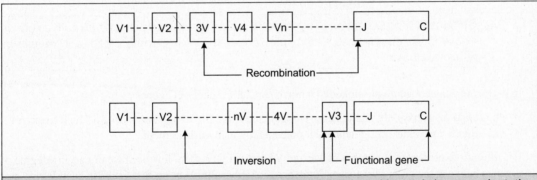

Fig. 9.7   A schematic representation of joining reaction involving a V gene in inverse orientation to the J segment could generate a functional V – J – C gene by inversion of the region between V and J.

The coexistence of productive and nonproductive rearrangements suggests the existence of a feedback loop to control the recombination process. A model of the same is illustrated in Fig. 9.8.

Generation of Antibody Diversity

Let us examine the different types of V and C genes to see how much diversity can be accommodated by the variety of the coding regions carried in the germ line. The structures of the two light Ig gene families of the human genome are summarized in Fig. 9.9 and 9.10.

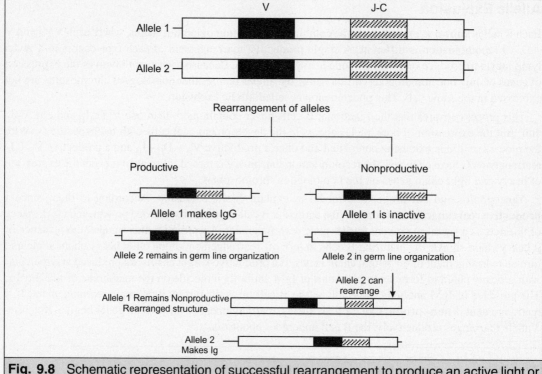

Fig. 9.8 Schematic representation of successful rearrangement to produce an active light or heavy chain suppresses further rearrangement of the same class ,and results in allelic exclusion.

In each case, many V genes are linked to a much smaller number of C genes:

- The kappa locus has only one C gene, which is preceded by 5 J segments (one of them inactive)
- The lambda locus has ~6C genes, each preceded by its own J segment.

It is difficult to estimate the number of Vκ and Vλ genes in the germ line because of varying degree of divergence between the germ line genes. There are probably <300 V germ line genes in each family and some of them are closely related and some distantly related, because of which a gene probe may bind to several genes simultaneously.

What is the mechanism of origin of V region diversity? To date seven mechanisms have been proposed to explain the generation of antibody diversity in humans and mouse. But the exact contribution of each of these mechanisms to the total antibody diversity is not known. It is estimated that a mammalian immune system on an average can generate 10^8 to 10^{11} different antibody specificities.

- Multiple germ-line V, D, and J gene segments
- Combinatorial V – J and V – D – J joining
- Junctional flexibility
- P-nucleotide addition
- N-Region nucleotide addition

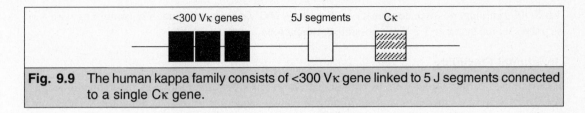

Fig. 9.9 The human kappa family consists of <300 Vκ gene linked to 5 J segments connected to a single Cκ gene.

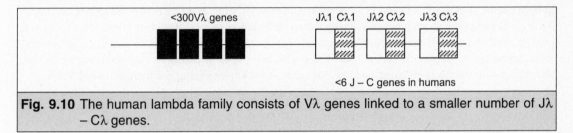

Fig. 9.10 The human lambda family consists of Vλ genes linked to a smaller number of Jλ – Cλ genes.

- Somatic hypermutation
- Combinatorial association of light and heavy chains

Multiple germ line V, D, and J gene segments

By combining any one of 300 Vκ genes with any one of 4 J segments, the mouse genome has the potential to produce some 1200 κ chains. A similar number of lambda chains can be produced. The Vκ genes occupy a large cluster on the chromosome, upstream of the constant region. The mouse kappa locus is similar in organization to the human. The lambda locus in mouse is much less diverse than the human locus. The main difference is that there are only two Vλ genes; each is linked to two J – C regions. Of the 4 Cλ genes, one is inactive and an estimated 13 D_H gene segments.

Combinatorial V – J and V – D – J joining

The random rearrangement of multiple germ line gene segments in somatic cells magnifies antibody diversity. The single locus of the heavy chain production consists of several discrete sections, whose structure in the human genome is summarized in Fig. 9.11.

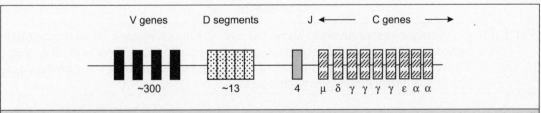

Fig. 9.11 Single gene cluster of human genome for heavy chain gene assembly contains all the information for the production of heavy chain.

The ability of any of the 300-1000 V_H gene segments to combine with any of the 13 D_H segments and any of the 4 J_H segments would give rise to enormous amount of diversity, that would be 300 X 13 X 4 =

1.6×10^4 minimum possible combinations. Similarly, 300 Vκ segments randomly combining with 4 Jκ segments would generate 1.2×10^3 possible combinations.

Junctional Flexibility

As mentioned earlier, the process of recombination involves both the joining of recombination signal sequences to form a signal joint and the joining of coding sequences to form a coding joint. The joining reaction is itself associated with changes in sequence that affect the amino acid coded at the V – J junction in light chains or at the V – D and D – J junctions in heavy chains. Base pairs may be lost or inserted at the V_H – D or D – J or both junctions during the recombination process. Deletion also occurs in V_L – J_L joining, but insertion at these joints is unusual. Junctional flexibility leads to many nonproductive rearrangements, as explained earlier, but it also generates several productive combinations encoding alternative amino acids at each coding joint. An example for kappa joining is illustrated in Fig. 9.12.

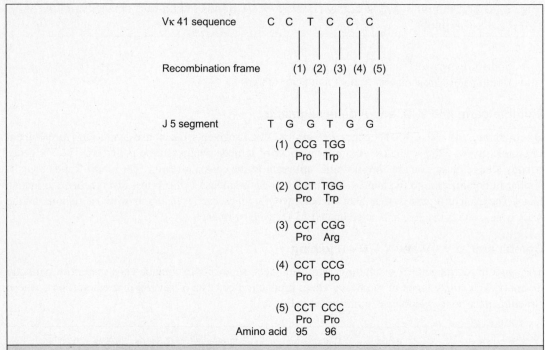

Fig. 9.12 A schematic presentation to show the use of alternative sites for recombination between aligned V and J segments sequences coding for amino acid 95 and 96. The recombination creates new codons. Similar events occur in V – J lambda and V – D – J heavy chain joining reactions.

The use of five potential frames for recombination generates three different amino acids at position 96, including one (arginine) not coded in the germ line. Since other Vκ and Jκ segments have different codons at these positions, great diversity becomes possible at the point of junction. The figure shows recombination between positions in the corresponding reading frames, but even greater diversity is possible because recombination can occur between any pair of points in the relevant regions of V and J. Some delete a codon from the somatic gene and other join the V – J region so that the J segment is out of phase and is translated in the wrong reading frame. The resulting gene is aberrant, since its expression is terminated by a nonsense codon in the incorrect frame. Similar although even greater diversity is generated in the joining reactions that involves the D segment of the heavy chain. The same problem exists of generating nonproductive genes by recombination events that place J and C out of phase.

P – nucleotide addition

Initial single strand break at the junction of a variable region gene segment and attached signal sequence, results in nucleotides at the end of coding sequences to turn back to form a hairpin loop. This loop is later cleaved by an endonuclease. Sometimes the cleavage occurs at a position that leaves a short single stranded region protruding out at the end of the coding sequences. These protruding sequences are referred to as **P – nucleotides,** subsequent addition of complementary nucleotides by repair enzyme results in palindromic sequences in the coding joint (Fig. 9.13). Variation in the sequence of the coding joint would occur with the variation in the position at which the hairpin is cut.

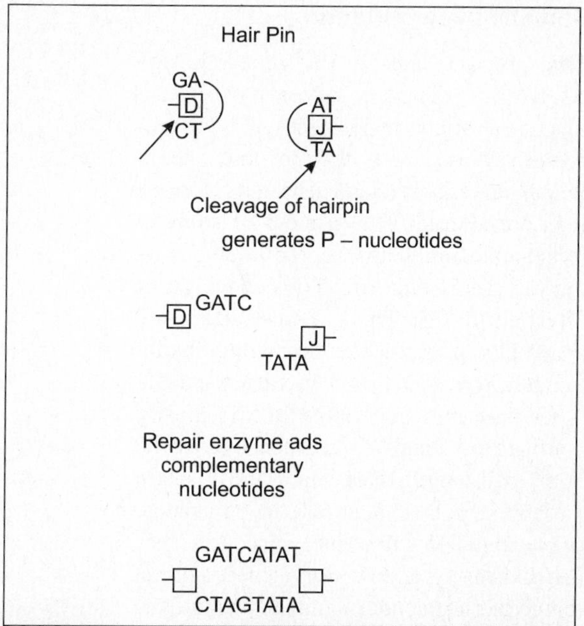

Fig. 9.13 A schematic representation showing P - nucleotide addition when single strand breaks occur in the coding sequence. (Break is shown by the arrows).

N-region nucleotide addition

Coding joints in the rearranged heavy chain variable region have been shown to contain short amino acid sequences that are not encoded by the V, D or J gene segments. At a free 3' end generated during the joining process is reacted upon by terminal deoxynucleotidyl transferase (TdT) (Fig. 9.14). Addition of new nitrogenous bases would lead to coding for new amino acids and these new bases are called **N-nucleotides**. Up to 15 N-nucleotides can be added to both the $D_H - J_H$ and $V_H - D_H J_H$ joints. This would lead to a complete heavy chain variable region encoded by a $V_H ND_H CJ_H$ unit. Since this diversity is confined to V – D – J coding joints, it is localized in the CDR3 of the heavy chain genes.

Combinatorial association of heavy and light chains

This is the final source of antibody diversity because the specificity of an antibody's antigen-binding site is determined by the variable regions in both its heavy and light chains, combinatorial association of H and L chains can generate diversity. In mice it has been roughly estimated that a minimum of 1.6×10^4 heavy chain genes and 1.2×10^3 light chain genes can be generated as a result of variable region gene rearrangements. Actual number of possible antigenic specificities is considerably higher because of unknown source of variations brought about by junctional flexibility, P-nucleotide addition, N-nucleotide addition and somatic hypermutation.

Somatic hypermutation

This process leads to the generation of additional antibody diversity once a functional variable region gene unit is formed. All this while it was thought that once a functional variable region gene unit is formed it is not altered. The process of somatic hypermutation leads to replacement of individual nucleotides in VJ or VDJ units with alternate bases. This process alters the specificity of the encoded immunoglobulin. Somatic hypermutation occurs at a rate of 10^{-3} per base pair generation and is mostly confined to VJ and VDJ segments. Since the combined length of H chain and L chain variable region is about 600 bp, an average of one mutation will be introduced for every cell division cycle. Recent evidences suggest that certain nucleotide motifs and palindromic sequences within the V_H and V_L may be especially prone to somatic hypermutation.

Class switching among constant region genes

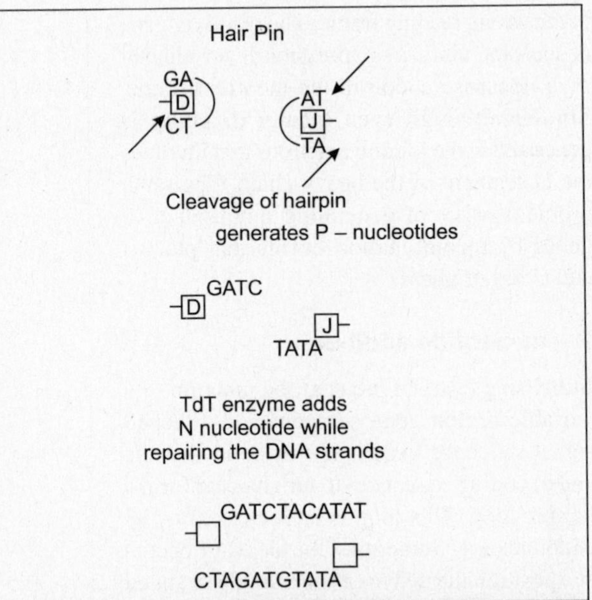

Fig. 9.14 A schematic representation showing N - nucleotide addition when single strand breaks occur in the coding sequence. (Break is shown by the arrows).

The type of C_H region defines the class of immunoglobulin. A B-lymphocyte generally produces only a single class of immunoglobulin at any one time, but the class (isotype) may change during the cell lineage. This is accomplished by a substitution in the type of C_H region that is expressed; the change in expression is called **class switching.** Switching involves only the C_H gene; the same V_H gene continues to be expressed. Thus a given V_H gene may be expressed successively in combination with more than one C_H gene. The same light chain continues to be expressed throughout the lineage of the B cell. Class switching therefore allows the type of effector response (mediated by the C_H region) to change, while maintaining the constant facility to recognize antigen (mediated by the V region).

Most B lymphocytes start productive life as mature cells engaged in synthesis of IgM. Cells expressing IgM have the germ line gene arrangement of the C_H gene cluster as shown in Fig. 9.11. The V – D – J joining reaction is sufficient to trigger expression of the Cμ gene. Changes in the expression of C_H genes are made in two ways. Some occur at the level of RNA processing (discussed later in this chapter). The majority occurs via further DNA recombination events, involving a system different from that concerned with V – D – J joining.

Cells expressing later C_H genes usually have deletions of Cμ and the other genes preceding the expressed C_H gene. Thus class switching may be accomplished by a recombination to bring a new C_H gene juxtaposition with the expressed V – D – J unit. The sequence of V – D – J – C_H units show that the sites of switching lie upstream of the C_H genes themselves. The switching sites are called **S regions.** Figure 9.15 depicts two successive switches.

In the first switch, expression of Cμ is succeeded by expression of Cγ1. The Cγ1 gene is brought into the expressed position by recombination between the sites Sμ and Sγ1, deleting the material between. The Sμ site lies between V – D – J and the Cμ gene. The Sγ1 site lies upstream of the Cγ1 gene. The region between

V – D – J and Cγ1 gene is removed as an intron during processing of the RNA. The linear DNA model imposes a restriction on the heavy gene locus: once a class switch has been made, it becomes impossible to express any C_H gene that used to reside between Cμ and the new C_H gene. In the example of Figure 9.15, cells expressing Cγ1 should be unable to give rise to cells expressing Cγ3, which has been deleted.

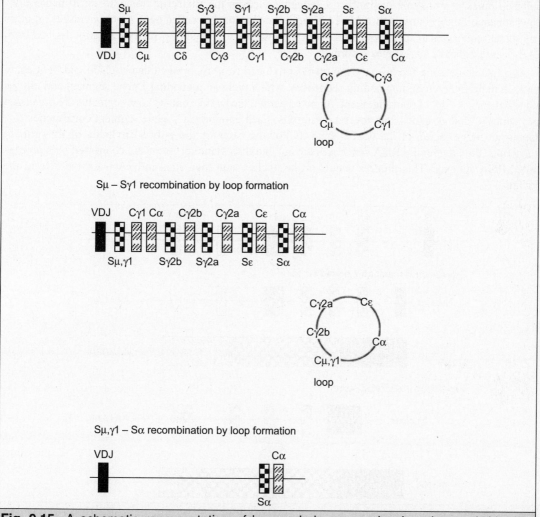

Fig. 9.15 A schematic representation of heavy chain genes showing class switching by recombination between switch regions (S), deleting the material between the recombining S sites. In this manner successive switches may occur.

In principle it should be possible to undertake another switch to any C_H gene downstream of the expressed gene. The figure shows a second switch to Cα expression, accomplished by recombination between Sα and the switch region Sμ,γ1 that was generated by the original switch. S regions lie ~2kb upstream of the C_H genes. Three distinct Sμ sites have been characterized; two of them show homology, but the other does not. Cytokines play an important role in class switching, which has been discussed in detail in Chapter 14.

Expression of Ig genes

As in other Eukaryotic genes, post transcriptional modification of immunoglobulin primary transcripts is required to produce functional RNAs. The first step in the RNA processing involves addition of 7-methylguanosine cap to the 5' end of the primary transcript. This helps in translation of mRNA on the polyribosomes. An enzyme recognizes a sequence cleaves the transcript some 15 to 30 nucleotides downstream of highly conserved AAUAAA sequence. An enzyme called poly-A polymerase recognizes this signal sequence and adds sequential adenylate residues to 3' end of primary transcript derived from ATP. A tail of about 250 residues is formed.

As explained earlier, the primary transcripts produced from rearranged heavy-chain and light chain genes contain intervening non coding sequences, which include noncoding J gene segment and introns not lost during V – D – J rearrangement. As noted earlier, the heavy chain C gene segments are organized as a series of coding exons and noncoding introns. Each exon of a C_H gene segment corresponds to a domain or hinge region of the heavy chain. Following capping and poly-adenylation of the primary transcripts, the intervening RNA sequences are cut and their flanking exons are connected by a process called RNA splicing. This process occurs in the nucleus and then final mRNA is exported from the nucleus.

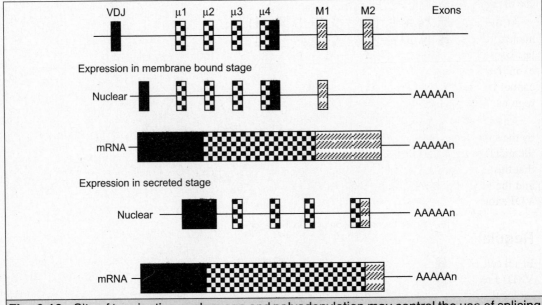

Fig. 9.16 Site of termination or cleavage and polyadenylation may control the use of splicing junctions so that alternative forms of the heavy chain gene are expressed.

RNA Processing leads to change in early heavy chain expression

The period of IgM synthesis that begins lymphocyte development falls into two parts, during which different versions of the μ constant region are synthesized.

As a stem cell differentiates into a pre B lymphocyte, an accompanying light chain is synthesized, and the IgM molecule (L2μ2) appears at the surface of the cell. This form of IgM contains the μm version of the constant region (m indicates membrane bound IgM). When the B lymphocyte differentiates further into a plasma cell, the μs version of the constant region is expressed. The IgM actually is secreted as a pentamer IgM$_5$J, in which J is a joining polypeptide that forms disulfide linkages with μ chains.

The μm and μs version of the μ heavy chain differs only at the C terminal end. The μm chain ends in a hydrophobic sequence that secures it in the B lymphocyte membrane. This sequence is replaced by the shorter hydrophilic sequence in μs; this substitution allows the μ heavy chain to pass through the membrane. The μm and μs chains are coded by different mRNAs. The two mRNAs share an identical sequence up to the end of the last constant domain. Then they differ; μm has 41 more codons followed by a nontranslatable trailer; and μs has 20 codons followed by a different nontranslatable trailer. The genomic sequences shows that the terminal regions of μm and μs are coded in different exons. The relationship between the structure of the gene and mRNAs is illustrated in Fig. 9.16.

At the membrane bound stage, splicing together six exons produces the constant region. The first four code for the four domains of the constant region. The last two M1 and M2 code for the 41 residue hydrophobic C terminal region and its nontranslated trailer.

At the secreted stage, joining only the first four exons generates the constant region. The last of these exons extend farther than it did at the previous (membrane) stage; it brings in the last 20 codons and its nontranslated trailer. The difference between the two mRNAs therefore hinges on whether a splicing junction within the exon for the last constant domain is spliced to M1 and M2 or is ignored. How is the use of this splicing site is controlled? To explain this a plausible model has been put forward.

At the membrane bound stage, the nuclear RNA has a polyadenylated end after M2. Because the nuclear RNA contains the acceptor splicing site at the beginning of M1, it uses the splicing site within the last constant exon. At the second stage, the nuclear RNA ends at an earlier site, after the last constant exon. Because no subsequent exons are present in the nuclear RNA, the splicing site within the exon cannot be utilized. A similar transition from membrane to secreted forms is found with other constant regions. The conservation of exon structures suggests that the mechanism is the same.

An exception to the rule that only one immunoglobulin types synthesized by any one cell is presented by the simultaneous production of IgM and IgD in mature B lymphocytes. The two immunoglobulins are identical except for the substitution between μ and δ constant regions in the heavy chain. It seems likely that this is the outcome of alternative pathways for RNA processing. The δ constant region is close to μ and the lack of switch site between them; if transcription sometimes continues through the region, the VDJ exon could be spliced to the series of μ exons (Fig. 9.17).

Regulation of Ig Gene Transcription

In a B cell immunogobulin genes are expressed at different rates during different developmental stage. The V (D) J recombination reaction, which serves as the basis for generating the vast repertoire of antibody molecules, occurs only in lymphoid cells and like other biological processes, is mediated by *cis*-acting elements and *trans*-acting factors. Three major classes of *cis*-regulatory sequences in DNA regulate transcription of immunoglobulin genes.

- **Promoters:** They promote initiation of RNA transcription in a specific direction. They are relatively short sequences extending up to 200 bp upstream from the transcription initiation site.
- **Enhancers:** They are specific nucleotide sequences situated some distance upstream or downstream from a gene that activates transcription from the promoter sequence in an orientation-independent manner.
- **Silencers:** These nucleotide sequences are responsible for downregulation of transcription, operating in both directions over a distance.

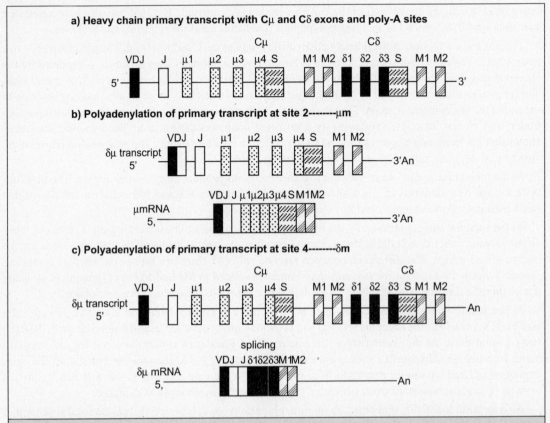

Fig. 9.17 Expression of membrane forms of μ and δ heavy chains by alternative RNA processing.

The locations of the three types of regulators of gene action in germ line immunoglobulin DNA are shown in Fig. 9.18.

Each V_H and V_L gene segment has promoter located just 25 to 35 bp upstream from the initiation site and it is AT rich region, called TATA box. RNA polymerase II binds to the TATA box and starts transcribing the DNA from the initiation site.

It is likely that enhancer elements operate both by opening chromatic structure, thus making recombination sites more accessible to the enzymatic machinery and by attracting the auxillary proteins required for rearrangement. Several lines of evidence indicate that local RNA transcription may be correlated with the recombination process. For ex. Un-rearranged gene transcripts are observed prior to or concomitant with the rearrangement event. It is observed that, enhancers also induce demethylation, which in turn permits gene rearrangements.

Both light (κ) and heavy (μ) chain genes harbor two large enhancers, one located in the J – C intron (Where C is the constant region) and the other 3' to the constant region. In the κ locus, these elements appear to work co-operatively since deletion of each enhancer individually is known to impair rearrangement while the removal of both suppresses this reaction. λ light chain enhancers are located 3'

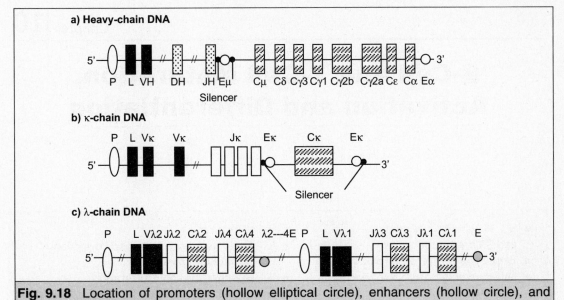

a) Heavy-chain DNA

P L VH DH JH Eμ Cμ Cδ Cγ3 Cγ1 Cγ2b Cγ2a Cε Cα Eα
Silencer

b) κ-chain DNA

P L Vκ Vκ Jκ Eκ Cκ Eκ
Silencer

c) λ-chain DNA

P L Vλ2 Jλ2 Cλ2 Jλ4 Cλ4 λ2---4E P L Vλ1 Jλ3 Cλ3 Jλ1 Cλ1 E

Fig. 9.18 Location of promoters (hollow elliptical circle), enhancers (hollow circle), and silencers (solid black circles) in mouse heavy chain, κ-chain and λ light chain germ line DNA.

of Cλ4 and 3' Cλ1. Silencers have not been identified in λ chain DNA but it exists in heavy chain and κ-chain DNA flanking the enhancers.

Enhancer elements in the immune system can direct the process of gene arrangement and, in this way, generate receptor diversity. Through interaction with *trans*-acting factors, these complex sequences form a molecular machine which is centrally located in each locus and can mediate a sequence of structural events that brings about rearrangement: DNA methylation; the opening of chromatin, juxtapositioning of the V, D and J genes; and finally, the recombination reaction themselves.

Exercise

1. Explain the genetic model for immunolgobulin structure (10 marks)
2. Describe the organization ofimmunoglobulin genes (20 marks)
3. Give a detailed account of gene rearrangements in variable region (20 marks)
4. Explain: (20 marks each)
   (a) Mechanism of variable region DNA rearrangements
   (b) Generation of antibody diversity
   (c) Expression of Ig genes
   (d) Regulation of transcription of Ig gene
5. Write notes on: (15 marks each)
   (a) Mechanism of class switching   (b) Junctional flexibility

Chapter 10

B-Cell and T-Cell Maturation, Activation and Differentiation

- B-Cell Maturation, Activation and Differentiation
- Bone Marrow Microenvironment
- Selection of Immature Self-Reactive B Cells
- Overview of the Major Pathways of BCR Signaling
- Formation of T and B Cell Conjugate
- T– Cell Maturation, Activation and Differentiation
- The Role of the Thymic Environment in Early T Cell Development
- TCR Coupled Signal Transduction
- IL-2 Signaling and the Activation of Proliferation of T Cells
- T Cell Clonal Anergy
- Evidence For Transcriptional Repression in Anergy
- γδ T Cells and their Function

- B Cell Maturation
- Ig – Gene Rearrangements and Formation of Pre-B Cell Receptors
- B-Cell Activation and Proliferation
- Role of Btk in B Cell Development and Signaling
- B – Cell Coreceptor Complex
- Role of th Cells in Humoral Response
- B – Cell Differentiation
- T – Cell Maturation
- Discrete Stages in Early T Cell Development
- Thymic Selection of the T Cell Repertoire
- T Cell Activation
- Redox Signaling Mechanism in T Cell Activation
- Co-Stimulation in T Cell Responses
- Altered Peptide Ligands as Antagonists or Partial Agonists
- Superantigen-Induced T Cell Activation
- Differences In Costimulatory Signals Among Antigen Presenting Cells

B-CELL MATURATION, ACTIVATION AND DIFFERENTIATION

Development of B cells from committed progenitors to terminally differentiated plasma cells and memory B cells is a multistep process, involving the ordered expression of a large number of genes. For the convenience sake, this entire process can be divided into three broad stages:

- Generation of mature, immunocompetent B cells (maturation),
- Activation of mature B cells by interaction with antigen,
- Differentiation of activated B cells into plasma cells and memory B cells.

Maturation of B cells occurs in the bone marrow microenvironment, which involves orderly sequence of Ig gene rearrangements and the developmental progression in the absence of antigen. Therefore, this stage of development of B cells is called **antigen-independent phase.**

Immature B cells, characterized by the expression of membrane bound immunoglobulin, mIgM and mIgD with single antigen specificity leave the bone marrow and migrate to the periphery where they traverse a transitional stage to become resting mature B cells or **naive B cells.** These naive cells that have not encountered the antigen, will circulate in the blood and lymph and are carried to the secondary lymphoid organs like spleen and lymph nodes. At this stage if a B cell encounters an antigen, which binds to its membrane bound IgM and IgD, the cell will undergo activation. Activation of B cell leads to its proliferation and differentiation leading to the formation of antibody secreting plasma cells and memory B cells. Antigen committed B cells will undergo affinity maturation, where class switching of immunoglobulin gene occurs. Since peripheral B cells for their development require antigen for activation and differentiation, it is called **antigen-dependent phase.**

B-CELL MATURATION

Maturation of B cells is a continuous process, which occurs all throughout the life of an individual. In the embryonic condition, fetal liver, yolk sac and fetal bone marrow are the major sites of B cell maturation and after birth, maturation of B cells occurs in the bone marrow.

Bone Marrow Microenvironment

The development of B cells begins from lymphoid stem cells, which differentiate into B cell lineage called **progenitor B cell** (pro-B cell). The earliest marker that defines cells committed to the B cell lineage is the CD45R in human's, the isoform of B220 of mice, and a transmembrane tyrosine phosphatase. Pro-B cells proliferate within the bone marrow and differentiate in to **precursor-B cells** (pre-B cells). The pre-B cells require microenvironment provided by the stromal cells of bone marrow. Stromal cells secrete various cytokines, most importantly, IL-7 as well as they interact with pro-B and pre-B cells directly. These two processes are essential for the development of the B cells. The cell adhesion molecules like VLA-4 on pro-B cells and VCAM-1 on stromal cells help in the interaction. Once this interaction is established, other molecules like c-Kit on the pro-B cells and stem cell factor (SCF) on the stromal cell establish contact and induce tyrosine kinase activity. As a result pro-B cells will start dividing and differentiate in to pre-B cells expressing a receptor for IL-7. Stromal cells secrete IL-7, which binds to pre-B cell receptors and downregulates the adhesion molecule contact so as to release the pre-B cells from the stromal cell contact. Detached pre-B cells continue to proliferate with the help of IL-7 stimulation and undergo maturation (Fig. 10.1).

Ig – Gene Rearrangements and Formation of Pre-B Cell Receptors

Further development and maturation of B cell depends on Ig gene rearrangements. The mechanisms involved in Ig gene arrangements have already been explained in Chapter 9. In the late pro-B cells heavy –chain D_H to J_H gene rearrangements takes place followed by V_H to $D_H J_H$ rearrangement (Fig. 9.2-9.5). Only after the completion of heavy-chain gene rearrangement the cell is called pre-B cell. From here on, the continuation of development of pre-B cell in to **immature B cell** requires a productive light-chain gene rearrangement. In the late pro-B cell, disulfide linked CD79a (Igα)-CD79b (Igβ) heterodimers as invariant signal transducing units together with calnexin. In the pre-B cell, heavy chain gene expresses

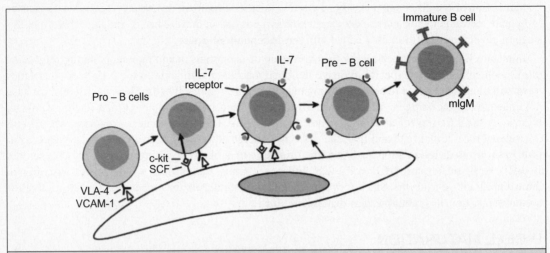

Fig. 10.1 Stromal cells in the bone marrow are required for maturation of progenitors of B cells into precursors of B cells.

μm (an immunoglobulin heavy chain) in association with **surrogate light chains VpreB** and λ5 and with Igα/Igβ, which constituted pre-B cell receptor (pre-BCR). Expression of the pre-BCR is essential for allelic exclusion at the heavy chain locus. This allelic exclusion depends on membrane expression of membrane μ chain (μm) but does not require λ5. Transition of cells from the pre-B to immature B cells stage is accompanied by productive VJ gene rearrangements allowing expression of conventional light chains. Immature B cells express Igα/Igβ and a mature mIgM and probably the earliest cells in the B cell lineage to exhibit antigen specificity. These cells progress to a transitional stage where they express low levels of mIgD containing receptors in addition to mIgM (Fig.10.2).

As mentioned earlier, at pro-B cell stage recombinase enzymes RAG-1 and RAG-2 make their appearance together with terminal deoxynucleotidyl transferase (TdT), which play an important role in heavy-chain, light-chain gene rearrangements. TdT expression is turned off at pre B cell stage, when light-chain gene rearrangement takes place, which does not need TdT whose function is mainly insertion of nucleotides at D_H-J_H region, which is not there in light-chain. Further development of B cells leads to the formation of **mature B cells** with fully expressed mIgM and mIgD on their membrane.

Molecular mechanism underlying Igα/Igβ signaling in B cell development

The fact that pro-B cells, Pre-B cells and mature B cell all contain Igα/Igβ dimers suggests these proteins function as universal transducers for these receptors. Mutant mIgM containing YS to VV mutations (using single letter code for amino acids) in the transmembrane domain is expressed on the surface without being associated with Igα/Igβ. This partial BCR does not support B cell development unless the μm carboxy terminal tails are fused to cytoplasmic domains of Igα or Igβ. These and other studies have demonstrated that rescue of development by these chimeric receptors requires the conserved ITAM tyrosine that interacts with Src and Syk family kinase. Thus, development requires the membrane disposition and ITAM signaling function of the Igα or Igβ. Importantly, Pax-5 is expressed at all B cell stages suggesting an important role in development and maintenance of B cells. By performing loss and gain of function experiments, it has been possible to identify four additional Pax-5 target genes, one of which is Igα.

Interestingly mice lacking Igα exon five, which encodes most of the ITAM, are arrested in the immature cell stage. This strongly suggests that signaling by both Igα and Igβ is required to support development of mature B cells, but that signaling through Igβ is sufficient to generate immature B cells. Syk is required for both of these steps in development, indicating that it is a necessary component of both operative signaling pathways.

Selection of Immature Self-reactive B Cells

It is estimated that 90% of the B cells produced each day die without ever leaving the bone marrow. This is due to stringent selection procedures that operate once the cell reach immature stage with high IgM and low IgD expression. This loss is called **negative selection.** Immature B cells migrate to the periphery, where high level expression of mIgM may further ensure increased sensitivity to negative selection upon recognition of autoantigens (self-antigens) found only in the periphery. In the bone marrow also B cells expressing autoantibodies (mIgM) against self-antigens will be subjected to clonal deletion.

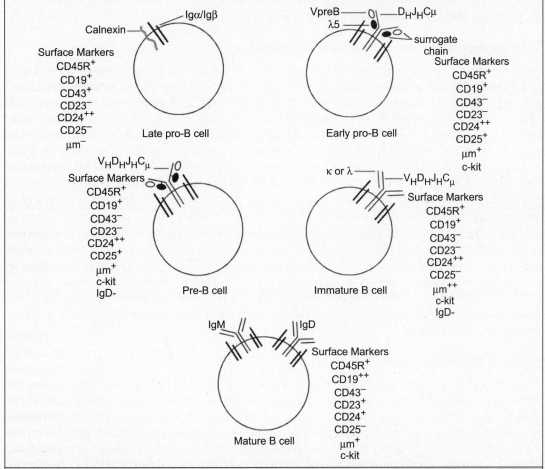

Fig. 10.2 Schematic diagram showing different stages of development of B cell and the membrane receptor molecules.

Negative selection

It has been well established that the cross-linking of mIgM on immature B cells leads to cell death. This has been demonstrated experimentally by treating immature B cells with monoclonal antibody (mAb) against μ constant region. mAb is known to cross-link with mIgM and results in death or apoptosis of immature B cells. Similar process is thought to occur in the bone marrow when the immature B cells encounter the self-antigens.

B-CELL ACTIVATION AND PROLIFERATION

Once the mature B cells loaded with low mIgM and high IgD activity is exported from the bone marrow, subsequent development proceeds in the periphery, i.e. in the spleen and the lymph node. Here they require antigen for the further development, otherwise naive B cells die within few weeks time. Therefore, latter part of the development of B cells is called antigen driven activation and clonal selection. This leads to the formation of antibody secreting plasma cells and memory B cells. Antigen driven activation of B cells goes through two different methods on the basis of antigen involved. It is classified in to **thymus dependent (TD) and thymus independent (TI)** process.

Thymus dependent and independent antigens

B cell response to TD antigens require direct contact with T_H cells, where as antigens that activate B cells in the absence T_H cell are called TI antigens. TI antigens are of two types: type 1 antigens are bacterial cell wall components including lipopolysaccharides (LPS). Type 2 TI antigens are bacterial cell wall polysaccharides with repetitive units conjugated to polymeric proteins, e.g. bacterial flagellins. Most type 1 TI antigens are strong mitogens, that are they are polyclonal activators of B cells regardless of their antigenic specificity. Some type 1 TI antigens at high concentration can stimulate as many as 35% B cells to produce antibodies. On the contrary, at lower concentration of type 1 TI antigens, only B cells specific for epitopes of the antigen will be activated. For ex. LPS of gram-negative bacteria, at low concentration stimulates specific antibody production, whereas at high concentration it is polyclonal B cell activator, stimulating proliferation and differentiation of large population of B cells.

Type 2 TI antigens activate B cells by cross-linking mIg receptor, but it also needs cytokines derived from T_H cells for efficient proliferation and class switching of immunoglobulin genes, even though direct contact with T_H cell does not occur. It is observed that response to TI antigen is generally weak and does not lead to immunological memory. In addition to this IgM is the only predominant antibody produced indicating lack of class switching mechanism. Therefore, T_H cell dependent immune response by B cells assumes significance because it helps in generation of memory B cells, affinity maturation and class switching to other isotypes.

Origin of activating signals

There are two type signals responsible for driving naive B cells to enter into proliferative stage and differentiate into antibody producing cells. **Competence signals** drive the naive B cells from Go into early G1 stage, rendering B cells competent enough to receive the next set of signals. **Progression signals** drive the cells from G1 to S, cell proliferation and ultimately differentiation. TI and TD antigens involve two different ways of competence signaling events, accordingly they are designated as **signal 1** and **signal 2.** TI antigens being multivalent in nature induce strong stimulation of B cells by cross-linking mIg molecules, which acts as signal 1. In addition type 1 TI antigens also contain an additional component that provides signal 2 (Fig. 10.3). Apparently type 2 TI antigens show extensive cross-linking with mIg receptor, generates an extensive competence signal, which itself will lead to progression signal leading to progression of B cells. Type 1 TI antigen seems to need an additional signal in the form of cytokine to enter into progression stage.

TD antigens are either divalent or oligovalent and soluble antigens, thus induce weak signal 1 when they bind to mIg on the B cell. In this case additional signal 2 is provided by the interaction of CD40 on the B cell and CD40L on the T_H cell (Fig. 10.3). B cells activated in this manner start producing cytokine receptors on their membrane and respond to the cytokines secreted by the T_H cells to proliferate and differentiate.

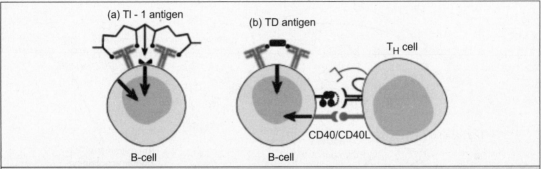

Fig. 10.3   Schematic diagram depicting the type of competence signals provided by TI and TD antigen for the activation of B cells.

Signal transduction from the B cell antigen-receptor

Proliferative expansion and differentiation are triggered through the pre-BCR and BCR complex in pre-B cells and mature resting B cell, respectively. At the opposite extreme, apoptosis is triggered in immature B cells upon excessive clustering of newly expressed receptors as mechanism for elimination of autoreactive membrane immunoglobulin (mIgM) expressing B cells. Strong BCR ligation in mature B cells has also been shown to inhibit V(D)J recombination at the mIg locus, while weak ligation promotes recombination-presumably to generate higher affinity antibodies. Finally BCR serves as a specific receptor to efficiently internalize antigen for processing and peptide presentation to helper T cells. In fact, signals through the BCR have recently been reported from the extensive research work carried out throughout 1990s in different labs. BCR signals are also responsible for reorganize antigen processing compartments in B cells to promote presentation of antigen internalized by mIg. Understandably, the B cell has devised a complex network of BCR signaling cascade to perform such a diverse array of functions.

Cross-linking of BCR complex (Fig. 10. 4) induces protein tyrosine pohosphorylation of the cytoplasmic domains of Ig-α and Ig-β suggested their involvement in signal transduction. The YXXL turned out to be a critical sequence element within the Ig-α and Ig-β cytoplasmic domains, termed the **immunoreceptor tyrosine-based activation motif (ITAM)**. While protein tyrosine kinases (PTKs) are intrinsic to growth factor receptors for transducing growth signals, ITAMs provide antigen-receptors with specific binding sites for nonreceptor PTKs.

Aggregation of mIg molecules through the binding of multivalent antigen induces phosphorylation of the ITAMs on Ig-α and Ig-β by Src family tyrosine kinases (Lyn, Fyn, Blk and or Lck). Phosphorylation of the ITAMs on Ig-α and Ig-β appears to mainly occur at the membrane-proximal tyrosine with only a

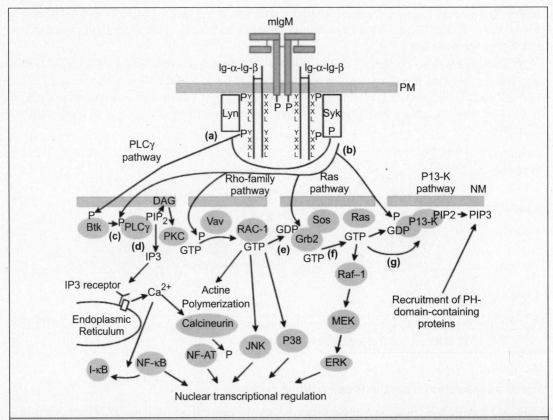

Fig. 10.4   A schematic presentation of the major intracellular signaling pathways activated by aggregation of the BCR. Major interconnections between the four major signaling cascades and their downstream effects leading to nuclear transcriptional regulation events are depicted. The BCR complex is composed of mIgM in association with Ig-α/Ig-β heterodimers. **(a)** Tyrosine residues in Ig-α/Ig-β ITAM motifs (YXXL) are phosphorylated-**P** by Src-family PTKs (Lyn). Tyrosine can then bind tandem SH2 domains of Syk; **(b)** Syk is then activated by phosphorylation. The concerted tyrosine phosphorylation events carried out by the PTKs Lyn, Syk and **(c)** Btk trigger **(d)** the activation of PLCγ to hydrolyze PIP2, **(e)** the Vav GEF to activate Rho-family GTPases (Rac-1; RhoA and Cdc42 are not shown) by displacing GDP with GTP, **(f)** the Sos GEF to activate Ras by displacing GDP with GTP and **(g)** Ras-mediated activation of PI3-K to phosphorylate PIP2 to PIP3. **(h)** Downstream effector cascades induce the nuclear translocation of the activated MAPKs (ERK, JNK and p38), NF-κB (after dissociation from the inhibitor, I-κB) and NF-AT (after dephosphorylation) where they regulate nuclear transcription events.

SOURCE: CAMBELL, K. S. *Curr. Opin. Immunol.* **11**: 256-264, 1999.

subset of ITAMs phosphorylated at both tyrosine residues. Phosphorylation of both tyrosine residues in the ITAM, however, creates a specific binding site for the tandem Src-homology (SH2) domains of the cytosolic PTK, Syk (See Fig. 10.4). Syk recruitment by the BCR is a key event that activates a plethora of down-stream signaling pathways-including phsophorylation, protein recruitment, activation of GTP-binding molecular switches, second messenger generation and gene transcription. Signals generated through Syk have also been shown to be important for BCR-mediated antigen presentation. Lyn contributes as an important positive effector through optimal activation of Syk, it also initiates negative feed back through direct tyrosine phosphorylation of the inhibitory receptors FcγRIIB1 and CD22. Co-localization with FcγRIIB1 and CD22 receptors suppresses BCR signaling responses by recruiting **SHIP (SH2 domain-containing inositol polyphosphate 5-phophatase)** and **SHP-1 (SH2 domain-containing protein tyrosine phosphatase [PTP-1])** respectively.

Overview of the Major Pathways of BCR Signaling

Several major signal events are triggered upon clustering of the BCR on mature resting B cells as outlined in Fig. 10. 4. These include activation of phospholipase C (PLCγ), the Rho family of GTPases, RAS and phosphatidylinositol-3 kinase (PI3-K). BLNK/SLP-65: a adaptor protein that links many signaling events.

Other B cell adaptors

CD19 has also been touted as a transmembrane adaptor molecule. PI3-K activation have been shown to be strongly potentiated by recruitment to phosphorylated tyrosine residue within the cytoplasmic domain of CD19. In addition, tyrosine-phsophorylated CD19 can recruit Vav and promote downstream activation of PIP5-K (Phosphotidylinositol-4-phosphate –5-kinase) to expand the PIP2 pool. Recent studies implicate the BCR-associated a4 protein as an important regulatory linker. The a4 protein can bind directly to, and regulate the catalytic activity of, the serine/threonine phosphatase, protein phosphatase 2A (PP2A). Association with a4 appears to regulate PP2A substrate recognition since it was shown to either inhibit or activate phosphatase activity, depending upon the phosphorylated substrate assayed.

Mechanism of MAPK activation by BCR

In addition to ERK activation mediated through BLNK/SLP-65, the kinase can be activated through pathways dependent upon either the adaptor protein, Shc, or PKC. Syk can tyrosine-phosphorylate Shc at two sites, which efficiently drives the assembly of Grb2-Sos complexes at the plasma membrane.

As with signaling pathway, negative feedback mechanisms are critical to shut down MAPK activities. The Rap family of GTPase inhibitor proteins directly counteracts Ras signaling by binding to and inhibiting Raf-1 kinase. Recently it has been found that BCR signaling can activate Rap1 through a DAG-dependent pathway. This GTP-binding molecular switch may directly impinge upon the stimulation of ERK by the BCR.

Critical role-played by PI3 – K in BCR signaling

PI3 – K is rapidly activated in parallel with PLCγ upon BCR cross –linking. Both enzymes are recruited to the plasma membrane to act upon the same substrate, PIP2. PLCγ cleaves PIP2 to generate IP3 and DAG whereas PI3 – K catalyzes the addition of a specific phosphate on the inositol ring to generate phosphatidylinositol 3,4,5-triphosphate (PIP3). PIP3-mediated plasma membrane recruitment of both PLCγ and Btk is essential for their activation. The activation of Btk requires both transphosphorylation on Tyr551 by membrane-associated Src-family PTKs and autophosphorylation on Tyr223. In addition, co-recruitment to the membrane interface brings Btk into direct contact with PLCγ where the PTK acts in concert with Syk and Src-family PTKs to tyrosine-phosphorylate the phospholipase. PIP3 binding by PLCγ is also believed to present the phospholipase directly to the PIP2 substrate. Recent evidence indicates that the regulatory influences of PI3 – K and Btk on PLCγ might greatly impact upon gene transcription events that are initiated through calcium mobilization. The role of Btk was recently shown to be essential for inducing prolonged calcium elevation by the BCR through enhanced IP3 production.

Role of Btk in B Cell Development and Signaling

Bruton's tyrosine kinase (Btk) was initially identified as the target of mutation responsible for X-linked agammaglobulinemia (XLA) in humans. Patients with XLA are unusually susceptible to pyogenic bacterial infections and enteroviral disease; plasma cells are absent and all classes of serum Ig are profoundly reduced. These features stem from an intrinsic defect in B cell development: peripheral B cells are rare and exhibit an immature phenotype, but the number of pre-B cells expressing cytoplasmic Igμ chain in the bone marrow is not significantly reduced, suggesting impaired cellular proliferation or increased cell death at the pre-B to B cell transition.

The xid (X-linked immunodeficiency of B cell function) mouse phenotype is distinct from XLA. Although humoral responses to a subset of T cell independent (TI) antigens are absent, xid mice are able to respond to most T cell dependent (TD) antigen. Peripheral B cells are present, albeit somewhat reduced in number, and are skewed towards an immature phenotype, with an over-representation of $IgM^{low}IgD^{high}$ class. Survival of peripheral B cells is diminished and the peritoneal B-1 B cell (CD5 B cell) population is absent. In serum the amount of IgM and IgG3, the major products of the B-1 population, are reduced. Thus, whereas xid mice suffer defects in B cell maturation and function they do not exhibit the substantial block in early B cell development observed in patients with XLA. In the past few years' considerable progress has been made in understanding of the regulation of Btk activity and the identification of downstream consequences of Btk action.

Effects of Btk deficiency on immune responsiveness and B cell development

At least 13 XLA-associated missense mutations, distributed throughout the Btk coding region, have been characterized to date. The xid mutation, R28C (in single letter amino acid code), resides at a conserved site within the PH domain. Detection of a similar mutation, R28H, in patients with XLA suggested that the distinction between the XLA and xid phenotypes was not the result of an allelic difference. The effect of Btk deficiency on central B cell development in the mouse is subtle. B cells from xid mice fail to proliferate in response to B cell receptor cross-linking by anti Ig antibodies and are hyporesponsive to lipopolysaccharides. B cell proliferation and induction of B7 in response to engagement of CD40 by CD40 ligand are also defective, as are responses to IL-5 and IL-10. In addition, B cell proliferation and expression of MHC class II molecules in response to CD38 cross-linking in the presence of IL-4 are impaired in B cells from xid mice. Btk-deficient B cells exhibit a constellation of signaling defects similar to those associated with xid: the proliferative response to anti-IgM antibodies is absent and responses to dextran-conjugated anti-IgD antibodies, LPS or CD40 engagement are reduced.

B-Cell Coreceptor Complex

This has been discussed in greater detail in Chapter 12, under separate heading. Please refer to the respective section in the chapter for the details.

Role of T$_H$ Cells in Humoral Response

Activation of B cells by soluble protein antigens requires involvement of TH cells, where binding of antigen to mIg does not induce an effective competence signal. Therefore, an additional molecule interaction on the membrane of B and T cells is required to bring out an effective activation response. In addition, B cell proliferation requires cytokines. The probable sequence of events involved in B cell activation by TD antigen is illustrated in Fig. 10.5.

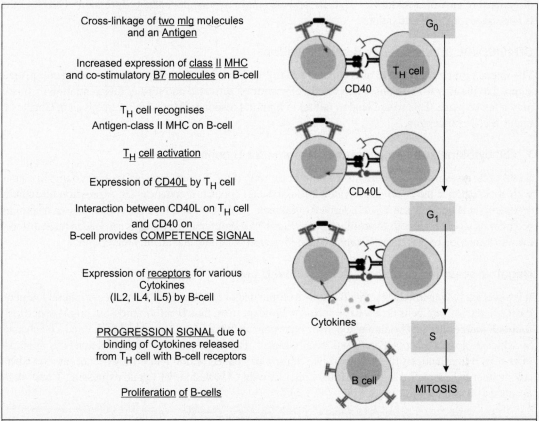

Cross-linkage of two mlg molecules and an Antigen

Increased expression of class II MHC and co-stimulatory B7 molecules on B-cell

T$_H$ cell recognises
Antigen-class II MHC on B-cell

T$_H$ cell activation

Expression of CD40L by T$_H$ cell

Interaction between CD40L on T$_H$ cell and CD40 on B-cell provides COMPETENCE SIGNAL

Expression of receptors for various Cytokines (IL2, IL4, IL5) by B-cell

PROGRESSION SIGNAL due to binding of Cytokines released from T$_H$ cell with B-cell receptors

Proliferation of B-cells

Fig. 10.5 Schematic representation of sequence of events involved in B cell activation by thymus dependent antigen.

Formation of T and B Cell Conjugate

Once the antigen binds to mIg receptor on B cells, the antigen is internalized by endocytosis and processed in the endocytic vesicles into peptides (See Fig. 13.4). Binding of antigen to B cell receptor mIg also results in signal transduction leading to sequence of events in the cytoplasm and gene action to upregulate the production of certain membrane associated molecules such as class II MHC, co-stimulatory molecule B7 and the receptors for the growth factors and cytokines. Enhanced expression of B7 and class II MHC molecule on B cells increases its ability to function as an antigen-presenting cell for T$_H$ cell activation. Class II MHC molecules carry processed antigenic peptides in the groove, which is presented to T$_H$ cell through MHC II-peptide-TCR interaction, leading to T cell activation. It is estimated that for the processing of antigenic peptides following internalization and present them on B cell class II MHC molecule generally takes about 30 to 60 min. It is observed that, when the antigen concentration is very high, macrophages and dendritic cells serve as APCs and when the antigen concentration is very low i.e. 100 to 10000 times lower than what is required for presentation by macrophages and dendritic cells, B cell serve as APC. T – B cell conjugate is formed only when the B cell presents the processed antigenic peptide on its class II MHC molecule to T_H cell through TCR. This contact between T and B cell is essential and it leads to the directional release of cytokines by T_H cells, and also the activation dependent expression of CD40L, that is necessary for B cell activation.

CD40/CD40L interaction for B cell activation

The interaction between CD40 of B cell and CD40L of T cell is very essential for providing competence signal 2 to the B cells, without which the B cells wont be activated and further differentiation of B cells may not take place. This would lead to failure in humoral response. More details are given in Chapter 12 under B cell coreceptors.

T_H cell cytokine induced progression signal for B cells

B cell proliferation and differentiation would occur only if the T_H cell derived cytokines come in contact with B cells. Once the B cell is activated through T cell contact, it enhances the expression of cytokine receptors on B cells. Three T_H cell derived cytokines, IL-2, IL-4, and IL-5 have been shown to provide progression signal for B cells to proliferate (See Fig. 10.6). Proliferation of B cells can lead to three different events: formation of plasma cells, memory B cells, class switching and affinity maturation.

Negative selection of mature, self-reactive B cells

It is a process by which self-reactive B cells are eliminated or rendered inactive in the peripheral lymphoid tissue. Some self-antigens do not have access to bone marrow, thus B cells expressing mIgM specific for such self-antigens cannot be eliminated in the bone marrow. Thus immune system has devised a mechanism by which these self-reactive B cells will be eliminated. The major pathway of elimination is by apoptosis of B cells if their antigen-receptor is triggered for a prolonged period and if they do not interact with T cells within a short period of time or if they interact with CD40L and Fas ligand expressing T cells in the absence of B cell receptor triggering.

Sites for induction of humoral response

Initiation of humoral immune response begins in the microenvironment of the lymph node. Initial activation of both B and T cells is known to occur in paracortex area of the lymph node (Fig. 4.9). In the lymph node B cells are mostly found in cortex area from where they migrate to T cell rich zone. B cells that have antigen bound to their mIg will internalize the antigen and present it in association with class II MHC. Such antigen-presenting B cells will try to interact with T_H cells and on establishing contact with T_H cells undergo activation. Once B cell activation takes place, small foci of proliferating B cells will be formed at the edge of the T cell rich zone and reach a maximum size within 3 to 4 days after the antigen entry in to the body. A few days after the formation of foci within the lymph nodes, a few activated B cells and some T_H cells migrate from the foci to primary follicles, forming the **germinal centers.** In the germinal center intense proliferation of B cells takes place, they are called **centroblasts**. Centroblast ultimately give rise to small centrocytes, which do not divide but express membrane Ig. Centrocytes establish contact

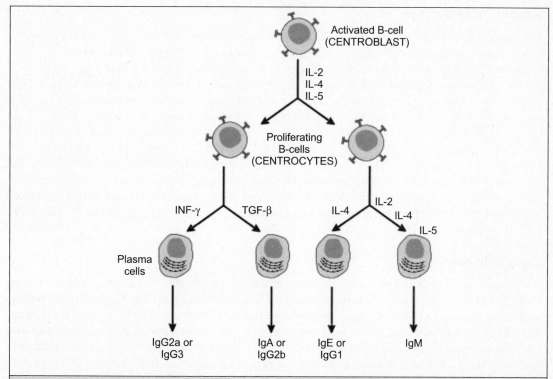

Fig. 10.6 Schematic representation of role of cytokines in proliferation and class switching of B lymphocytes.

with macrophages and follicular dendritic cells, which are presenting antigens on class II MHC on their surface. The area becomes densely packed with lymphocytes called basal light zone. Centrocytes possessing membrane IgM bind to antigen presented by follicular dendritic cells and undergo differentiation to form two types of progeny: small memory B cells and large plasmablasts. The plasmablasts leave the germinal center and migrate to the medulla region where they transform into plasma cells and begin to secrete antibody molecules. A large majority of centrocytes does not establish contact with antigen presented by follicular dendritic cells. These cells die by apoptosis.

B-Cell Differentiation

Three important B cell differentiation events take place in the germinal centers: affinity maturation, class switching and formation of plasma cells and memory B cells. These events require signals provided by T_H cells or follicular dendritic cells.

Affinity maturation

This event in the B cell differentiation is the result of two processes: somatic hypermutation and antigen selection of high affinity clones.

Somatic hypermutation

The antigen-activated centroblasts undergo proliferation and simultaneously undergo somatic hypermutation of the heavy and light-chain variable region genes ((Chapter 9). As a result of somatic hypermutation, deletions, insertions and point mutations are introduced into the V, D, and J segments of rearranged immunoglobulin genes. These mutations are restricted to complementarity-determining regions (CDRs). Most interesting aspect of somatic mutation is that it does not occur until the primary response peaking well into the second week following primary antigen challenge. Thus, somatic mutations are located predominantly in the secondary antibodies. Both activated T_H cells and germinal centers are required for the somatic mutation to take place. Since somatic mutation is a random event, it will generate few cells with high affinity receptors and many cells with low affinity or no affinity receptors. Those cells with high affinity receptors go through **positive selection**. These cells with their high affinity mIg receptor bind to antigens presented by follicular dendritic cells on their class II MHC molecules. This contact saves these cells from apoptotic death, due to high level of expression of Bcl-2 by the B cells, which inhibits apoptosis.

Class switching

As discussed in Chapter 9, class switching allows an antibody molecule to retain the specificity but the biological effector activities of the molecule change. Class switching allows any V_H domain to associate with the constant region of any isotype. As mentioned earlier, humoral response to TD antigens is associated with extensive class switching, whereas the response to TI antigens is dominated by production of only IgM. For the class switching, interaction between CD40 on the B cells and CD40L on the T_H cells is essential. Significance of this association is given detail in Chapter 12. It is observed that type 1 TI antigens do not induce class switching, whereas type 2 TI antigens induce class switching but predominantly produce IgM. In the humoral response to type 2 TI antigens, cytokines like IL-4, IFN-γ and TGF-β known to be involved in the class switching. Microenvironment of the secondary lymphoid organs is known to play an important role in class switching, like Peyer's patches or mesenteric lymph nodes are committed to produce IgA. On the other hand, plasma cells originating in spleen, peripheral lymph nodes, or tonsils are mainly committed to IgG production (Fig. 10.7).

Generation of plasma cells and memory cells

The centroblasts can directly differentiate into both memory B cells and plasma cell. The question has been whether a positive factor pushes the cells into a pathway or if a negative signal prevents cells from entering a pathway. A recent experiment demonstrated that CD40 ligand represents a key negative signal that prevents centroblasts entering into terminal plasma cell differentiation. As long as CD40 ligand is provided centroblasts remain as it is in the presence of IL-2 and IL-10. Upon withdrawal of the CD40 ligand, centroblasts rapidly differentiated into plasma cells (Fig. 10.7). The inhibitory effect of CD40 ligand on B cell differentiation has been confirmed by other human B cell culture systems.

Regulation of naive and memory B cell differentiation

Some immunologists are of the opinion that the majority of memory B cells do not undergo further somatic mutation within GC upon stimulation. This observation supports the so called "decreasing potential hypothesis" suggesting that memory T and B cells generated after each round of stimulation acquire a decreased potential to generate new memory cells and an increased potential to undergo terminal

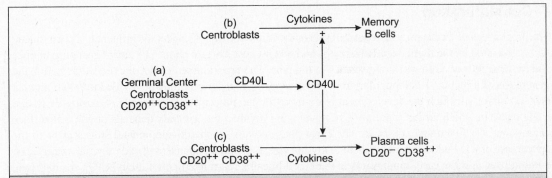

Fig. 10.7   Schematic representation of CD40L directed differentiation of germinal center B cells towards the memory B cell or plasma cell pathway. **(a)** CD20++CD38+ germinal center B cells undergo strong proliferation and give rise to centrocytes of CD20+CD38+ after three days of culture with CD40L and cytokines IL-2 and IL-10. **(b)** These centrocytes predominantly give rise to CD20++CD38-memory cells after another four days of culture with CD40L, IL-2 and IL-10. **(c)** if CD40L is withdrawn after four days of culture, these cells predominantly give rise to plasma cells. This experiment indicates that the CD40L represents a suppressor of centrocytes terminal differentiation.

SOURCE: LIU, Y. J., ET AL *Curr. Opin. Immunol.* **9**: 256-262. 1997.

differentiation into effector cells. Culturing isolated human naive B cells and memory cells with IL-2 and IL-10 and different concentrations of CD40L directly tested this hypothesis. This experiment showed that memory B cells underwent terminal differentiation into plasma cells more readily than did naive B cells. Memory B cells 5 to 8 fold more plasma cells and 3 to 4 fold more secreted Ig. By contrast naive B cells gave rise to a larger number of nondifferentiated activated B cells. The novel feature of memory B cells may confer two important capacities to the immune system: the rapid generation of a large number of effector cells to efficiently eliminate pathogens; and the prevention of over-expression and chronic accumulation of one particular memory B cell clone which would freeze the peripheral B cell repertoire.

T-CELL MATURATION, ACTIVATION AND DIFFERENTIATION

The character that distinguishes the antigen recognition ability of T cell from B cell is MHC restriction. The progenitors of T cells in the thymus as well as the peripheral T cells need the MHC molecules for their activation. T cells also undergo maturation by a selection process and during maturation only MHC restricted and nonself-reactive T cells undergo maturation. The final stages of T cell maturation follows two different pathways on the basis of MHC restriction. Those T cells restricted by class I MHC develop into CD8$^+$ T cells, and those restricted by class II MHC give rise to CD4$^+$ T cells. Mature peripheral T cell activation occurs through the interaction of T cell receptor (TCR) with MHC-antigenic peptide complex presented by antigen-presenting cell (APC) or target cell (virus infected or cancerous cell). If the TCR-antigen-MHC interaction is of low affinity type, T cells would involve co-receptors and other accessory membrane molecules to enhance the stimulation and signal transduction. T cells activated in this manner undergo proliferation and differentiation to form various types of effector T cells and memory T cells.

T-Cell Maturation

The progenitors of T cells migrate from the bone marrow into the thymus under the influence of chemotactic factors secreted by the thymic epithelial cells, and this process starts at about 11th day of gestation in mice and in the eighth or ninth week of gestation in humans. The programmed series of events that lead to the generation of a mature T cell population with a diverse TCR repertoire may be divided into two phases: an early phase, in which the development of thymocytes can proceed in the absence of mature TCR, and a late phase in which further maturation of developing thymocytes critically depends on the cell surface expression of a functional $\alpha\beta$ TCR. The early phase covers all the developmental stages prior to the appearance of $CD4^+ CD8^+$ (double positive) thymocytes. It includes expansion of early thymic immigrants, commitment of these early immigrants to the T cell lineage, rearrangement of their TCR γ, δ and β loci, selection of cell with functional TCR-β rearrangements, allelic and possibly isotypic exclusion (i.e. the expression of only one TCR-β chain and only one type of TCR-$\alpha\beta$ or $\gamma\delta$, per cell) and the commitment decision between $\gamma\delta$ and $\alpha\beta$ T cell lineage.

Discrete Stages in Early T Cell Development

On the basis of their expression of CD4 and CD8 accessory molecules, developing thymocytes are usually subdivided into four sub-populations that correspond to discrete developmental stages: **double negative, double positive, single negative-single positive, and triple negatives**. The most immature thymocytes lack TCR-CD3 expression and reside in the $CD4^-CD8^-$ population, which are designated as **triple negatives** (TNs). This population comprises only about 1 to 2% of all thymocytes, passes through a series of differentiation stages defined by distinct cell surface markers (Fig. 10.8). These stages ultimately lead to the co-expression of CD4 and CD8 and to the generation of $CD4^+$ and $CD8^+$ **double positive** (DP) thymocytes, essentially all of which carry one functionally rearranged TCRβ allele. The most useful markers that distinguish developmentally relevant subsets within the TN population have turned out to be CD25 (IL-2 receptor α chain), CD44 (phagocyte glycoprotein-1/Pgp-1) and c-kit (tyrosine kinase receptor for stem cell factor).

The most immature thymocytes within the TN subset are c-kit$^+$, CD44$^+$ and CD25$^-$ (Fig.10.8a). These cells express low levels of CD4 on their cells surface and are therefore, in the strictest sense, not really 'triple negative'. The cell surface phenotype of low CD4s is not yet fully committed to the T cell pathway, all of their T cell receptor genes are still in germ line configuration and, upon intravenous transfer, they can develop into B cells, natural killer cells and thymic dendritic cells. Upon down regulation of CD4 and upregulation of CD25, low CD4s become c-kit$^+$CD44$^+$CD25$^+$ TNs (Fig. 10.8b). At this developmental stage they lose the capacity to develop into B cells but, interestingly, they retain their precursor activity for the formation of thymic dendritic cells.

At least four decisive events in early T cell development take place at this maturational stage. First, rearrangement of TCRγ, δ, and β chain genes are initiated and essentially completed. These rearrangements seem to occur irrespective of whether CD44$^{-/low}$CD25$^+$ cells subsequently follow the $\alpha\beta$ or $\gamma\delta$ developmental pathway, because all three types of rearrangements are found in mature T cells of both lineages. Second, the cells become fully committed to the T lineage; for instance CD44$^{-/low}$CD25$^+$ pre-T cells can no longer generate thymic dendritic cells. Third, those cells that produce a functional TCRβ chain, because they have managed to rearrange one of their TCRβ alleles in-frame, are selected for further maturation, a process that has been termed β-**selection**. Cells that undergo β-selection enter the cell cycle, expand rapidly and progress to the next developmental stage. In contrast, cells that fail to experience β-selection, because both TCRβ alleles are rearranged in a nonproductive fashion, remain

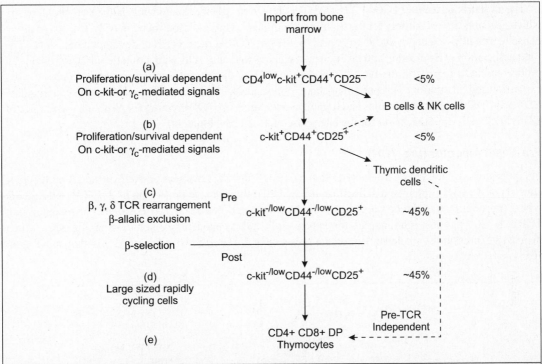

Fig. 10.8 Schematic illustration of early T cell development in mice. The figure shows the four discrete developmental stages (a–d) within the triple negative thymocyte population which are defined by surface expression of CD44, CD25 and c-kit (CD117). Survival and/or maintenance of populations-(a) and (b) depend on signals transmitted through c-kit or a γc containing receptor. Percentages give the approximate proportion of each respective subset. Thick arrows define the major developmental pathway; thin arrows define minor, alternative pathways leading to B, NK and thymic dendritic cell production. The dashed arrow leading to NK cells indicate that population-(b) can give rise to NK cells. A dashed horizontal line indicates the boundary represents a developmental checkpoint, which allows only those cells, which have productive TCRβ rearrangement and can thus express functional pre-TCER complex to progress (β-selection). Dashed thick arrow indicates a pre-TCR independent very inefficient pathway, which allows few thymocytes to reach CD4$^+$CD8$^+$ stage. In the absence of pre-TCR derived signal (e), the pathway seems to bypass the stage –(d) of rapidly dividing cells, giving rise to DP thymocytes, which have not undergone β-selection and in part they still express CD25.

quiescent and eventually die unless they have the potential to develop γδ T cells (because maturation of γδ T cells does not require β-selection). Finally successful expression of a functional TCRβ chain in CD44$^-$CD25$^+$ pre-T cells suppresses rearrangement at the second TCRβ locus, a phenomenon known as **allelic exclusion**.

The most striking feature of CD44$^{-/low}$CD25$^-$ TNs, however, is their extraordinarily high rate of proliferation, which accounts almost entirely for the thymic cell numbers. This enormous burst in cell division is a direct consequence of β-selection, and is triggered by the pre-TCR at the preceding developmental stage. The tight association of β-selection and proliferation ensures that only cells with a functional TCRβ chain can proliferate and progress to the next developmental stage, thereby preventing useless precursors from expansion and maturation. This precursor stage represents the final stage. They spontaneously upregulate CD4 and CD8 accessory molecules and transform into large sized DP thymocytes. With the appearance of CD4$^+$CD8$^+$ cells, the stage is set for the late phase of T cell development.

Pre-T cell receptor (pre-TCR)

This receptor is expressed on thymocytes that lack CD4 and CD8 markers on their surface. This receptor consists of the CD3 protein and a disulfide-linked heterodimer made of β-chain of the TCR and a 33 kD type I transmembrane glycoprotein (gp33), which is called pre-Tα (pTα) covalently associated with TCRβ. It belongs to the immunoglobulin superfamily and is encoded by a non-rearranging gene, which means its expression is not dependent on the presence of RAGs. The structure of pTα is shown in Figure 10.9.

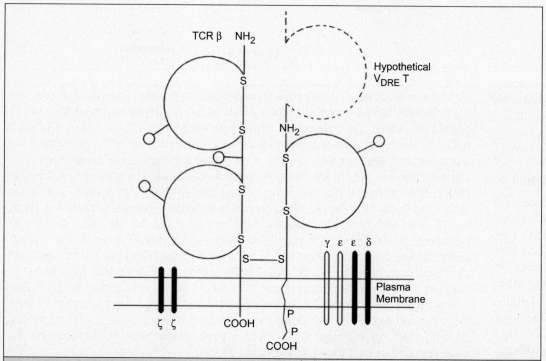

Fig. 10.9   Schematic structure of the pre TCR heterodimer or possible heterodimer. Immunoglobulin-like domains are shown as circles. S – S symbolizes disulfide bridge. CD3 receptor is made up of γ, ε, ε, δ, ζζ responsible for signal transduction.

Source: FEHLING, H. J. AND VON BOEHMER, H. *Curr. Opin. Immunol.* 9: 263-275, 1999.

In the thymus, pTα seems to be expressed in all immature TN stages with the possible exception of the c-kit$^+$CD44$^+$CD25$^-$ sub-population as, for unknown reasons. The identification of pTα as a partner chain for TCRβ in immature TN thymocytes provides the basis of an attractive hypothesis put forward by Von Boehmer to explain the crucial role of TCRβ in early T cell development; in immature TN thymocytes, which in general have not rearranged the TCRα locus, newly formed TCRβ chains may associate with pTα to form a functional pre-TCR complex: this could then trigger intense pre-T cell proliferation and maturation to the DP stage. The overall result of this pre-TCR-mediated selection is:

- The efficient generation of a large pool of DP thymocytes with TCRβ chains and selection of these thymocytes for further maturation.
- Suppression of further rearrangement of TCRβ chain genes so that allelic exclusion of β chain will occur.
- Development of CD4$^+$CD8$^+$ double positive thymocytes.

Signal transduction in the pre-TCR

Several lines of evidence indicate the involvement of the lymphocyte-specific tyrosine kinase p56^{lck} in the transmission of pre-TCR-mediated signals. PTα is endowed with a significantly larger cytoplasmic tail than all conventional TCR molecules. In mice, it contains amino acid motifs that could serve as phosphorylation sites for protein kinase C and as docking sites for molecules with Src homology (SH3-domains). This has led to speculation that the cytoplasmic portion of pTα may actively participate in signal transduction. Amino acid sequence in the extracellular Ig-like domain has 80% resemblance between mice and human, whereas it is different after the transmembrane region. Human pTα cytoplasmic tail comprises about 114 amino acids versus only 30 amino acids in mice. Recent study in pTα-deficient mice, which express a tail-less pTα showed that cytoplasmic portion of pTα is not essential for pre-TCR signaling, because of significantly increased number of DP thymocytes in pTα-deficient mice. Another recent report indicates that a cAMP-dependent signal transduction pathway can interfere with signals delivered through pre-TCR-CD3-p56^{lck} complex.

Single positive T cell development

Once a specific signal is transmitted through pre-TCR, it halts further β-chain gene rearrangement and induces expression of both CD4+ and CD8+ (double positive-DP) thymocytes. At this stage, even though RAG-1 and RAG-2 genes are transcriptionally active, TCRα chain gene rearrangement does not take place. DP thymocytes undergo extensive proliferation, which contributes to T cell diversity by generating a clone of cells with a single TCRβ chain rearrangement. Each of the cells within this clone can then rearrange different α-chain genes allowing for greater diversity.

DP thymocytes that express αβ TCR CD3 complex and survive thymic selection now chose two different pathways to develop either single positive (SP) CD4$^+$ thymocytes (10%) or single positive CD8$^+$ thymocytes (5%) of total thymocyte population. The single positive thymocytes migrate to the periphery.

The Role of the Thymic Environment in Early T Cell Development

A recent search for developmentally important surface molecules on thymic epithelial cells has suggested a role for CD81, a member of the transmembrane-4 superfamily which comprises a group of cell-surface proteins that are characterized by the presence of four hydrophobic, presumably membrane spanning domains. Addition of anti-CD81 specific monoclonal antibody to fetal thymic organ culture blocked the development of DP and SP αβ thymocytes almost completely. Another recent antibody inhibition study has provided evidence for the involvement of CD27, a lymphocyte-specific member of the tumor necrosis factor (TNF) receptor family, in early T cell development. The tyrosine kinase c-kit (CD117), which acts as a receptor for SCF, is expressed at high levels on immature low CD4s and CD44+CD25+ thymocytes. SCF is found in the thymus as a transmembrane protein on the surface of stromal cells and as a secreted soluble molecule generated by differential splicing. Mice carrying null mutation in the c-kit gene have revealed an approximately 40-fold reduction in cell numbers of the three earlier TN (triple negative) thymocyte populations.

Thymic Selection of the T Cell Repertoire

Thymocytes that undergo productive TCR gene rearrangement are put through selection process, which would involve **positive selection** or **negative selection.** The positive selection would ensure αβ TCR expressed on the T cell of an individual, will bind to self-MHC. Those cells, which fail to undergo positive selection are eliminated within the thymus. Those thymocytes, which show high affinity receptors for self-MHC molecules will undergo death by apoptosis or **self-tolerance**. Both processes are necessary to generate mature T cells that are self-MHC restricted and self-tolerant. In the thymic environment, stromal cells, epithelial cells, macrophages and dendritic cells are thought to play a role in positive and negative selection. Stromal cells are known to express high levels of class I and class II MHC molecules.

Positive selection

It involves an interaction between immature DP (CD4+CD8+) thymocytes with thymic epithelial cells. Thymocytes interact with epithelial cells through their TCR, which establishes the contact with class I and class II MHC expressed on thymic epithelial cells. Those thymocytes, which fail to establish such contacts undergo apoptosis. During positive selection, high amount of RAG-1, RAG-2 and TdT proteins will be expressed, which facilitates rearrangement of α chain genes, thereby resulting TCR heterodimer of αβ chains will be used for self-MHC recognition. Only those thymocytes whose αβ TCR hetrodimer recognizes a self-MHC molecule are selected for survival. If a thymocyte fails to express αβ TCR heterodimer that fails to recognize the self-MHC, then the cell will die by apoptosis (Fig. 10.10).

Negative selection

The MHC restricted population of positively selected thymocytes shows two type of TCR affinity to self-MHC. Some cells will show low affinity and some others show high affinity. Those thymocytes, which show high affinity with self-MHC molecules will undergo negative selection by interaction with bone marrow-derived dendritic cells or macrophages in the medulla of thymus. During the negative selection process, thymocytes with high affinity TCR will interact with dendritic cells or macrophages presenting self-MHC alone or self-MHC + self-antigen (Fig. 10.10). The exact mechanism behind negative selection is not known, but the selected cells are observed to undergo death by apoptosis. Tolerance to self-antigens is thereby achieved by eliminating self-reactive T cells and only allowing maturation of T cells that are specific for foreign antigens and altered self-molecules.

Probable mechanism involved in T cell apoptosis

Recent work on TNF receptor superfamily expressed on T cells, which includes FasL, TNF, CD40L, CD30L and CD30 have been implicated in negative selection and apoptosis of T lymphocytes. CD30 and

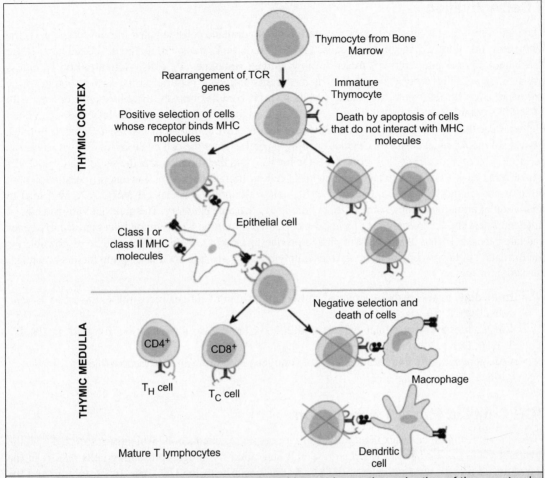

Fig. 10.10 Diagrammatic representation of positive and negative selection of thymocytes in the thymus.

CD40 pathways shown to be involved in negative selection, where as the Fas and TNF pathways are found to play a more crucial role in apoptosis of peripheral T cells. The role of CD40L in negative selection is thought to be indirect, because CD40 is not expressed on T cells. Engagement of CD40 expressed on thymic epithelial cells by CD40L may lead to the induction of a costimulatory molecule, which directly participates in the apoptotic process of negative selection.

Following the activation of Fas and TNF receptor type I by their respective ligands, a cascade of proteases is activated. Protease activity seems to be required for all forms of apoptosis although the initial apoptotic events are different with apoptotic stimuli.

Yet there are many unanswered questions like how the signals from the same receptors in T cells can either result in apoptosis, differentiation or T cell activation.

T Cell Activation

The major event that is involved in the generation of humoral and cell-mediated immune response is the activation and clonal expansion of T_H cells. The activation of T_C cells will not be discussed here (Refer to Chapter 13) but attention will focus on how antigen stimulates T_H cells. Activation of T_H cell is initiated by an antigen-presenting cell, which presents antigenic peptide on its surface bound to the groove of class II MHC molecule. Class II MHC-peptide complex on APC established the contact with TCR-CD3 complex of T_H cell resulting in activating signals, which involves at least 100 individual elements and the number is probably much higher (See Table 10.1). Interaction of these elements initiates cascade of biochemical events that induces resting T_H cell to enter the cell cycle Go to G1, which results in expression of high affinity autocrine receptor for IL-2 and the T_H cell starts the secretion of IL-2. IL-2 is referred to as T cell growth factor, helps in T_H cell proliferation, progression and differentiation in to effector and memory T cells. Interaction of T_H cell with antigen on class II MHC-APC will lead to activation of numerous genes, some of them belong to oncogene category. The gene activation occurs at different intervals, accordingly they have been classified into three types: Immediate genes, early genes and late genes. Each has its own role to play in producing certain proteins, which will be responsible for the formation of new receptors or act as transducing factors and some act transcription factors or nuclear activation factors.

- **Immediate genes** are those activated within half an hour of antigen recognition. Ex. c-Fos, c-Myc, c-Jun, NFAT, NF-κB.
- **Early genes** are those, which express within 1 to 2 hr of antigen recognition. Ex. IL-2, IL-2R, IL-3, IL-6, IFN-γ.
- **Late genes** express more than 2 days after antigen recognition and are responsible for secretion of various adhesion molecules

TCR Coupled Signal Transduction

TCR is a multisubunit complex that consists of clonotypic αβ chains noncovalently associated with the invariant CD3-γ, -δ, -ε and TCRζ chains. T cell activation by antigen-presenting cells results in the activation of protein tyrosine kinases (PTKs) that associate with the CD3 and TCRζ subunit and the coreceptors CD4 or CD8. It has now been firmly established that members of the Src, ZAP (ξ-associated protein)-70/Syk, Tec and Csk families of nonreceptor PTKs play a crucial role in T cell activation.

Activation of PTKs following TCR engagement results in the recruitment and tyrosine phosphorylation of enzymes such as phospholipase Cγ1 (PLCγ1) and Vav as well as critical adaptor proteins such as LAT (linker for activation of T cells), Src-homology domain (SH2)-containing leukocyte protein 76 (SLP-76) and cbl. These proximal activation events lead to reorganization of the cytoskeleton as well as transcriptional activation of multiple genes leading to T lymphocyte proliferation, differentiation and/or effector function. Following is the brief account of those findings made during the past year that have significantly improved the understanding of proximal TCR signaling events (Fig. 10.11).

Redox Signaling Mechanism in T Cell Activation

Lymphocytes with high levels of GSH (reduced glutathione) are more likely to enter the cell cycle and reduction in GSH levels appears to favor prooxidant state that leads to apoptosis. There are numerous

Table 10.1 T cell activation signaling components

Ligands	
MHC class II	Major histocompatibility complex II
CD86/CD80	Transmembrane glycoproteins (found on APCs) responsible for stimulation of CD28/CTLA4
IL-2	Interleukin-2
TNF	Tumor necrosis factor
FasL	Fas ligand
Receptors	
TCRα	T cell receptor α
TCRβ	T cell receptor β
CD3γ	The γ-chain of the CD3 component of TCR
CD3δ	The δ-chain of the CD3 component of TCR
CD3ε	The ε-chain of the CD3 component of TCR
ζ	The zeta chain of the TCR
	The eta chain of the TCR
CD4	An accessory coreceptor of TH cell that binds to MHC class II
CD28	A coreceptor of TH cell that binds to B7 of APC
IL-2Rα	Interleukin-2 receptor α
IL-2Rβ	Interleukin-2 receptor β
IL-2Rγ	Interleukin-2 receptor γ
TNFR	Tumor necrosis factor receptor
Fas	The membrane receptor that triggers apoptosis (also known as APO-1 or CD95)
ITAM	Immunoreceptor tyrosine-based activation motif
Transducers	
lck	A member of the Src family-a nonreceptor tyrosine kinase
fyn	A member of the Src family-a nonreceptor tyrosine kinase
itk	T cell specific tyrosine kinase
ZAP-70	ζ-associated protein tyrosine kinase
Syk	Spleen tyrosine kinase
CD45	A transmembrane tyrosine protein phosphatase
CSK	C-terminal src kinase
PLCγ1	Phospholipase Cγ1
SHP	SH2-containing protein tyrosine phosphatase
SIP	SH2 containing inositol polyphosphate 5-phosphatase
Precursors	
PITP	Phosphatidylinositol transfer protein
PI	Phosphatidylinositol
PIP	Phosphatidylinositol 4-phosphate
PIP$_2$	Phosphatidylinositol 4,5-biphsosphate
PI 4-K	Phosphatidylinositol4-kinase
PIP5-K	Phosphatidylinositol 4-phsophate 5-kinase
SM	Sphingomyelin

Contd.

Table 10.1 (Contd.)

Signaling cassettes	

IP3/Ca^{2+} pathway

IP$_3$	Inositol 1,4,5-triphosphate
IP$_3$RI	IP$_3$ receptor type I
IP$_3$RII	IP$_3$ receptor type II
IP$_3$RIII	IP$_3$ receptor type III
IP$_3$ 3-K	Inositol 1,4,5-triphosphate 3-kinase
IP$_3$ 5-pase	Inositol 1,4,5-triphosphate 5-phosphatase
Ca^{2+}	Calcium
SOC	Store operated channel
GKCa	Ca^{2+}-activated potassium channel
CAML	Calcium-signal modulating cyclophilin ligand
SERCA	Sarco/endoplasmic reticulum Ca^{2+} ATPase
PMCA	Plasma membrane Ca^{2+} ATPase

DAG/PKC pathway

DAG	Diacylglycerol
DAG kinase	Diacylglycerol kinase
PS	Phosphatidylserine
PKCα	Protein kinase C-α
PKCε	Protein kinase C-ε
PKCζ	Protein kinsae C-ζ

PI 3-kinase pathway

PIP$_3$	Phosphatidylinositol 3,4,5-triphosphate
PI 3-K (p85)	Phosphatidylinositol 3-kinase (regulatory subunit)
PI 3–K (p110)	Phosphatidylinositol 3-kinase (catalytic subunit)
PIP$_3$ 5-pase	Phosphatidylinositol 3,4,5-trophosphate 5-phsophatase
PKB	Protein kinase B (also known as Akt)
FRAP	FKBP12-rapamycin associated protein
P70^{rsk}	70-kD ribosomal S6 kinase
P85^{rsk}	85-kD ribosomal S6 kinase

ras/MAP kinase pathway

ras	A small GTP binding protein
mSOS	mammalian son of sevenless
SHC	SH2 domain-containing protein (an adaptor protein for ras activation
GRB-2	Growth factor receptor-bound protein2
GAP	GTPase activating protein
raf-1	Cellular homologue of the V-raf oncogene (a serine/threonine protein kinase)
MEK	MAPK/ERK kinase
MAPK	Mitogen-activated protein kinase

JAK/STAT pathway

JAK1	Janus kinase 1
JAK3	Janus kinase 3

Contd.

Table 10.1 (Contd.)

Signaling cassettes	
STAT3	Signal transducer and activator of transcription 3
STAT5	Signal transducer and activator of transcription 5

Redox signaling

ROIs	Reactive oxygen intermediates
GSH	Glutathione (reduced state)
GSSG	Glutathione (oxidized state)

Sphingomyelin pathway

Ceramide	A second messenger released from Sphingomyelin
Smase	Sphingomyelinase
CAP	Ceramide activating protein kinase

Cytoplasmic and nuclear effectors

NFAT$_c$	Nuclear factor of activated T cells (cytoplasmic component)
NFAT$_n$	Nuclear factor of activated T cells (nuclear component)
CAM	Calmodulin
CAMK IV/Gr	Ca^{2+}/calmodulin-dependent protein kinase type IV/Gr (the Gr stands for granule because this Enzyme is also strongly expressed in brain

Granule cells

CN	Calcineurin
Ub	Ubiquitin
Proteasome	A multi-subunit complex responsible for Degrading ubiquitin-protein conjugates
IκB	Inhibitor of NF-κB
NF-κB	Nuclear transcription factor κB
c-Jun	Protooncogene-a transcription factor (a component of AP-1)
c-Fos	Protooncogene-a nuclear transcription factor (a component of AP-1)
c-myc	Protooncogene-a nuclear transcription factor
REF-1	Redox factor-1
FRK	Fos regulating kinase (target of the ras/MAP kinase cassette)
JNK1	c-Jun kinase 1
JNK2	c-Jun kinase 2
Bcl-2	B-cell lymphoma/leukemia-2 gene
Bcl-x	B-cell lymphoma/leukemia-x gene
p21	A 21kD inhibitor of cyclin dependent kinases
p27^{kip1}	A 27kD inhibitor of cyclin dependent kinases
cyclin E	A cell cycle protein that functions late in G1 to control onset of DNA synthesis
Cdk2	Cyclin dependent kinase-2 (a threonine/serine protein kinase)
CAK	Cyclin dependent kinase activating kinase
ICE	Interleukin-1β-converting enzyme
Rb	Retinoblastoma gene

Source: BERRIDGE, M. J. Crit. Rev. Immunol. **17**: 155-178, 1997.

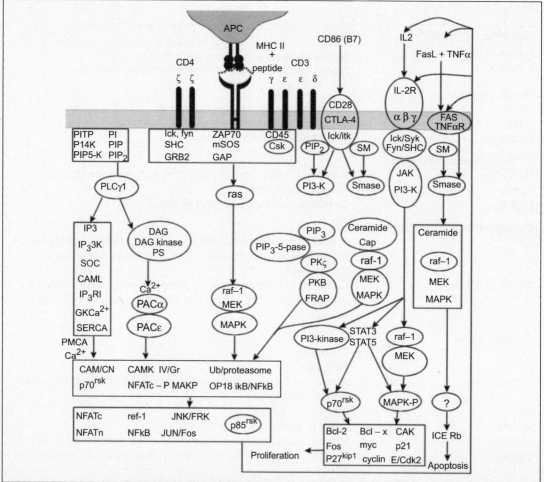

Fig. 10.11 A spatiotemporal map of T cell activation. The sequence begins (top left) with the antigen bound to MHC II interacting with the TCR and culminates many hours later (bottom right) in either proliferation or apoptosis. During this sequence of events, information is passed from one signaling component to the next via a number of pathways that have receptors, precursors, transducers, signaling cassettes, and cytoplasmic and nuclear effectors. For simplicity, those components that are functionally related have been grouped together into boxes. Description of abbreviations is given in Table 11.1.

Source: BERRIDGE, M. J. *Crit. Rev. Immunol.* **17:** 155-178, 1997.

TCR signaling pathways that have cysteines, which have to be reduced to transmit proliferative signals and is done by GSH.

1. The interaction between lck and the short cytoplasmic domains of CD4 and CD8 depend upon four cysteines. lck has a CXXC sequence in its N-terminal region that interacts with CXCP sequence in CD4.

2. Tyrosine phosphatase such as CD45 has a critical cystein in the active site that functions as a phosphate acceptor.
3. A number of transcription factors, ex. AP-1, NF-κB are under redox control in that their DNA-binding domains contain a single highly conserved cysteine that has to be reduced for activation to occur. A nuclear redox factor 1 (Ref-1) is thought to be responsible for ensuring that the critical cysteine remains reduced.

It seems likely that reducing conditions favor proliferation by ensuring that critical cysteines required at a number of signaling steps are kept in a reduced state. The finding that the level of GSH is abnormally low in the lymphocytes from HIV-1 infected patients has highlighted the significance of redox signaling mechanism.

IL-2 Signaling and the Activation of Proliferation of T Cells

One of the primary functions of the TCR complex is to initiate the IL-2-mediated autocrine loop responsible for completing the activation of proliferation (Fig. 10.14). The IL-2R (receptor) is made up of three separate subunits (α, β, and γ). X-linked severe combined immunodeficiency (X-SCID) results from the defects in the γ-subunit, which is a common component of other cytokine receptors like IL-4R and IL-7R. Because the three IL-2R subunits lack intrinsic enzyme activity, they act by recruiting both protein serine/threonine kinase and nonreceptor tyrosine kinase (ex. lck, fyn, Syk, JAK1 and JAK3). One consequence of binding these kinases is that the receptor becomes phosphorylated and the activated complex begins to transmit information via number of signaling cassettes (Fig. 10.11). Important signaling precursors are the signal transducers activators of transcription (STATs), which relay information directly to the nucleus. Upon activation, JAK and JAK3 are recruited to the IL-2R complex, where they function to phosphorylate various sites on the IL-2Rβ and IL-2Rγ chains that then bind in the STATs. The JAKs then phosphorylate the STATs, which then travel to the nucleus to activate transcription. IL-2 is also responsible for activation of genes such as fos, myc, and Bcl-2.

Co-stimulation in T Cell Responses

Co-stimulation can be defined as a stimulus necessary for optimal T cell activation delivered jointly to T cell along with the TCR signal. TCR stimulation in the absence of adequate co-stimulation fails to generate T cell responses and may result in the induction of anergy. It is now widely believed that naive T cells require two distinct signals for activation and subsequent proliferation into effector cells:

- **Signal 1:** It is generated by interaction of an antigenic peptide with the TCR-CD3 complex
- **Signal 2:** It is a antigen-nonspecific co-stimulatory signal provided by interaction between CD28 on the T cell and B7 on the APC.

CD28 is the primary T cell co-stimulatory receptor, and upon interaction with its ligands B7.1 (CD80) and B7.2 (CD86) it enhances T cell proliferation. B7 molecule is the member of the immunoglobulin superfamily and it has a single variable domain and a single constant domain. Both B7 molecules have similar extracellular domains but different cytosolic domains (Fig.10.12).

Recently it has been shown that the interaction of CD40 on B cells and CD40L on activated T cells upregulates B7 expression on B cells, thereby increasing T cell co-stimulation. B7 is not only seen on B cells but also on other antigen presenting cells like dendritic cells and activated macrophages. B7 has two types of ligands on T cells like CD28, which is stimulatory and CTLA-4 (cytotoxic T lymphocytic

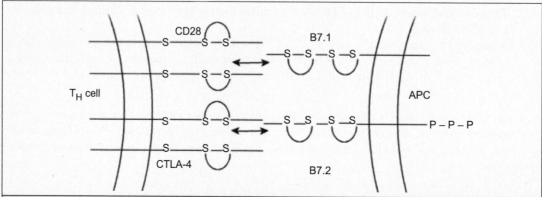

Fig. 10.12   Schematic representation of co-stimulatory signal molecules and their involvement between T_H cell and antigen presenting cell.

antigen-4), which is inhibitory. CTLA-4 is expressed only on activated T cells at a lower level but it binds to B7 molecule with 20 fold higher affinity than CD28. The interaction of B7 and CD28 leads to enhanced proliferation of T cells, production of IL-2 secretion and induces the expression of the anti-apoptotic protein Bcl-x_L.

Recent evidences indicate that CTLA-4 acts as a inhibitory co-stimulation molecule and is responsible for regulation of T cell activation. CTLA-4 blockade has been reported to enhance T cell response in vivo. The absence of CTLA-4 protein is known to cause T cell lymphoproliferation, resulting in spleenomegaly and lymphadenopathy. Thus, CTLA-4 appears to be an essential molecule for maintaining peripheral T cell homeostasis.

During ongoing immune response, there is a marked expansion of antigen-specific T cells. Upon clearing the antigen, the effector T cell population must be controlled. A number of molecules have been demonstrated to be important for this regulation by mediating activation-induced cell death, including Fas-FasL and tumor necrosis factor TNFR (TNF receptor). On the basis of its pattern of cell surface expression, it has been proposed that CTLA-4 acts at this stage of T cell proliferative responses, and participates solely in the process of downregulating ongoing immune responses.

Alternatively, recent data suggest that CTLA-4 plays a role in regulating the initiation of T cell responses. In the presence of MHC-peptide ligand complexes sufficient for adequate TCR-CD3 signaling, differential temporal and spatial expression of physiologically relevant levels of B7/CD28/CTLA-4 will determine the outcome of the antigen-specific T cell encounter with the APC displaying the MHC-peptide complex. Under conditions of limiting B7 ligands, CTLA-4-mediated signals will predominate and inhibit T cell responses. As CTLA-4 has a much greater avidity than CD28 for B7, only low protein levels of CTLA-4 would be required. In the presence of adequate TCR signaling and increased expression of B7, initially on dendritic cells and subsequently on activated B cells, CD28 mediated co-stimulation would predominate, however, and induce a T cell proliferative response. As a result of T cell activation and IL-2 production, there would be optimal induction of CTLA-4 expression. Increased focal expression of both the B7 protein, as a result of the increased synthesis and the clustering induced by CD28 binding, and of CTLA-4, as a result of increased synthesis and intracellular trafficking to the cell surface, would facilitate B7-CTLA-4 interactions, thereby the CTLA-4-mediated inhibitory signals would eclipse the stimulatory signals and lead to downregulation of the T cell response.

Altered Peptide Ligands as Antagonists or Partial Agonists

It has been observed that, the interaction of peptide-MHC complex with TCR of T cell does not always lead to activation of T cells. Certain experiments carried out with altered peptide-MHC complex and its effect on T cell activation have revealed that, some peptides can act as partial activating signals (**partial agonist peptides**) and some peptides totally block activating signal (**antagonist peptides**). The peptides are altered by single amino acid substitution, such that the **altered peptide ligand** has alteration in the region that binds to TCR i.e. epitope, and no alteration in the region that binds to MHC groove i.e. agretope. The T cell recognizes this subtle difference in peptide but the MHC molecule fails to recognize this difference.

This suggests that altered peptides interfere with proper signaling events even though they establish contact with TCR, such as lack of production of cytokines, phosphorylation of certain receptors or protein domains, etc. It is presumed that certain pathogens produce altered peptide ligands as a way to escape from the T cell recognition and immune attack. Probably high rate of mutation of HIV-1 may induce production of altered peptides during its life cycle in the human body, which allows its infection to continue unabated.

T Cell Clonal Anergy

Recognition of and antigenic peptide presented by class II MHC molecule of and APC by the T_H cell through its TCR may either result in activation of T_H cell leading to clonal expansion or T_H cell may enter into a nonresponsive state called clonal anergy. Induction of T cell clonal anergy was first demonstrated by stimulating $CD4^+$ T_H1 clones either with peptide antigens and chemically fixed cells APCs or with purified MHC class II molecules in planar lipid membrane. These forms of TCR engagement in the absence of costimulatory signals failed to activate T cells to produce IL-2, but they did stimulate the cells to enter a proliferative unresponsive state called anergic state in which restimulation with antigen and normal APCs elicited hardly any IL-2 response. In the anergic state IL-2 production decreased 20-50 fold. The production of other cytokines was also affected, but to a varying degrees: IL-3 and/or granulocyte-macrophage colony-stimulating factor (GM-CSF) production was decreased 10 folds, IFN-γ production was halved, whereas IL-4 production in T_H0 clones was unaffected. The molecular basis for profound block in IL-2 production has subsequently been shown to occur at the level of transcription of the IL-2 gene and it also involved a failure of a transcription factor, activator protein (AP-1). During the past year, substantial progress has been made in understanding the signal transduction pathways that are inhibited in the anergic state and the nature of the changes that lead to a block in AP-1 function. In addition, evidence has emerged for a *cis* dominant repression mechanism that also functions in anergic cells to dampen IL-2 transcription.

Evidence for Transcriptional Repression in Anergy

Negative regulatory element (NRE-A) located at the enhancer region has been shown to play an important role in induction of anergy. The protein that binds to enhancer site, Nil-2-a is a member of the zinc finger E box binding protein (ZEB) repressor family. The level of Nil-2-a is increased substantially in anergic T cells, and CD28 signaling antagonizes this increase. Therefore, the current model for the anergic effect on IL-2 gene transcription involves multiple components acting on the IL-2 promoter. First, there is the failure to produce and activate the positive acting AP-1 transcription factor c-Fos-JunB following TCR stimulation. Second, there is the presence of three negative regulatory factors, Nil-2-a, the inactive AP-1 and the AP-1 like protein, which act in concert to repress transcription of the IL-2 gene.

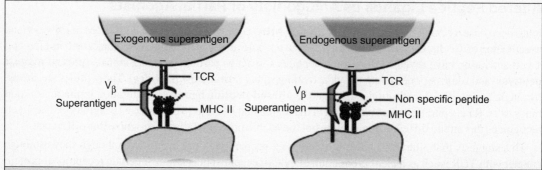

Fig. 10.13   Cross-linkage of T-cell receptor and class II MHC molecules mediated through superantigen. Note Exogenous superantigens are soluble bacterial proteins. Endogenous superantigens are membrane embedded proteins.

Superantigen-induced T Cell Activation

Superantigens are bacterial or viral proteins that bind simultaneously to Vβ region of the TCR and α chain of class II MHC molecule. There are two categories of superantigens: exogenous and endogenous, which are capable of cross-linking TCR and class II MHC provide an activating signal resulting in activation of T cells and proliferation (Fig. 10.13).

Exogenous antigens are soluble antigens secreted by bacteria and they belong to variety of exotoxins of gram-positive bacteria, ex. exfoliative dermatitis toxin, staphylococcal enterotoxin, streptococaal pyrogenic toxin, toxic-shock syndrome toxin.

On the other hand endogenous superantigens are cell-membrane proteins encoded by certain mammalian viruses. Mouse mammary tumor virus produces 4 different types of superantigens called minor lymphocyte stimulating determinants.

Certain superantigens can not only bring about T cell activation but also maturation of T cells in the thymus. These superantigens bind to TCR Vβdomain of the thymocytes and when these thymocytes interact with thymic stromal cells, it leads to deletion of these thymocytes. Sometimes, such deletions by superantigens may reach a massive proportion, which is called "holes in the repertoire" characterized by absence of T cells with Vβ domain.

T – Cell differentiation

Naive T cells have been thought to survive only about 5 to 7 weeks in the absence of antigen stimulation, but some are of the opinion that they have considerably longer life span. It is estimated that each naive T cell recirculates from the blood to the lymph nodes and back again every 12 to 24 hrs. During recirculation the naïve T cells reside in secondary lymphoid tissue such as lymph nodes.

Generation of effector T cells and memory T cells

Primary response will be initiated if a naive T cell encounters an antigen-MHC complex on an appropriate APC or target cell. This leads to activation of T cells and the activated cells enlarge in size and give rise to blast cells. Blast cells have high rate of cell division and they divide 2 to 3 times per day and for 4 to 5 days, generating large population of clones or progeny cells, which differentiate into memory or effector T cells.

The various effector T cells and their specialized functions have been dealt in Chapter 3 and more details are given in Chapter 13. Effector T cells have a short life span ranging from few days to a few weeks. There is remarkable difference among effector and naive T cells with respect to cell surface markers, which contributes to their recirculation ability.

$CD4^+$ effector T cells give rise to two different sub-populations, characterized by the type of cytokine they secrete. One subset is called T_H1 subset secretes IL-2, IFN-γ and TNF-β and these cells are responsible for activation of cytotoxic T cells and they are also involved in delayed type hypersensitivity. The other subset T_H2 secretes IL-4, IL-5, IL-6 and IL-10 and serves as effector helper cell for B cell activation.

The memory T cells are derived from naive T cells as well as from effector T cells after they have encountered the antigen. Memory T cells is responsible for generating secondary response and they are thought to be long lived. Like naive T cells, memory T cells are resting cells with cell division activity arrested at Go stage. Memory T cells are activated by macrophages, dendritic cells, and B cells, whereas naive T cells are activated only by dendritic cells. Memory T cells are known to express wide variety of cell adhesion molecules at a higher level than the naive cells. These molecules are known to enhance their ability of interaction with APCs.

Differences in Costimulatory Signals among Antigen Presenting Cells

For the complete T cell activation, only professional antigen presenting cells (APCs) like dendritic cells, macrophages and B cells can deliver the necessary signals in the form of costimulation as well as simultaneous presentation of antigen on class II MHC molecules. As has been already explained the chief costimulatory molecules expressed on APCs are the Ig family B7.1 and B7.2 molecules (see Fig. 10.12). There is difference among professional APCs as regard display of antigen and delivery of costimulatory signals. The resting macrophage expresses hardly any class II MHC molecules or B7 molecules. Therefore they are not able to activate naive T cells and they are poor activators of effector and memory T cells. Macrophages are activated only after phagocytosis of bacterial antigens or bacteria, which upregulates their expression of class II MHC and B7 molecules as well as cytokine production. Thus, activated macrophages are the common APCs of effector and memory T cells. On the other hand, dendritic cells are most potent antigen presenting cells, because they express class II MHC and B 7 molecules constitutively at very high levels. Thus, dendritic cells play an important role in activation of naive, effector and memory T cells. B cells also serve as antigen presenting cells and involve in T cell activation, but without endocytosis of antigen they are unable to express B7 molecules. Only after receptor-mediated endocytosis, the resting B cells are activated otherwise, resting B cells express only antigen receptor and class II MHC molecules on their surface. Thus, resting B cells are unable to activate naive T cells, although they can activate effector and memory T cells. Activated B cells upregulate the expression of class II MHC and B7 molecule, therefore they are capable of activating naive T cells as well as effector and memory T cells.

$\gamma\delta$ T Cells and their Function

They constitute about 0.5-10% of human peripheral blood lymphocytes and 1-3% of T cell population in lymphoid organs of the mouse. They are most abundant in intestinal cryptal patches (Peyer's patches), skin and pulmonary epithelium. Intestinal epithelial lymphocytes (IELs) express $\gamma\delta$-TCR-CD3 complex as well as express CD8 molecule. The skin $\gamma\delta$ T cell population is called dendritic epidermal cells (DECs) express Thy-1, the earliest T cell marker together with $\gamma\delta$-TCR-CD3 complex, but fail to express CD4 or CD8. $\gamma\delta$ T cells in different epithelial tissue known to express different Vγ and Vδ gene segments. Unlike αβ T cells, which recirculate extensively, γδ T cells are mostly confined to the epithelial tissue remain fixed in these tissue sites. Like antibodies, the γδ T cells TCR appears to have a broader specificity for antigens, binding to nonpeptide antigens as well as peptide antigens. γδ T cells can mediate tumor cell lysis in non-MHC restricted manner indicates that they may function like NK cells. They are known to respond to heat shock proteins like mycobacterial PPD (purified protein derivatives) and the cells expressing these proteins under extreme stress like viral infection, cancer and inflammatory responses. Therefore, it is strongly presumed that γδ T cells are responsible for elimination of damaged cells as well as microbial invaders. One proposal is that, since these cells are confined to the primary epithelial lining of skin, lung and intestine, they are responsible for first line of defense against any microbial invaders through these system and they provide immune surveillance in the epithelial cell milieu. Hence they are the chief contributors of innate immune response at body surfaces.

Exercise

1. Describe the process of (15 marks each):
    (a) B cell maturation
    (b) Activation of B lymphocytes
    (c) Differentiation of B cells

2. Give schematic representation of BCR signaling mechanism and explain the important steps involved in signaling (15 marks)

3. Write notes on Role played by: (10 marks each)
    (a) Btk in B cell development
    (b) T and B cell interaction in B cell development
    (c) CD40/CD40L interaction
    (d) Somatic hypermutation
    (e) Class switching
    (f) B cell selection

4. Write short notes on: (5 marks each)
    (a) Generation of plasma cells and memory cells
    (b) Regulation of naïve and memory B cell differentiation
    (c) Sites for induction of humoral immune response

5. Give a descriptive account of (15 marks each):
    (a) T-cell maturation
    (b) T-cell activation
    (c) T-cell differentiation

6. Give a brief account of: (10 marks each)
    (a) Thymic selection of T-cell repertoire
    (b) Co-stimulatory molecules in T cell response
    (c) T cell anergy
    (d) Super antigens induced T-cell activation

Chapter 11

T-cell and B-cell Receptors

- Structure of T-cell Receptor
- TCR Multigene Families
- T-cell Receptor Complex (TCR – CD3)
- T Cell Accessory Membrane Molecules
- Ternary TCR-peptide-MHC Complex
- B-cell Receptors

☐ ☐

The T cell receptor (TCR) differs from the B cell antigen binding receptor in two important ways. First, the T cell does not secrete its receptor as B cell does. Second, the TCR is specific not only specific for antigen alone but also for antigen in association with MHC. TCR is found to be heterodimer made up of either α and β or γ and δ chains. The genomic organization and the mode of generation of diversity of each chain of TCR are found to be similar to that of the B cell receptor's (BCRs) immunoglobulin chains (mIgM and mIgD). In addition to this TCR is found on the membrane of T cells in association with signal transducing complex called CD3. This signal-transducing complex has a similar role like that of Ig-α and Ig-β complex of the BCR.

Structure of T-cell Receptor

Study of amino acid sequences of $\alpha\beta$ and $\gamma\delta$ TCR heterodimer revealed that, their domain structure is almost similar to immunoglobulins (Fig. 11.1). Therefore, TCRs are classified as immunoglobulin superfamily. Each domain has 65 to 70 amino acids and an intrachain disulfide bond. The amino terminal domain in both chains show marked sequence variation but the sequence of the other part of chain is conserved. The variable and constant domains of the TCR are structurally similar to the V and C domain of the immunoglobulin. TCR variable region has three hypervariable regions, which are similar to CDRs in immunoglobulin light and heavy chain. The two chains of the TCR are held together by a single disulfide bond at the lower end followed by a transmembrane region of 21 to 22 amino acids. The transmembrane region of both the chains contain positively charged amino acids, which enable the chains of the heterodimer to interact with CD3 signal transducing complex. At the carboxy terminal end of the TCR chain has 5 – 12 amino acids, which extends into cytoplasm. The hypervariable region of TCR consisting of three CDRs is the antigen-binding site, of which CDR1 and CDR2 contact primarily the α-helical region of the MHC. The antigenic peptides held in the cleft of the MHC molecules are found to interact with CDR3 located in the center of the antigen-binding site of TCR (Fig.11.1).

TCR Multigene Families

Germ line DNA is known to contain four TCR multigene families, each encoding one of the receptor chains of heterodimer molecule. As in the Ig genes, functional TCR is produced by gene rearrangements in V and J segments in the α and γ-chain families and V, D, and J segments in the β and δ-chain families. In humans, α and δ-chain genes are located on chromosome 14 and β and γ-chain genes are located on chromosome 7.

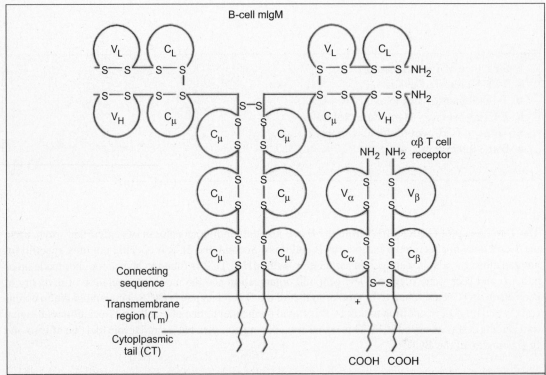

Fig. 11.1   Diagrammatic illustration of structural similarity between the ab TCR and membrane bound IgM of B cell.

The human germ line DNA contains about 50 Vα and 70 Jα segments and a single Cα segment. The δ-chain gene family contains about 3 Vδ gene segments, 3 Dδ, and Jδ segments and a single Cδ segment. The δ-chain gene family is located between Vα and Jα segments. The β-chain gene family contains 57 Vβ and 13 Jβ and 2 Dβ, Cβ each. In the β-gene family there are two repeats each containing 1Dβ, 6 or 7 Jβ, and 1 Cβ. The γ-chain gene family consists of 14 Vγ, 5Jγ and 2 Cγ. In the γ-gene family also there are two repeats each containing 2 or 3 Jγ and 1Jγ (Fig. 11.2). In all most all respect TCR multigene family of mouse resembles the human, although the number of segments differs.

Variable region gene rearrangements

The organization of the gene segments in the germ line DNA encoding α and β chains of the TCR is generally analogous to that of the immunoglobulin germ line DNA. α and γ chain, like the immunoglobulin

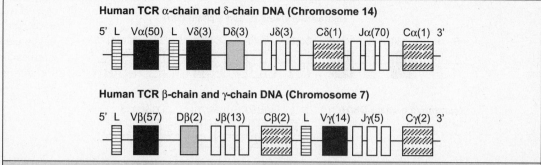

Fig. 11.2 Germ-line organization of human TCR α, β, γ, and δ-chain gene segments. Each C gene segment is composed of a series of exons and introns, which are not shown.

L chain is encoded by V, J, and C gene segments. β and δ chain, like the immunoglobulin H chain, is encoded by V, D, J and C gene segments. Rearrangements of the TCR

α, β, δ, and γ chain gene segments results in VJ joining for α and γ chains, and VDJ joining for the β, and δ chains (Fig. 11.3). Unlike the immunoglobulins, which are membrane bound or secreted, the αβ or γδ heterodimers are expressed only in membrane bound form. Therefore, no differential RNA processing required to produce membrane or secreted forms.

Immunoglobulin heavy chain C gene segment has multiple C genes encoding different isotypes with different effector function, whereas C gene segment of TCR is much simpler. TCR α-chain DNA has only one C gene segment; the β-chain has two C gene segments, but their protein products have no functional differences.

Mechanism of TCR DNA rearrangements

The mechanism of rearrangement of germ-line DNA for TCR is found to be similar to that of mechanism used in Ig gene rearrangements. In TCR germ line also, conserved heptamer and nonamer recognition signal sequences (RSSs), containing one-turn (12 bp) or two-turn (23 bp) spacer sequences have been identified flanking each V, D, and J gene segment (see Fig. 9.2-9.5 in chapter 9). Like the pre-B cells pre-T cells express the recombination-activating genes (RAG-1 and RAG-2) or recombinase. The recombinase recognizes the heptamer and nonamer recognition signals and catalyzes V – J and V – D – J joining during TCR gene rearrangement by the same deletional or inversional mechanisms that occur in Ig genes (see Fig. 9.2-9.5). Rest of the steps like transesterification, hairpin loop formation, double strand break etc occurs similarly as explained in Chapter 9 for immunoglobulin genes.

Allelic exclusion of the TCR genes

Similar to Ig genes, rearrangement of the TCR β-chain genes exhibits allelic exclusion. Once a productive rearrangement occurs for one β-chain allele, the rearrangement of the other β allele is inhibited. Allelic exclusion appears to be less stringent with α chain genes. Therefore, more than one α chain is occasionally expressed on the membrane of a T cell. Researchers are of the opinion that of the two different αβ TCRs, only one is likely to be self-MHC restricted and therefore functional.

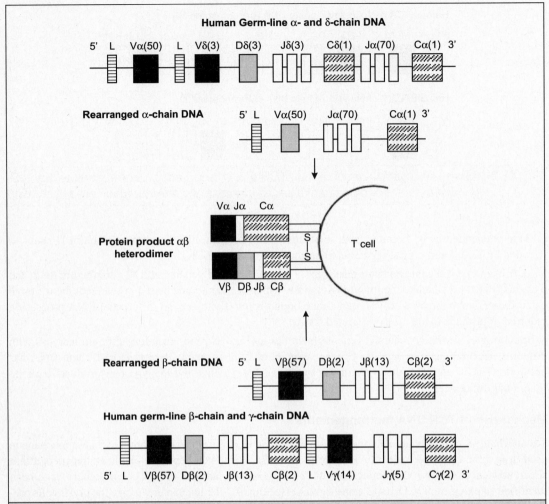

Fig. 11.3 Schematic representation of gene rearrangement to yield a functional gene encoding the αβ T cell receptor.

Structure of rearranged TCR genes

The variable region of TCR is encoded by rearranged VDJ and VJ sequences and the combinatorial joining of V gene segments appears to generate CDR1 and CDR2, whereas junctional flexibility and N-region nucleotide addition generates CDR3. The rearranged TCR genes also contain a short leader (L) exon upstream of the joined VJ and VDJ sequences. As the nascent polypeptide enters the endoplasmic reticulum, the amino acid sequences encoded by leader exon are cleaved. The general structure of rearranged TCR genes is shown in Fig. 11.4. The constant region of each TCR chain is encoded by C gene segment that has multiple exons, corresponding to connecting region, transmembrane region, and cytoplasmic tail.

Generation of TCR diversity

Mechanism of generation of TCR diversity is same as that of Ig gene, but more diversity among TCRs are produced as compared to antibodies because of type of gene rearrangement available for TCR gene segments. Combinatorial joining of variable-region gene segments generates large number of random gene combinations for all the TCR chains. For. Ex. In mouse 100 Vα and 5 Jα gene segments can generate 5×10^3 possible VJ combinations for the TCR α chain. Similarly, 25 Vβ, 2Dβ and 12Jβ gene segments can give 6×10^2 possible combinations. Random association of 5×10^3 Vα combinations with 6×102 Vβ combinations can generate a minimum of 3×10^6 possible combinations for the $\alpha\beta$ TCR.

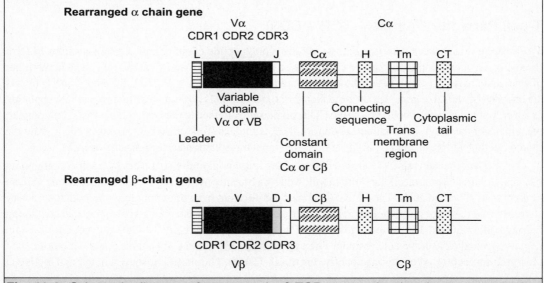

Fig. 11.4 Schematic diagram of rearranged $\alpha\beta$-TCR genes showing the exons encoding various domains of the $\alpha\beta$-TCR.

The location of one-turn and two-turn recognition signal sequences in TCR β and δ-chain DNA differs from that of Ig heavy chain DNA. Because of this, in TCR germ line DNA, **alternative joining of D gene segments** can occur by following one-turn and two-turn joining rule (see Fig. 9.5). Therefore, it is possible for a Vβ gene segment to join directly with a Jβ or Dβ gene segment, generating VJβ or VDJβ unit. Alternative joining of δ-chain gene segments generates similar units; in addition one Dδ can join with another, giving rise to VDDJδ and in humans VDDDJδ. This mechanism has not been observed in Ig heavy chain gene recombination, therefore it can generate remarkable additional diversity in TCR genes.

Junctional flexibility in TCR gene rearrangement has also been observed as it occurs in Ig genes. This flexibility generates many nonproductive rearrangements, but it can also increase the diversity by encoding several alternative amino acids at each junction (Refer to Fig. 9.12, 13, & 14). P-region nucleotide addition and N-region nucleotide addition can also occur with TCR gene rearrangement. One of the difference between Ig gene N-nucleotide addition and TCR is that, N-region nucleotide addition occurs only in Ig heavy chain genes, whereas it occurs in all the genes encoding TCR chains. As many as 6 nucleotides can be added by this mechanism at each junction, generating up to 5461 possible combinations assuming random selection. Estimates suggests that the combined effects of P- and N- nucleotide addition and joining flexibility can generate as many as 10^3 possible amino acid sequences in the TCR junctional regions alone.

The CDR1 and CDR2 region of the TCR is encoded by the V gene segments, are known to have limited diversity as compared to CDR3, which has even greater diversity than that of immunoglobulins. CDR3 diversity is generated by junctional diversity in V – D – j joining, joining of multiple D gene segments and the introduction of P and N nucleotides at the V – D – J and V – J junctions. Unlike Ig genes, TCR genes do not seem to undergo extensive somatic mutation. That is the functional TCR genes generated during T cell maturation in the thymus are generally the same as those found in the mature peripheral T cell population.

T-cell Receptor Complex (TCR – CD3)

T cell receptor associates with CD3-a five invariant polypeptide chain complex that associates to form three dimers: a heterodimer of γ and ε chains (γε), a heterodimer of δ and ε chains (δε) and a homodimer of two zeta chains (ζζ) or a heterodimer of zeta and eta chains (ζη) (Fig. 11. 5). The ζ and η chains are encoded by the same gene, but differ in their carboxyl terminal ends due to differences in RNA splicing of the primary transcript. About 90% of the CD3 complexes examined to date incorporate the ζζ homodimer; the remainder has the ζη heterodimer. Therefore, TCR complex is four dimers consisting or αβ or γδ for the ligand binding and γε, δε, and ζζ or ζη of CD3 for signal transduction and expression of TCR.

The γ, δ, and ε chains of CD3 are members of the immunoglobulin superfamily, each containing an immunoglobulin like extracellular domain followed by a transmembrane region and a cytoplasmic domain of more than 40 amino acids. The ζζ and ζη chains are different from their counterparts; both have a very short external region of only 9 amino acids, a transmembrane region and a long 113 amino acid containing tail segment in ζζ and 155 amino acids in ζη. The transmembrane region of CD3 polypeptides contain negatively charged aspartic acid residue. The cytoplasmic tails of the CD3 chains contain a motif called the **immunoreceptor tyrosine-based activator motif** (ITAM). This motif is also seen in Igα and Igβ B cell

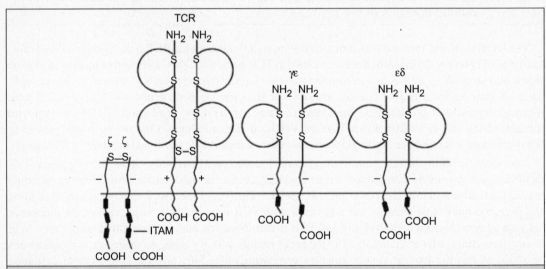

Fig. 11.5 Schematic diagram illustrating TCR-CD3 complex.

receptor and Fc receptor of IgE and IgG. ITAM interacts with tyrosine kinases and plays an important role in signal transduction. In CD3, the γ, δ, and ϵ chains contain a single copy of ITAM, whereas ζ and η chains contain three copies.

T Cell Accessory Membrane Molecules

In addition to CD3, there are other accessory molecules, which play an important role in antigen recognition, T cell activation, signal transduction and some enhance ability of T cell binding with antigen presenting cells.

CD4 and CD8 coreceptors

On the basis of these two receptors T cells are classified. $CD4^+$ T cells are called T helper cells, responsible for antigen recognition in association with class II MHC, whereas $CD8^+$ T cells recognize antigen in association with class I MHC and these cells called cytotoxic cells. CD4 is a 55kD monomeric membrane glycoprotein, made up of four extracellular (D1–D4) immunoglobulin like domains, a hydrophobic tranmembrane region, and a long cytoplasmic tail containing three serine residues, which can be phosphorylated. CD8 is generally $\alpha\beta$ heterodimer and less frequently $\alpha\alpha$ homodimer. Both $\alpha\beta$ chains of CD8 are glycoproteins of approximately 30 to 38 kD. A disulfide bond holds the two chains of the CD8 together. Each chain of CD8 consists of a single extracellular immunoglobulin-like domain, a hydrophobic transmembrane region and a cytoplasmic tail continuing 25-27 residues, several of which can be phosphorylated. A schematic diagram of CD4 and CD8 receptors of T cell is shown in Fig. 11.6.

Both CD4 and CD8 are called as **co-receptors** because both are responsible for establishing contact with MHC molecule and signal transduction. The extra cellular domain of CD4 binds to $\beta2$ domain of class II MHC molecule, whereas CD8 binds to the $\alpha3$ domain of MHC Figs. 6.4 and 6.6 in Chapter 6). This interaction increases the avidity of the interaction between TCR and a peptide-MHC complex, which is augmented by 100 fold by CD4 and CD8. The signal transduction property of CD4 and CD8 is mediated through their cytoplasmic tails and both are associated with the protein tyrosine kinase Lck, which is similar to Lyn kinase of B cell co-receptor.

Recent evidences indicate that during antigen recognition TH cell TCR molecule first binds to a dimer of the class II MHC and the membrane distal domain of CD4 then binds to $\beta2$ domain of the class II MHC molecule forming a ternary complex TCR, CD4 and MHC (Fig.11.7). Once CD4 binds to MHC molecule, CD4 undergoes conformational change, enabling its membrane proximal domains to interact with membrane proximal domains of adjacent CD4 molecule that has complexed with TCR and MHC molecule in the same manner. This gives rise to tetrameric structure on the membrane (Fig. 11.7). This complex formation is highly essential for signal transduction. It is not known whether CD8 interactions with class I MHC molecule forms similar tetrameric structure or not.

Other accessory membrane molecules

In addition to CD4 and CD8, T cells are known to possess several other accessory membrane molecules such as CD2, LFA-1, CD28, and CD45R. These molecules do not interact with peptide MHC complex, instead they bind to other legands present on the antigen presenting cells or target cells (Table 11.1).

These interactions strengthen the association between a T cell and an antigen presenting cell or a target cell. Once the T cells are activated, the strength of adhesion between these molecules and their respective ligands is shown to increase, thereby prolonging the association between the cells. Figure 11.8

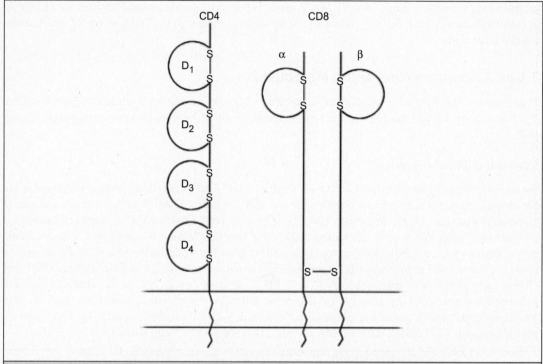

Fig. 11.6   Schematic diagram of general structure of CD4 and CD8 co-receptor.

schematically illustrates the interaction between various T_H and T_C cell accessory membrane molecules and their ligands on antigen presenting cells and the target cells.

Ternary TCR-peptide-MHC Complex

Interactions involved in forming Ternary complex

For the recognition of peptide and MHC molecule, both α and β chains of the TCR heterodimer have been shown to make an equal contribution. One chain is not specific for peptide recognition and the other chain is specific for MHC recognition. In addition to this, it is well known that the same V region of α and β chains recognize both peptide class I MHC complexes and peptide class II MHC complexes. This indicates there is no separate specific V region sequence for class I and class II MHC molecules. It is not still clear about the relative contribution of TCR-MHC contact and TCR-peptide

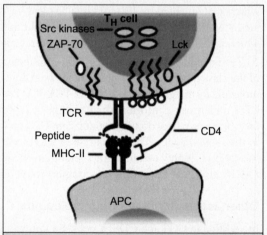

Fig. 11.7   A diagrammatic representation of interaction involving ternary complex of TCR, CD4 and class II MHC, where T_H cell is interacting with an antigen presenting cell.

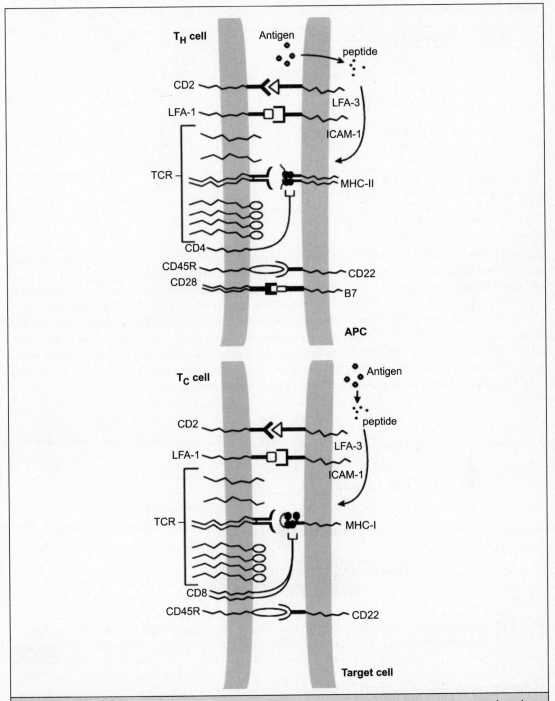

Fig. 11.8 Schematic illustration of the interaction between the T cell receptors and various accessory molecules with their ligands on an antigen presenting cells or target cell.

Table 11.1   Selected T cells accessory molecules and their ligands, and functions performed.

Accessory Molecule	Ligand or Receptor
CD4	Class II MHC*
CD8	Class I MHC*
CD2 (LFA-2)	CD58 (LFA-3)*
LFA-1 (CD11a/CD18)	ICAM-1 (CD54)#
CD28	B7@
CTLA-4	B7+
CD45R	CD22*
CD5	CD72+

*Act as Adhesion molecules, signal transduction and member of Ig superfamily
Act as adhesion molecules and more or less belong to Ig superfamily
@Act as signal transduction molecule as well as belong to Ig superfamily
+Act as only signal transduction molecules

contacts for the formation of trimolecular complex. The high degree of TCR specificity for both antigenic peptides and MHC molecules must be achieved through the diversity of the variable region of the T cell receptor. Figure 11.9 schematically illustrates the current model of the interaction between a T cell receptor, antigenic peptide, and MHC molecule. The peptide-binding region of the T cell receptor belongs to CDR3, while CDR1 and CDR2 interact with MHC molecules. It has already been discussed in Chapter 6 with regard to MHC molecule and the peptide-binding site. It is α1 and α2 domains of the class I MHC and α1 and β1 domains of class II MHC molecules. These same molecules with antigenic peptide bound to them will be responsible for interaction with TCR. The site on an antigenic peptide that interacts with a TCR is called **epitope,** and the site that interacts with and MHC molecule is the **agretope.**

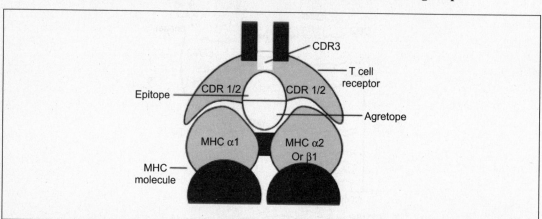

Fig. 11.9   Diagrammatic representation showing the various sites in a T cell receptor, antigenic peptide and MHC molecule that interact in TCR-peptide-MHC trimolecular complex.

Self MHC restriction of the TCR

T cells are capable of recognizing antigens only when it is presented on the membrane of a cell by self-MHC molecules. This attribute is called **self-MHC restriction.** It is distinct from the recognition of antigen by the B cells. Extensive work of Zinkernagel and Doherty on mice proved the fact that antigen recognition by T cells is specific not only for MHC molecules but also for a viral antigen presented on an infected cell. In 1966 they were awarded Nobel prize for this work. Two models were proposed to explain the MHC restriction of the TCR. **The dual-receptor model** proposed that a T cell as having two separate receptors, one for antigen and one for class I or class II MHC molecules. The **altered-self model** proposed that, there was a single receptor capable of recognizing foreign antigen complexed to self-MHC molecule. The second model predicts that a single receptor recognizes the alteration in MHC molecules induced by their association with foreign antigens.

Alloreactivity of T cells

MHC molecules function as histocompatibility antigens, therefore graft-rejection reaction occurs from the direct response of T cell to MHC molecules. MHC molecules in random breeding individuals are known to be highly polymorphic within the same species and each species is known to have a unique set of histocompatibility antigens. Therefore, T cells respond to allogenic grafts and the MHC molecules contributing to this allogenic graft rejection are called **alloantigens**. $CD4^+$ T cells are known to respond to class II alloantigens and $CD8^+$ T cells to class I alloantigens. The alloreactivity of T cells to alloantigens comes from the micropeptides of the donor carried in the groove of the MHC molecules of donor cells as well as the MHC domains and its interaction with TCR is known to trigger the alloreaction by activating T cells leading to graft rejection.

B-cell Receptors

For a long time immunologists were puzzled about how mIg molecule of B lymphocytes mediates an activating signal after contacting an antigen. Major reason of this puzzle was, all the mIg isotypes are known to have a very short cytoplasmic tails: the mIgM and mIgD cytoplasmic tails contain only 3 amino acids; mIgA tail has 14 amino acids; mIgG and mIgE tails have 28 amino acids each. In each case it was thought that cytoplasmic tails being too short are unable to carry out signal transduction of associate with cytoplasmic molecules. It is only when the other molecules in association with mIg receptors were discovered the puzzle was unraveled. The **B cell receptor (BCR)** is transmembrane protein complex composed of mIg and a disulfide linked heterodimer called Ig-α/Ig-β. It is evident now that, two molecules of this heterodimer are in association with one mIg and they are present on either side of mIg molecule to form a single BCR (Fig. 11.10).

The Ig-α chain has long cytoplasmic tail containing 61 amino acids and Ig-β tail has 48 amino acids. The cytoplasmic tails of Ig-α and Ig-β are known to interact with intracellular signaling molecules, thereby facilitating signal transduction and activation of B cells.

Co-receptors of B lymphocytes

A paradigm in lymphocyte activation is that co-receptor molecules modify stimulation by the antigen receptor. These co-receptors respond to a variety of ligands and may both enhance and inhibit antigen receptor signals. The integration of input from antigen receptor and co-receptor is thought to allow the lymphocyte to mount a response appropriate to the source of the antigen and the lymphocyte environment. In B lymphocytes, the co-receptors CD5, CD19-CD21, CD22, FcγRIIB (CD32) and CD40 modulate the response to antigen (Fig.11.11).

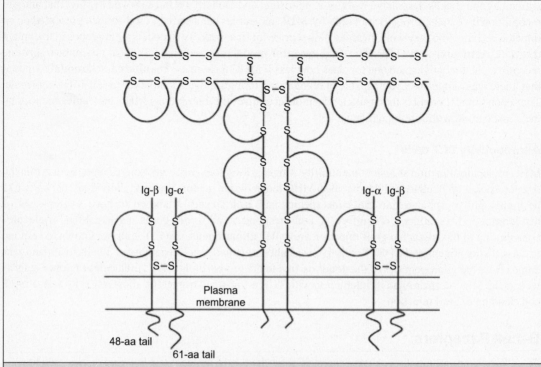

Fig. 11.10 Diagrammatic illustration of B cell receptor complex.

CD19 receptor

It is a B cell restricted 95kD glycoprotein present throughout the B cell lineage until plasma cell differentiation takes place. It has been observed that co-ligation of CD19 with antigen receptor (AgR) decreases the threshold for AgR dependent stimulation by at least two order of magnitude. CD19 gets tyrosine phosphorylated upon AgR ligation and is associated with the signaling proteins phsophatidylinositol 3-kinase (PI3-K), Len, Fyn and Vav. It is observed that CD19 deficient mature B cells show an impaired response to T cell dependent antigens; mice with this deficiency have an accompanying lack of both germinal center formation and affinity maturation of serum antibodies. There is also a reduction in the self-renewing CD5$^+$B-1 subpopulation (B-1a) of B cells in the peritoneal cavity, which suggests that CD19 is required for optimal expansion and maintenance of this population.

CD19 is found to be part of a complex containing CD21 (complement receptor 2 [CR2], CD81 (target of antiproliferative antibody [TAPA-1] and in some cells the membrane protein Leu13. It has become clear from studies using CD19-deficient and CD21-deficient mice that the CD19-CD21 signaling pathway plays an important role in T cell dependent responses. CD19-CD21 signaling not only lowers the threshold for antigen mediated B cell activation but also modulates CD40-mediated T cell help. Signaling via CD21 is found to be co-stimulatory for anti-CD40 stimulated splenic B cell growth and the two signals together lead to enhanced B cell differentiation. The enhancement of AgR sensitivity and co-stimulation of CD40 signal are found to be important during the early stages of B cell proliferation in the T zone foci and germinal centers, when both antibody affinity may be low and the number of antigen specific T cells limiting. CD19 may also play a role in enhancing B cell to T cell contact. It is observed that, ligation of VLA-4 and VLA-5 induces tyrosine phosphorylation of CD19 (Fig.11.11).

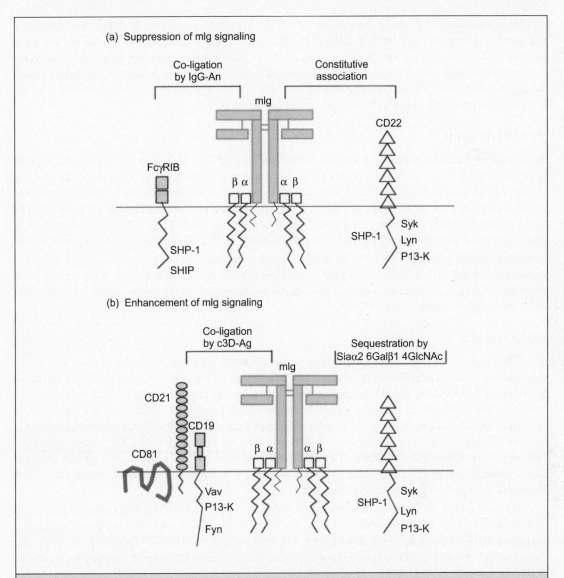

Fig. 11.11   Possible roles of B-lymphocyte co-receptors in mIg signaling. **(a)** Suppression of mIg signaling-FcγRIIB co-ligation with mIg by IgG-antigen (Ag) complexes exerts an inhibitory effect on mIg signaling through its association with the inositol polyphosphate 5-phosphatase SHIP and/or the tyrosine phosphatase SHP-1. **(b)** Enhancement of mIg signaling. Co-ligation of CD19-CD21-CD81 complex to mIg by C3d (CD21 ligand)-Ag recruits positive signal transduction effectors, which synergize with mIg to augment B cell activation.(SOURCE:O' ROURKE, L., TOOZE, R. AND FEARON, D. *Curr. Opin. Immunol.* **9:** 324-329, 1997).

One of the common features observed in CD19, CD21 and Vav-deficient B cells is the significant reduction in the number of CD5⁺B-1 cells (B-1a cells). Interestingly, peritoneal B-1a cells are known to produce little or no calcium flux in response to AgR or CD19 ligation alone but do show a synergistic response upon AgR and CD19 co-ligation. In contrast, CD5 is found to be a negative regulator of AgR signaling in B-1 cells. Stimulation of peritoneal B-1 cells via the AgR known to induce apoptosis whereas CD5 deficient B-1 cells proliferate in response to AgR ligation.

FcγRIIB receptor

B cell proliferation induced by AgR ligation is inhibited by FcγRIIB-AgR co-cross linking except in the presence of IL-4. The significance of this pathway *in vivo* was determined by analysis of the humoral response to antigen challenge in FcγRIIB-deficient mice. FcγRIIB-deficient mice display a slightly elevated immunoglobulin level in response to both thymus dependent and thymus independent antigens. The mechanism of negative signaling by FcγRIIB may involve Src homology (SH2) domain containing phosphotyrosine phosphatase (PTP) SHP-1 (hematopoietic cell PTP [HCP], SHPTP1, PTP1C) (Fig. 11.11).

Inhibition of B cell proliferation by FcγRIIB is found to be impaired in motheaten mice, which do not express functional SHP-1. A 13 amino acid tyrosine phosphorylated immunoreceptor tyrosine inhibitory motif (pITIM) in the cytoplasmic domain of FcγRIIB is considered to bind to the carboxy terminal SH2 domains of SHP-1 and activate SHP-1.

CD22 receptor

It is a B-lymphocyte restricted member of the immunoglobulin superfamily (IgSF), is a member of the sialoadhesin family of adhesion molecules and a co-receptor for mIg. In humans, surface CD22 is restricted to resting B lymphocytes and is lost after *in vitro* activation and in mice, surface CD22 is found on all subsets of mature B cells including IgA positive memory B cells and is not lost after *in vitro* activation. In some human cell lines, such as Daudi, Ramos, and Raji, CD22 is upregulated from cytoplasmic stores to the site of mIg stimulation. Rapid upregulation followed by degradation of CD22 might provide a mechanism for transient desensitization of mIg. Human and murine CD22 differ in their affinity for sialic acids: whereas human CD22 binds to α 2-6 linked N-acetyl neuraminic acid (NeuAc), murine CD22 only recognizes N-glycolyl neuraminic acid (NueGc).

CD22 associated with plasma membrane and is rapidly tyrosine phosphorylated after mIg or CD22 cross-linking. Tyrosine phosphorylated CD22 recruits a number of intracellular signaling molecules, including SHP-1, Lyn, Syk, PI3-K and PLC-γ1. The reported ability of CD22 to coprecipitate with Lyn, Syk, PLC-γ1 and PI3-K has suggested, however, that CD22 is also involved in assembling a positive signaling complex (Fig. 11.11).

CD40 receptor

CD40-CD40L (CD154) belongs to the emerging receptor-ligand families composed of type I, type II transmembrane proteins respectively. Receptor-ligand pairs, which belong to these families, include tumor necrosis factor (TNF) and its receptor (TNFR), CD27-CD70, CD30-CD30L and Fas (CD95)-FasL. Studies on CD40 signal transduction have now yielded several mediators and pathways involved in this cellular activation mechanism. Most of the studies have been performed with B cells, but there are other cells that express CD40 and that alternative pathways may very well be operational in other cell types.

In recent years it has been established that members of the TNFR family associate intracellularly with different families of signaling molecules, including the "death domain" family and the TNFR-associated factor (TRAF) family. Using the two-hybrid system, such protein-protein interactions have been demonstrated for TNF1, TNF2, Fas, CD30 and CD40. Interestingly, there is no cross reactivity between the extracellular ligands of the TNFR family, the intracellular ligands seem to be much more promiscuous and form a complex network of homodimers and heterodimers (Fig 11.12).

In vitro demonstration of function of CD40 in B-lymphocytes

CD40 activated B cells enter into proliferative state, which is further enhanced by the addition of cytokines like IL-4, IL-13 or IL-10 and their combinations. Cytokines can also induce CD40 activated B cell to

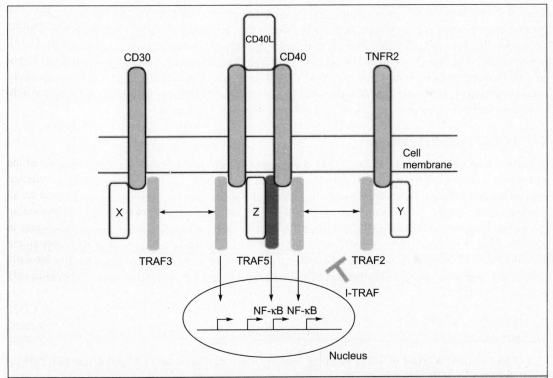

Fig. 11.12 Schematic representation of the molecules involved in CD40 signal transduction. X, Y, and Z represents as yet unidentified molecules associated with the signaling complexes of TNFR members. TRAF2 and TRAF3, which are indicated by the hatched figures, associate with CD40, but are also shared by other members of TNFR family (TNFR2 and CD30) as indicated by double-headed arrow). TRAF5 can also induce NF-κB activation. Activation processes are initiated when the CD40 receptor becomes cross-linked by the interaction with CD40L. Intracellular association TRAF2 and I-TRAF results in inhibition of TRAF2 mediated signal transduction. Thin vertical arrows represents signal transduction pathways leading to NF-κB activation. (SOURCE: KOOTEN, C. V. AND BANCHEREAU, J. *Curr. Opin. Immunol.* **9**: 330-337, 1997).

secrete immunoglobulins, with IL-10 inducing the secretion of large quantities of immunoglobulins as a consequence of inducing plasma cell differentiation. A combination of IL-10 and transforming growth factor β (TGF-β) induces IgA production in CD40 activated B cells, and either IL-4 or IL-13 induces CD40 activated B cells to switch towards IgG4 and IgE production. CD40 activated B cells show increase in size and increased level of expression of cell surface molecules. CD40 activation of B cells also results in the induction of Fas expression and renders cells susceptible for Fas-induced apoptosis. In fact, together with BCR cross-linking, these three receptors (Fas, CD40 and BCR) generate a complex network of positive and negative signals whereby the response of the B cell, activation or death, is determined by its differentiation stage.

In vivo function of CD40-CD40L interactions (Hyper IgM syndrome)

It is a X-linked immunodeficiency occurs due to genetic alteration of CD40L. The disease is characterized by a severe impairment of T cell-dependent antibody responses and a lack of memory B cells and circulating antibodies like IgG, IgA, and IgE. Patients with hyper IgM syndrome have an enhanced susceptibility to opportunistic infections, such as *Pneumocystis carini* (pneumonia) and *Cryptosporidium* (diarrhea). The disease characteristics indicate a role for CD40-CD40L interactions in cell-mediated immune responses. Patients with hyper IgM syndrome lack germinal centers in their lymphoid organs. In accordance, somatic mutations within V, D, and J transcripts are not found in circulating B cells.

CD40-CD40L role in immunity

Administration of antibodies to CD40L has been shown to prevent the establishment of autoimmune symptoms in various murine models. Administration of anti-CD40L antibodies also known to prevent the development of graft-versus-host disease that occurs as a major complication of allogenic bone marrow transplantation. Furthermore, a combination of allogenic B cells and anti-CD40L antibody considerably decreases the host reactivity of both CD4$^+$ and CD8$^+$ T cells thereby allowing efficient transplantation of allogenic pancreatic islet β cells. Anti-CD40L antibodies markedly extend the survival of cardiac allograft in both naïve and sensitized hosts when administered at the time of transplantation. Long term acceptance of skin and cardiac allograft can be obtained by a simultaneous blocking of the CD40 and CD28 pathways.

Exercise

1. Give detailed account of T cell receptor complex and write in detail TCR genes and their role in diversity of TCR. (20 marks)
2. Write notes on: (10marks each)
   (a) T cell accessory membrane molecules
   (b) Describe B cell receptor complex
   (c) Interaction of TCR with MHC complex
   (d) B cell accessory membrane molecules
   (e) Role of CD40 in B lymphocytes
   (f) TCR multigene family
   (g) TCR gene rearrangement
   (h) Ternary TCR-peptide-MHC complex

Chapter 12

Antigen Processing and Presentation

- Self-MHC Restriction of T Cells
- Cytosolic Pathway of Antigen Presentation
- Endocytic Pathway of Exogenous Antigen Presentation

□ □

It all depends on where the antigen enters the body. If they penetrate the tissues they will end up in lymph nodes. Antigens encountered in upper respiratory tract or intestine is trapped by mucosal associated lymphoid tissue, and the antigens in the blood initiate the reaction in spleen. Macrophages, that roam the body ingesting the extracellular materials they find, degrade them to produce peptides and presenting the peptides as antigens. These antigen presenting cells (APCs) travel from site of infection to the lymph node, where they recruit lymphocytes for the immune response: in effect APCs are like messengers from the front lines of battle. T-cell recognition of antigen requires that peptides derived from foreign antigen be displayed within the cleft of a MHC molecule on the membrane of APC. The sequence of events involved in the formation of peptide-MHC complexes would require degradation of antigen into peptides and the process is called **antigen processing.** In the cytoplasm of APC the degraded peptides then associate with MHC molecules and then the peptide-MHC complexes are transported to the membrane and displayed on the APC membrane, which is called **antigen presentation**.

Viruses, many other bacteria and protozoan parasites such as those that cause malaria, sleeping sickness and leishmaniasis are not easily thwarted. They establish their infections inside the host cells, where antibodies cannot reach. To rebuff these organisms, another arm of the immune system comes to play an important role. The host cells carry MHC molecules on their surface and in infected cells these MHC molecules will be displaying small peptides derived from the intracellular parasites. Such peptide-MHC complexes form the antigen, which will be recognized by antigen receptors on cytotoxic T cells. Generally class I MHC molecules bind to peptides derived from the cells infected by parasites and such antigens are called **endogenous antigens**. Endogenous antigens could be even normal cellular proteins. Class II MHC molecules bind to peptides derived from processed antigens of bacteria or viruses or other disease causing parasites. These antigens are internalized by phagocytosis or endocytosis and processed within the phagosome or endosome (Chapter 4) and the processed antigen is displayed on the cell surface of APC by class II MHC, which is called **exogenous antigen** processing.

SELF-MHC RESTRICTION OF T CELLS

Self-MHC restriction of $CD4^+$ and $CD8^+$ cells occurs only when the self-antigens are presented on the membrane of a cell in association with self-MHC molecules. In 1970, many reports appeared in various scientific journals explaining the self-MHC restriction in T-cell recognition. For ex. Rosenthal and Shevach showed that, antigen presented by macrophage of the same MHC haplotype were only capable of stimulation of proliferation of T_H cells. In their experiment, macrophages obtained from guinea pig-strain 2 were mixed with an antigen and incubated. This stimulated the macrophages to process the antigen and present it with class II MHC molecule on their membrane. These antigen pulsed macrophages were mixed with T cells obtained from Strain 2, strain 13 and strain 2 X strain 13 cross bred F_1 progeny and the magnitude of T cell proliferation was measured. The results showed that strain 2 pulsed macrophages activated T cells of strain 2 and F1 progeny T cells but not strain 13 T cells. These experiments confirmed the fact that, the $CD4^+ T_H$ cell is activated only by antigen pulsed macrophages of same strain or share class II MHC alleles. Therefore, antigen recognition by $CD4^+ T_H$ cells is class II MHC restricted.

In 1974, Zinkernagel and Doherty demonstrated self-MHC restriction of $CD8^+$ T cells. In their experiment, mice were immunized with lymphocytic choriomeningitis (LCM) virus. After a latent period of two weeks or so, T_C cells from the spleen of the mice were isolated and incubated with LCM-infected target cells of the same mice or different mice. They found that the T_C cells were capable of killing only syngeneic virus infected target cells. Later experiments showed that the T_C cells and virus infected target cells must share class I MHC molecule encoded by the K or D region of the gene. Therefore, antigen recognition by $CD8^+ T_C$ cells is class I MHC restricted.

Role of antigen presenting cells

Separate studies conducted in the laboratories of E. R. Unanuae, first at Harvard and later at Washington University, and of H. M. Grey at National Jewish Center of immunology and Respiratory medicine in Denver provided evidence that to stimulate an immune response, extracellular proteins must be first endocytosed and broken into peptides by an antigen-presenting cell (APC). These peptides then bind to class II MHC molecule and appear on the cell surface of the APC. MHC peptide complex is recognized by T_H cell. This sequence of events-the ingestion of antigen, fragmentation into peptides and binding of peptide to MHC molecule is called antigen processing, which occurs only in APC. Unanuae and Ziegler observed that T_H cell activation by APCs can be prevented by treating the APCs with paraformaldehyde prior to antigen exposure. It was observed that, if the APCs are allowed to ingest antigen and then 1 to 3 hr later fixed with paraformaldehyde, T_H cell activation still occurred.

In another experiment, Shimonkevitz showed that internalization and processing of antigens could be bypassed if the APCs are readily exposed to peptide digests of an antigen. In this experiment, glutaraldehyde treated APCs are exposed to partially digested ovalbumin or intact ovalbumin. The digested ovalbumin still interacted with APCs inspite of them being fixed in glutaraldehyde. This interaction led to stimulation of ovalbumin specific T_H cells, where as intact ovalbumin failed to do so. This experiment proves the fact that antigen processing is a metabolic process and it is essential for stimulation of T_H cells through class II MHC molecule.

Class I MHC molecules are also involved in antigen processing and presentation. As A. R. M. Townsend of John Radcliffe Hospital in Oxford, England learned that, cytotoxic T lymphocytes identify virally infected cells by looking for viral peptides presented by class I MHC molecule. Further work of T. J. Braciale of Washington University and M. J. Bevan of Scripps Research Institute established that all the peptides naturally presented by class I MHC molecules are derived from proteins in a cell's cytoplasm.

Antigen presenting cells

Almost all cells expressing class I or class II MHC molecules on their surface can present peptides on their MHC molecule to T cells. The cells that display peptides (antigen) associated with class I MHC molecule to $CD8^+$ T_C cells are called as **target cells.** Virtually all nucleated cells express class I MHC molecule on their membrane and the cell could function as target cells presenting endogenous antigens to the TC cells. Target cells could be altered self-cells (transformed or cancerous) or those infected by the pathogens. The cells that display peptides associated with class II MHC molecule to $CD4^+$ T_H cells are called **antigen-presenting cells** (APCs). The APCs are classified in to two types: **professional** and **nonprofessional** APCs.

(a) **Professional APCs**

Dendritic cells macrophages and B-lymphocytes belong to this category.

- Dendritic cells constitutively express high levels of Class II MHC molecules and show co-stimulatory activity. They can activate naive T_H cells. They are most effective of the APCs.
- Macrophages get activated only through the process of phagocytosis of microorganisms or antigens and then express class II MHC molecules as well as co-stimulatory molecules such as B7 membrane molecule.
- Antigen molecules should activate B cells before they express co-stimulatory molecules, but they constitutively express class II MHC molecules.

(b) **Nonprofessional APCs**

Skin fibroblasts, brain glial cells, pancreatic beta cells, thymic epithelial cells, thyroid epithelial cells and vascular endothelial cells belong to this category. They can be induced to express class II MHC molecules or co-stimulatory signal.

CYTOSOLIC PATHWAY OF ANTIGEN PRESENTATION

Intracellular, soluble protein antigens that are delivered into cytoplasm of a cell are degraded into peptides and class I MHC molecule presents these peptides to T_C cells. Viral endogenous antigens found in the cytoplasm of infected cell are degraded within the cytoplasm into peptides and presented on class I MHC molecules. The pathways chosen for endogenous antigen degradation for presentation with class I MHC molecule are the one utilized by the cell for normal turnover of intracellular proteins.

Results of different experiments indicate that the two kinds of MHC molecules sample antigens that are processed in different intracellular compartments. The ability of MHC molecules to bind to specific peptides and to participate in antigen processing and presentation is a consequence of their structure and synthesis.

Cytosolic proteasomes and peptide generation

All cells possess cytosolic proteolytic system, which is used for degradation of intracellular proteins into short peptides. A small protein, called ubiquitin specially tags those proteins that are targeted for degradation. Ubiquitin tagged proteins are broken down in special, multifunctional complex called **proteasome.** Proteasomes are large cylindrical structures found in many compartments of a cell. They are an amalgamation of several different proteases and they appear to be cells principal mechanisms for degradation of proteins that have either outlived their usefulness, been damaged or been folded incorrectly. Proteasome contains four rings of protein subunits with a central channel of 10-20 A^O. Degradation of proteins in proteasomes is ATP dependent process and it occurs in the central hollow of the proteasome, thus preventing proteolysis of other proteins within the cell cytoplasm.

J. J. Monaco of Medical College of Virginia has performed some of the most intriguing studies of proteasomes. He demonstrated that, genes belonging to MHC cluster encode the two subunits- LMP2 and LMP7 found in proteasomes. Increased levels of IFNγ induce these proteins. K. L. Rock and A. L. Goldberg of Harvard have recently shown that the inclusion of these subunits in a proteasome causes it to produce peptides that end in basic or hydrophobic amino acids-exactly the types to which most class I MHC molecules bind.

Transport of peptides from cytosol to RER

A transporter protein called TAP (transporters associated with antigen processing) into the rough endoplasmic reticulum (RER) by a process that requires the hydrolysis of ATP translocates the peptides generated in the cytosol by the proteasome.

TAP is membrane –spanning heterodimer consisting of two proteins: TAP1 and TAP2 (Fig. 12.1), each have one hydrophobic domain, which is thought to project through the membrane into the lumen of the RER and one ATP binding domain, which projects into the cytosol. TAP has the highest affinity for peptides containing 8 to 13 amino acid residues, which is the optimum length of peptide required for binding to class I MHC. Class I MHC molecule is uniquely designed so as to favor binding of hydrophobic or basic carboxyl terminal amino acids.

Assembly of peptides with class I MHC molecule

Class I MHC molecule consist of two protein components: one α chain and the other β2-microglobulin, which are synthesized on the polysomes along the RER. The assembly of these to individual components into stable class I MHC molecule requires the presence of another peptide called molecular chaperones.

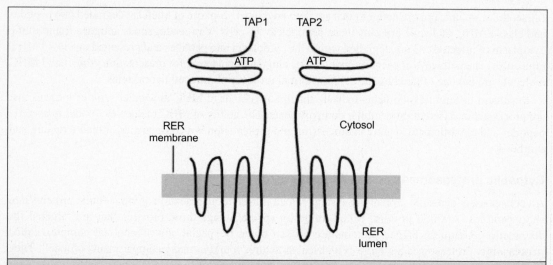

Fig. 12.1 Schematic diagram of TAP (transporter associated with antigen processing). A heterodimer (TAP1 and TAP2) anchored to the membrane of rough endoplasmic reticulum. Cytosolic domain has ATP bound to it.

The predominant molecular chaperone involved in class I MHC assembly is calnexin, which is found in the membrane of endoplasmic reticulum. Within the lumen of RER newly synthesized α chain of class I rapidly associate with β2-microglobulin in the presence of calnexin and assemble to from partially folded structure. The association of calnexin with the protein components of class I MHC (Fig. 12. 2) appears to inhibit proteolytic degradation of α chain.

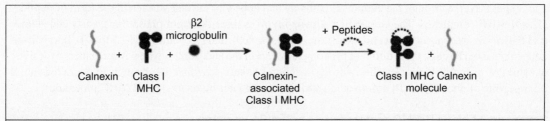

Fig. 12.2   Assembly, stabilization and association of newly formed class I MHC molecule by calnexin.

The calnexin associated class I MHC then physically associates with TAP protein, which helps in capture of the processed peptide of proteasomes by the class I MHC before the peptide is exposed to the luminal environment of RER. Association of class I MHC with peptide stabilizes it further, hence it dissociates from calnexin and TAP (Fig. 12. 3).

ENDOCYTIC PATHWAY OF EXOGENOUS ANTIGEN PRESENTATION

Most of the APCs internalize antigens by endocytosis (either receptor mediated or pinocytosis) because they do not have the ability of phagocytosis. For ex. B cells, internalize antigens effectively by receptor

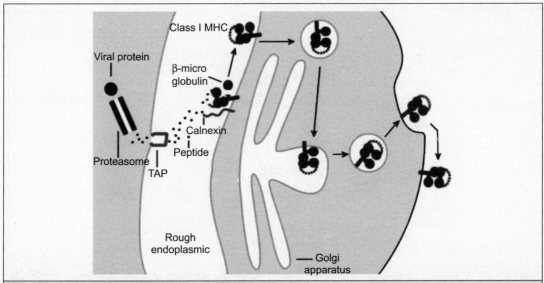

Fig. 12.3   A model of antigen presentation for endogenous antigens. Note the association of classes I MHC molecule with peptide.

mediated endocytosis through antigen specific membrane bound antibodies acting as receptors. On the other hand, macrophages internalize antigens by both processes, i.e. phagocytosis and endocytosis.

Peptide generation in endocytic vesicle

An internalized antigen is degraded into peptides within the endocytic or phagocytic vesicles and it takes 1 to 3 hr to traverse through the endocytic pathway and appear at the cell surface in the form of peptide-class II MHC complexes. The endocytic pathway involves three different pH settings: early endosomes (pH 6.0 to 6.5); late endosome or endolysosome (pH 5.0 to 6.0); and lysosomes (pH 4.5 to 5.0). Internalized antigen is passed through these different pH compartments of the endosomes, where it encounters hydrolytic enzymes of different kinds. By the hydrolytic action of these enzymes the protein id degraded into a oligopeptide of about 13 to 18 amino acid residues, which later binds to class II MHC molecules.

Transport of class II MHC molecule to endocytic vesicles

Given that the MHC class I and II molecules assemble inside the endoplasmic reticulum, it is surprising that they do not bind to the same peptides. Recent studies have shown that when class II MHC molecule synthesized within RER, it associates with another protein called the invariant (Ii) chain. The invariant chain prevents peptides from binding to class II molecules, either by directly interfering with peptide binding or by keeping the class II MHC molecules in a partially unfolded state. It also redirects class II MHC molecules along a path to the cell surface that class II MHC molecules and most other membrane surface proteins do not follow. It routes the class II MHC to the endocytic pathway through Golgi apparatus into endosome (Fig. 12.4).

Peter Cresswell of Duke University found that when class II MHC-Ii complexes move into endosomes, the movement of vesicles toward the surface stops for up to six hours. During this time, endosomal proteases digest the invariant chain, which frees itself from class II MHC and binds to other peptides in the vesicles. Many of those peptides are of course derived from extracellular sources. Finally the class II MHC-peptide complexes move out to the cell surface.

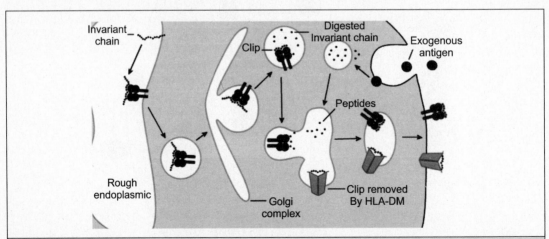

Fig. 12.4   A model of the antigen presenting pathway for exogenous antigens. Note the association of class II MHC with invariant (Ii) chain.

Assembly of peptides with class II MHC molecules

Another interesting point about the formation of class II MHC-peptide complex was learned by looking at certain mutant cells created by E. D. Mullins and D. A. Pious of the University of Washington. On the surface of these cells, the class II MHC molecules have an oddly floppy, easily denatured form. The appearance and behavior of these molecules resemble that of newly synthesized class II MHC molecules in RER. The floppy molecules were found to have bound to a set of peptides derived from one small region of the invariant chain. These peptides are called CLIP (class II –associated invariant chain peptide) remains bound to the class II MHC molecule after the invariant chain has been cleaved within the endosome while the class II MHC-Ii complex was traversing through the endosomal pathway. CLIP physically occupies the peptide binding cleft on the class II MHC molecule or that at least alters the structure of the class II MHC molecule to prevent other peptides from binding (Fig. 12.5).

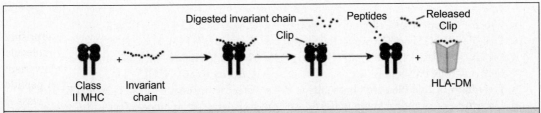

Fig. 12.5   Assembly and stabilization of class II MHC molecule. Within the endoplasmic reticulum the molecule binds to invariant chains which, prevents binding of peptides to class II MHC and dirests it to bind to endogenous antigens.

Digestion of invariant chain leaves CLIP. HLA-DM, an MHC-like molecule mediates exchange of CLIP with peptides within the endosomal compartment.

CLIP remains associated with class II MHC molecule until it is actively removed by HLA-DM, which is class II MHC-like molecule. HLA-DM is a heterodimer of α and β chains like class II MHC molecule, but unlike class II molecule it is not expressed at the cell membrane and instead it is confined to endosomal vesicles. In humans DMα and DMβ genes are located near TAP and LMP genes of MHC complex. As in the case of class I MHC molecule, peptide binding is required to maintain the stable structure of class II MHC molecules. One the peptide is bound; the class II MHC peptide complex is transported to the plasma membrane.

Exercise

1. Write briefly on the role of antigen presenting cells in antigen processing and MHC restriction of T cell (20 marks)
2. With illustrations, describe the cytosolic and endocytic pathway of antigen presentation (20 marks).
3. Write notes on: (10 marks each)
   (a) Cytosolic pathway of antigen presentation
   (b) Endocytic pathway of antigen presentation
   (c) Role of TAP, proteasome, calnexin and CLIP in antigen presentation

Chapter 13

Effector Responses of
Cell-Mediated and Humoral Immunity

- Effector Response of Cell-Mediated Branch
- Cell-Mediated Direct Cytotoxic Response
- Nk Cell-Mediated Cytotoxicity
- Delayed-Type Hypersensitivity
- Detection of Cell-Mediated Immunity
- Detection of Humoral Immune Response
- Immunological Memory
- Requirement For Cell-Cell Communication
- Properties of Effector T Cells
- Cytotoxic T Lymphocytes (CTLS)
- Antibody-Dependent Cell-Mediated Cytotoxicity (ADCC)
- Effector Response of the Humoral Branch
- Regulation of Immune Effector Response
- Factors Controlling the Long-Term Survival of Memory Cells

The cell-mediated and humoral immune responses serve different functions and involve different effector mechanisms for generating immunity. Secreted antibodies are the effectors of the humoral system, which can neutralize soluble antigens. Antibodies can also bind to membrane bound antigens of microorganisms and then activate complement system, leading to opsonization, lysis of the microorganisms and viral neutralization. Antibodies bound to particulate antigens or microorganisms can also facilitate Fc-mediated phagocytosis of the microorganisms. Cell-mediated branch has various effector cells, both antigen specific and nonspecific cells contribute to cell mediated immune response. Specific cells include $CD4^+$ T_H1 cells and T_H2 cells and $CD8^+$ T cells or T cytotoxic cells or cytotoxic T lymphocytes (CTLs). Non- specific cells include macrophages, neutrophils, eosinophils and natural killer (NK) cells. The cell-mediated branch is responsible for clearance of intracellular parasites, virus infected cells, transformed cells and foreign grafts, whereas humoral immune system serves mainly to eliminate extracellular bacterial antigens and bacteria. This chapter mainly deals with different types of effector mechanisms shown by cell-mediated and humoral immune system.

EFFECTOR RESPONSE OF CELL-MEDIATED BRANCH

The importance of cell-mediated immune response becomes evident when the system is defective, such as Di-George syndrome. In this disorder children will be born without a thymus and therefore lack T cell component of the cell-mediated immunity. These children are highly susceptible to viral infections and intracellular pathogenic infections, but they can easily cope with infections caused by bacteria because their humoral immune branch is perfectly normal. These children cannot even cope with attenuated vaccines, which could be life threatening. Cell-mediated immune response can be divided into two major categories on the basis of effector functions performed by the cells. One group involves effector cells with direct cytotoxic activity to lyse virally infected cells or tumor cells, but also indirectly regulate their own growth and function as well as that of other immune effector cells such as B lymphocytes, macrophages and granulocytes. The other group involves special group of $CD4^+$ T cells showing delayed type hypersensitivity reactions.

Properties of Effector T Cells

There are four types of effector T cells, which include $CD4^+$ T_H0, T_H1, and T_H2 cells and $CD8^+$ cytotoxic T cells. The classification of $CD4^+$ T_H cells is on the basis of their cytokine production profile as well as type of receptors and markers expressed by these cells. The effector T cells differ from the naive T cells in several characters, particularly, effector cells show increased expression of adhesion molecules, cytokines and membrane bound molecules, whereas naive T cells require activation signal molecules, and express other molecules at very low level.

Cell adhesion molecules

These molecules play an important role in T cell adhesion to antigen presenting cells or target cells infected with intracellular pathogen or transformed cells. Without these molecules T cells cannot be activated, because some of these adhesion molecules act as signal transducers. The effector T cells produce adhesion molecules like CD2 and the integrin LFA-1 in addition to possessing TCR on their membrane. CD2 and LFA-1 help in binding to LFA-3 and ICAMs expressed on antigen presenting cells and various target cells. When compared with naive T cells, the level of CD2 and LFA-1 expression on effector T cells is two folds higher, which helps them to bind more effectively with APC and target cells. First time when a effector T cell establishes the contact with APC or target cell, the interaction will be weak, but the TCR of the effector will be scanning the membrane of APC or target cell for MHC molecule with peptide complexed to it. If the TCR does not establish the contact with MHC-peptide complex, the effector T cell disengage itself from the APC or target cell and does not undergo activation. On the other hand, if the TCR comes in contact with MHC-peptide complex presented by APC or target cell, the contact becomes firmer and effector T cell undergoes activation, leading to the production of cytokines and more quantity of cell adhesion molecules. Increased expression of cell adhesion molecules increases the affinity of T cell with APC or target cell and the interaction will be prolonged. Macrophages expressing class II MHC-peptide complex will engage T_H1 effector T cells; B cells displaying class II MHC-peptide complex will engage T_H2 cells and the cytotoxic T cells will be engaged by class I MHC-peptide complex presented by target cells.

In addition, effector T cells express increased levels of homing receptors CLA, LPAM-1 and LFA-1, which facilitates these cells to enter tertiary lymphoid tissue and to the sites of inflammation. The naive T cells express different kinds of homing receptors, L-selectin, which binds to vascular addressins GlyCAM-1 and CD34 expressed on high-endothelial venules (HEV). In addition, effector T cells produce soluble as well as membrane bound effector molecules. The membrane bound effector molecules belong to tumor necrosis factor (TNF) family of membrane proteins like Fas ligand (major molecule for initiating apoptosis) is found on $CD8^+$ CTLs, TNF-β on T_H1 cells and the CD40L (ligand) on T_H2 cells. Each of this effector T cells also produce soluble effector molecules called cytokines, whose property and function has been discussed in greater details in Chapter 14. Soluble as well as membrane bound effector molecule play an important role in cell-mediated immune response.

CELL-MEDIATED DIRECT CYTOTOXIC RESPONSE

This is one of the method by which immune system eliminates foreign cells and the cells that have been infected by viruses or intracellular pathogens or transformed cells (cancerous cells). Cell mediated cytotoxic response involves two major mechanisms: those involving antigen-specific cytotoxic response mediated by cytotoxic T lymphocytes (CTLs) and those involving nonspecific cells such as macrophages and natural killer (NK) cells. Both these responses lead to killing of target cell and lysis. The target cells on which these effector mechanisms operate include allogeneic cells (foreign cells), cancerous cells, virus, bacteria, and protozoan infected cells, and chemical conjugated cells.

Cytotoxic T Lymphocytes (CTLs)

CTLs are formed from activation of $CD8^+$ T cells or T_C cells. These cells play an important role in recognition and elimination of virus infected and cancerous cells as well in graft rejection reactions. These cells are class I MHC restricted. Since almost all nucleated cells in the body express class I MHC, CTLs can recognize non-self peptide presented by class I MHC and eliminate the cell. For the convenience of understanding, CTL-mediated immune response can be divided in to two stages. Stage 1 involves activation and differentiation of naive T_C cells and stage 2 involves recognition of class I MHC-peptide complex on a target cell and destruction of target cell.

Stage 1. Activation and differentiation of CTLs

Naive $CD8^+$ T cells or T_C cells are referred to as **CTL precursors** (CTL-Ps), which are incapable of performing any function other than recognition of class I MHC-peptide complex on a target cell through its TCRs. For activation of CTL-P at least three signals are required. The signals include:

1. Antigen specific signal transmitted by class I MHC-peptide complex + TCR for the recognition of the peptide
2. Costimulatory signals transmitted by the interaction of CD28- of T_C cell and B7 of APC.
3. Cytokine induced signal, i.e. IL-2 interaction with high affinity IL-2R (receptor) on CTL-Ps leading to activation and differentiation of CTL-P into an effector CTL.

On antigen-mediated activation of CTL-Ps, they begin to produce IL-2R to which IL-2 secreted by proliferating T_H1 cells binds. IL-2 induces differentiation of activated CTL-Ps into effector CTLs. Memory CTL-Ps are capable of autocrine activation by producing their own IL-2. This indicates CTL-Ps are not only class I MHC restricted but also IL-2 restricted, without which they cannot undergo activation, which ensures that only antigen specific CTL-Ps are clonally expanded to acquire cytotoxic property (fig. 13.1).

The role of T_H1 cells in the generation of CTLs from naïve CTL-Ps is still debated. It is presumed that, within the lymphoid tissue, T_H1 cells and CTL-Ps may interact with common antigen presenting cell (Fig.13. 2). Such APCs may be presenting the processed viral antigen on class II MHC as well as antigenic viral peptides on class I MHC, and thus would be recognized by $CD4^+$ T_H cells and $CD8^+$ T_C cells.

Stage 2. Destruction of target cell

For the destruction of target cells, CTLs involve two major pathways:

(1) Interaction of CTLs membrane bound Fas ligand with FasR on the target cell surface
(2) Release of cytotoxic proteins such as granzymes and perforins from CTLs into target cells.

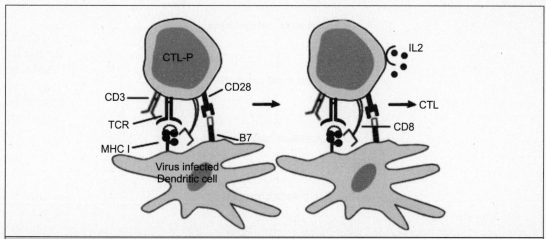

Fig. 13.1   Schematic illustration showing activation and proliferation of memory CTL-Ps by class I MHC restriction through APC and autocrine IL-2 stimulation.

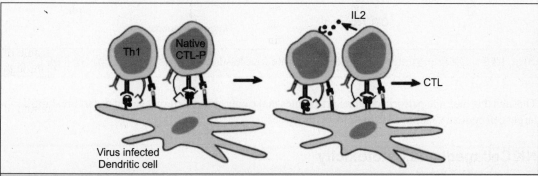

Fig. 13.2   Schematic illustration showing activation and proliferation of naïve CTL-Ps by class I MHC restriction through APC and IL-2 secretion from T$_H$1 cells.

The sequence of events involved in destruction of a target cell by CTL is given in a schematic form in Fig. 13.3.

Recent evidences suggest that the primary mode of destruction of target cell by CTL is by initiating apoptosis through Fas-FasL pathway. In addition to this, electron microscopic studies of CTLs have revealed that, CTLs store cytotoxic proteins in the form of granules in their cytoplasm and these proteins belong to two categories. One belongs to **perforins** involved in pore formation and the other belongs to **granzymes** or **fragmentins** responsible for hydrolysis or fragmentation of cellular products. Immediately following the CTL contact with target cell, Golgi stacks loaded with granzymes and granules loaded with perforins orient themselves and move towards the junction of cell contact (CTL-target cell). Then perforins monomers are released from the granules by exocytosis into the junctional space between the two cells. As the perforin monomers establish contact with target cell membrane, they undergo polymerization in the presence of Ca^{2+} ions and form cylinders with a pore size of 5 – 20 nm on the target cell membrane. By this time perforins have established a multiple pipeline channel between the CTL and target cell.

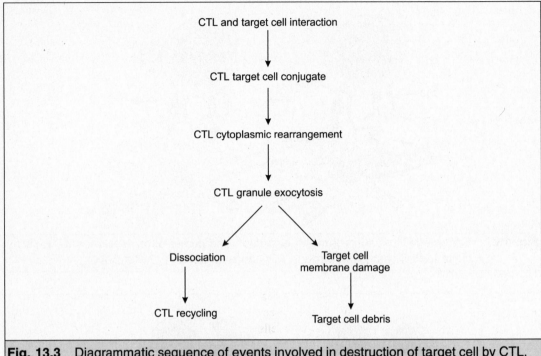

CTL and target cell interaction

↓

CTL target cell conjugate

↓

CTL cytoplasmic rearrangement

↓

CTL granule exocytosis

Dissociation   Target cell membrane damage

↓   ↓

CTL recycling   Target cell debris

Fig. 13.3 Diagrammatic sequence of events involved in destruction of target cell by CTL.

Through this multiple perforin channel granzymes make entry into the target cell and start breaking down target cell contents. Granzymes are mostly proteases.

NK Cell-mediated Cytotoxicity

NK cells belong to lymphocytic lineage and they are comparatively large in size with granules in their cytoplasm. They have important regulatory functions in both innate and acquired immune response. For instance, the production of IFN-γ by NK cells in response to IL-12 secreted by infected macrophages is essential for the elimination of certain intracellular pathogens. NK cell origin is from bone marrow like other hematopoietic cells, they are also derived from pluripotent hematopoietic stem cells. IL-2, IL-12, and IFN-γ prompt NK cell production, and their development may occur briefly in the fetal thymus but primarily it is extrathymic with critical steps occurring in the bone marrow. In humans 5 to 8% of all white blood cells or 10 to 15% mononuclear cells represent NK cells. Unlike T cells NK cells do not recirculate or have homing receptors and they are not found in thoracic lymph duct. NK cells are mainly found in secondary lymphoid organs and a small number is found in bone marrow. Several NK cell sub-population exists with minor difference in surface antigens and their biologic activity. Some act on circulating tumor cells and others act more effectively on solid tumors.

NK cells show early response, i.e. within 3 days of viral or bacterial infection. Their activity is stimulated by IFN-α, IFN-β and IL-12, levels of which increases remarkably in the blood in the course of viral and bacterial infection. This triggers NK cell activity and they provide first line of defense much before the T_C cells come in the picture. It would at least take 7 days for the activated and differentiated T_C cell to make its appearance in the infected person.

Lineage of NK cells is still debated, but they do posses certain membrane markers of T lymphocytes and some markers of monocytes and granulocytes. As has been stated earlier different NK cells express different sets of membrane molecules and accordingly they differ in function. Among the most commonly expressed membrane molecules by NK cells are Thy-1, CD2, 75 kD β subunit of the IL-2R, CD16 or FcγRIII. FcγRIII is a receptor for Fc region of IgG, therefore once in a while NK cells may also show antibody dependent cell mediated cytotoxicity (ADCC) reaction.

Mechanism of NK cell killing

NK cell kill the virus infected or tumor cells by the same mechanism as employed by CTLs, where cytoplasm of NK cells is also known to contain perforin and granzymes. NK cells also show target cell destruction by apoptosis. There are several significant differences between CTLs and NK cells. CTLs need activation before they produce granzymes and perforins, whereas NK cells possess them constitutively. Therefore, NK cells are constitutitvely cytotoxic. Target cell recognition by NK cells is not MHC restricted. NK cells do not express antigen specific TCR or CD3. NK cell response does not generate immunologic memory.

NK cell receptors

The NK cell cytotoxic activity against target cells is easily triggered through the engagement of many different surface receptors, as discussed below. Because healthy cells express some of the ligands for these activating NK receptors, activation of NK cells is under tight negative control through inhibitory receptors. Thus, the decision of killing or sparing a target cell results from a balance between positive and negative signals received by the NK cells. The major ligand identified so far for the NK inhibitory receptors is MHC class I molecule, a polymorphic set of molecules usually expressed by normal cells. On the basis of chemical nature NK cell receptors are classified into type I and type II and they are regulatory in nature.

Activation of NK cell function

Once NK cells have matured, many different surface molecules upon antibody-mediated cross-linking in vitro can trigger their cytotoxic activity. In some cases, a combination of signals from different receptors may be required to achieve NK cell activation. Activating molecules include integrins (lymphocyte function-associated antigen [LFA-1]), type I Ig like receptors (CD2, CD16, 2B4) and type II lectin-like receptors (CD69, NKR-P1).

Antibody-Dependent Cell-Mediated Cytotoxicity (ADCC)

The cells that have cytotoxic potential have been found to possess membrane bound Fc receptors for antibody molecules, which facilitates their interaction with cells readily bound by antibodies. The antibody molecule acts as a bridge between cytotoxic cell and the target cell, subsequently causing the target cell lysis due to activation of cytotoxic cell through Fc receptor. This type of cytotoxicity is called **antibody-dependent cell mediated cytotoxicity (ADCC)**.

The cells that can mediate ADCC are NK cells, macrophages, neutrophils, monocytes and eosinophils. Generally virally infected target cells are killed through ADCC reaction mediated by NK cells and macrophages. Schistosome infected target cells are killed through ADCC reaction mediated by eosinophils, neutrophils and mast cell. The ADCC killing of target cells by different cytotoxic cells involves different mechanisms. Neutrophils, eosinophils and macrophages on activation through Fc receptor, release lytic enzymes at the site of Fc-mediated contact and damage the target cells. In the process, neighboring normal cells may also get damaged. In addition activated monocytes, macrophages and NK cells may also release tumor necrosis factor (TNF) a toxic factor, affects the target cells. NK cells and eosinophils have perforins in their cytoplasm, therefore, target cell killing may also involve perforin-mediated membrane damage similar to the mechanism described for CTL-mediated cytotoxicity (Fig.13.4).

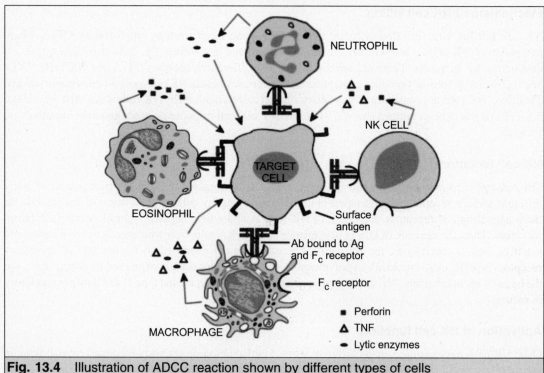

Fig. 13.4   Illustration of ADCC reaction shown by different types of cells

Delayed-Type Hypersensitivity

It mainly involves T$_H$ cells and causes localized inflammatory reaction due to secretion of cytokines and initiating infiltration of the area by inflammatory cells. This has been dealt in greater detail in Chapter 18-Hyeprsensitivity.

DETECTION OF CELL-MEDIATED IMMUNITY

Tests for T cell functions

Tests for T cell function can be done both *in vitro* as well as *in vivo*. Since monoclonal antibodies against T cell specific surface antigens are available and it is possible to culture T cells in the presence of IL-2, it has been possible to perform these tests in the laboratory in the case of suspected immune deficiency cases.

In vitro T cell function tests

(i) Phenotyping   T cells of different types can be identified with the help of monoclonal antibodies to stage specific T cell antigens. At different stages of maturation of T cells, specific monoclonal antibodies are used and different functional subsets of T cells are identified and quantified. It is possible to count $CD4^+$ and $CD8^+$ population of T cells for which immunofluorescence or immunoperoxidase staining method is used. In a normal individual, T helper cells ($CD4^+$) are 65% and T cytotoxic cells 35%. In the case of immunodeficiencies these numbers are altered.

(ii) Polyclonal activation of T cells   These tests are performed for the non-specific proliferation of T cells in the presence of mitogens like phytohemagglutinins (PHA). Cultured T cells are stimulated to undergo proliferation in the presence of PHA and monocytes. Monocytes provide IL-1 for the activation of T cells and stimulate them to undergo mitosis. Mitosis involves DNA synthesis, which can be measured by tritiated thymidine incorporation into the dividing cells. Another method to assay T cell proliferation is to monitor the level of IL-2 production in the culture, which is indicative of T cell activation and proliferation.

(iii) Test for T helper cells   T helper cell assay can be done by adding T cells of a patient to the culture of B cells and monocytes together with a mitogen called pokeweed mitogen (PWM). If the T helper cells are performing their normal duties, they should stimulate B cells to undergo maturation and differentiation by secreting cytokines and B cells should transform themselves into plasma cells, which ultimately results in production of antibody. Detection of antibodies in the medium is the indication of T helper cell function.

(iv) Mixed lymphocytic reaction (MLR)   X. Ginsburg and D. H. Sachs discovered this in 1965. When they mixed rat lymphocytes with mouse fibroblast cells, the rat lymphocytes proliferated and destroyed the mouse fibroblasts. This occurs due to HLA-DR antigens of two different individuals when not matched. When two different lymphocytes belonging to two different individuals are mixed together, due to HLA-DR incompatibility, the cells are stimulated to divide. Excessive DNA synthesis will occur in the stimulated lymphocytes, which is called **blast transformation.** This can be detected by increased uptake of tritiated thymidine by stimulated lymphocytes.

(v) Detection of NK cell activity   NK cells are detected by using specific monoclonal antibodies against NK cell receptors. NK cell killing activity in the non-specific, non-HLA dependent manner can be detected in the peripheral blood sample by stimulating them with IFN-γ and IL-12 and adding nonspecific tumor cells. Death of tumor cells would indicate NK cell killing activity.

In vivo tests for T cell function

These are performed by intradermal injection of common antigens like vaccinia virus, herpes simplex virus, and mumps virus antigens. Within 24 to 48 hrs a nodular reaction is detected and anergy to all antigens would indicate T cell defects. Anergy to all antigens is observed in AIDS and Hodgkins disease.

Detection of other cell activity other than T cells

The macrophage and neutrophil function like phagocytosis and killing of microorganisms and their response to lymphokines is performed in vitro to assess their activity.

I. Tests for chemotaxis of macrophages and neutrophils   This is performed by using a semipermeable membrane by putting on one side of the membrane the factors that are mitogenic or antigenic and on the other side known number of mcarophages or neutrophils. The measure of number of cells moving across the semipermeable membrane would indicate the response of cells in terms of chemotaxis.

II. Tests for phagocytosis Macrophages and neutrophils are incubated in a serum containing medium to which known counts of *Staphylococcus aureus* are added and after some time percentage of viable organisms in the medium are calculated by bacterial count. This would give an assessment of phagocytosis and intracellular killing. Similarly by adding latex particles it is possible to assess the phagocytic activity of macrophages and neutrophils.

EFFECTOR RESPONSE OF THE HUMORAL BRANCH

The Effector function of the humoral branch relies upon the production of large number of antibodies against epitopes of different types and foreign pathogens. Humoral response helps in elimination of extracellular pathogens by specific antibody production against different antigenic determinants or epitopes of a pathogen. The variety of functions performed by the antibodies to eliminate the pathogen from the body is as follows:

- Antibodies initiate complement-mediated lysis of the pathogen by activating the complements
- Antibodies bind to pathogens and bring about opsonization and facilitate phagocytosis mediated through Fc receptor on phagocytic cells
- Antibodies directly bind to bacterial toxins and neutralize them
- Antibodies facilitate cell-mediated cytotoxicity through their Fc receptor and help in killing the infected cell.
- Antibodies bind to viruses and prevent from proliferation

Humoral effector response in a person can be of primary or secondary type depending on the contact of the individual with the exogenous antigen (Fig. 13.5).

Primary response

It is characterized by the production of antibody secreting plasma cells and memory B cells from the first contact of an individual with exogenous antigen. Depending on the nature of the antigen, serum levels of antibodies vary. Most important of all, route of antigen entry, dose, and the species play an important role in antibody production (more details of this is dealt in Chapter 5). The primary response begins with a **lag phase**, during this phase naive B cell undergo clonal selection in response to antigen and differentiate in to plasma cells and memory cells (Fig. 13.5A). The lag phase lasts for 3 to 4 days and during this period no antibody is detected in the serum. The lag phase is immediately followed by logarithmic phase, where increase in serum antibody levels is observed for 4 to 10 days, which reaches a peak and than plateaus for a variable time and then declines. For soluble protein antigens the lag phase is little longer, often lasting about a week. The early primary response is characterized by the presence of IgM followed by IgG. The primary response can last for varying period depending on the persistence of antigen.

Secondary response

This occurs upon exposure to the same antigen, weeks, months or even years later. The memory B cells formed during the primary response and had entered into G_0 phase are now stimulated by the presence of same antigen. They undergo rapid proliferation and differentiation into plasma cells. There is of, course a short negative phase before the secondary response starts, which is characterized by activation,

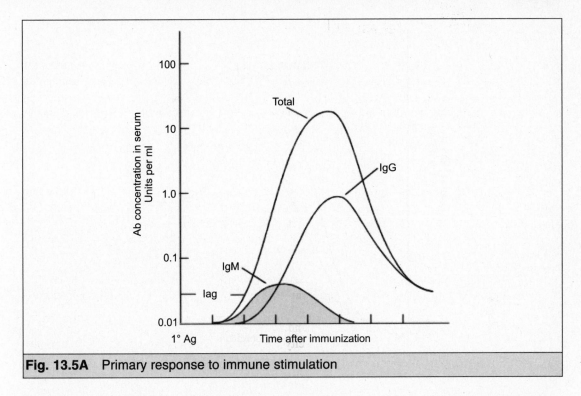

Fig. 13.5A   Primary response to immune stimulation

proliferation and differentiation of memory B cells. IgM produced during the secondary immune response is much lower when compared to primary response, whereas IgG levels will be two to four fold higher in the secondary response there by hastening the recovery and tackling the pathogen much earlier (Fig. 13.5B).

DETECTION OF HUMORAL IMMUNE RESPONSE

Tests for B cell function

It is performed by *in vitro* as well as *in vivo* methods.

In vitro tests for B cell function

These tests are done on peripheral circulating B cells.

(i) **Polyclonal activation**   Activation of B cells can be checked by non specific mitogens like pokeweed mitogen (PWM) or purified protein derivatives (PPD), which are T cell dependent antigens and T cell independent antigens include capsular material of pneumococci or Epstein-Barr virus. The test is performed by measuring the number of plasma cells or the quality of immunoglobulin produced in the medium after incubating the B cells in the culture medium with above antigens.

(ii) **Phenotyping**   B cell surface markers like γ, δ, α, μ and ε heavy chains are detected by using antibodies against each of these chains and immunofluorescence or immunoperoxidase staining method does the detection. The κ and λ chains can be also detected by same method.

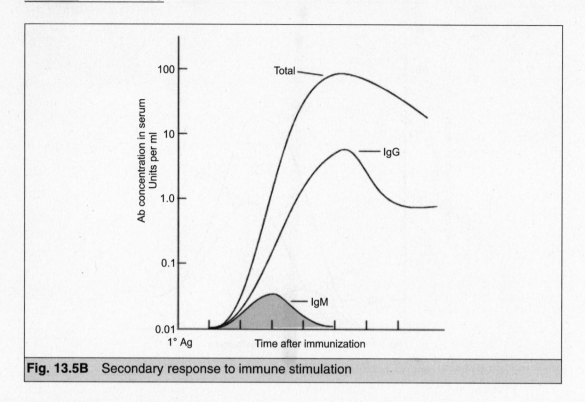

Fig. 13.5B Secondary response to immune stimulation

In vivo tests for B cell function

Measurement of levels IgG or IgM antibodies following immunization with a known antigen is the true test for humoral immunity. This test cannot be performed in infants and in bone marrow transplant recipients, where measurement of total IgG, IgM, IgA and IgE is necessary. In infants isohemagglutinins are measured to see the B cell response.

REGULATION OF IMMUNE EFFECTOR RESPONSE

An immune system can either respond to an antigen and develop immune response or enter into unresponsive state and develop tolerance. Both these responses rely upon the specific antigen recognition ability of T and B cells, which is carefully regulated. Any lapse in the regulatory mechanism would lead to catastrophic effect. Both cell-mediated and humoral branch of immune responses are well regulated. Each time an antigen is encountered, there is whole lot of screening of antigen is done and the immune system decides which branch to be activated, the intensity of the response and its duration. Various cytokines secreted by T_H1 and T_H2 cells also play an important role in regulation and determining which antibody isotypes are produced. Regulation of immune effector response can be dealt under:

- Antigen-mediated regulation
- Antibody-mediated regulation
- Immune complex mediated regulation
- Idiotype-mediated regulation
- Neuroendocrine regulation

Antigen-mediated regulation

In this case immunologic background of an individual plays an important role. Probably the individual is encountering the antigen for the first time and it is a naive response, than it would be different from an individual that had already encountered antigen earlier. Earlier exposure to an antigen makes an individual either tolerant to antigen or may have immune memory cells. In some cases antigenic competition may regulate the immune response. This can be demonstrated by injecting mice with two different types of antigens at two different times. Prior immunization of animals with sheep RBCs (SRBCs) severely impairs the response against horse red blood cells (HRBCs). It is presumed that competing antigens may interfere with antigen presentation and activation of T_H cells or immune response to a competing antigen may induce certain cytokines that may downregulate the response against the other.

Antibody-mediated

It relies upon feed back regulation as it happens in other biochemical reactions. Antibody exerts feed back regulation on its own production, which is also called **antibody-mediated suppression**. Because of this reason, infants are not immunized with measles and mumps vaccines before 1 year of age. The reason being, passively gained maternal antibodies will be circulating in the blood at a very high titer up to 6 months after birth. If an infant is immunized with mumps or measles vaccine at this time, child may fail to develop humoral immune response as well as immune memory cells.

Immune complex mediated regulation

Antigen-antibody complexes have been shown to exert regulatory response on immune system either by enhancing or by inhibiting the immune system. Direct evidences in connection with this are not available, but it is presumed that immune complexes deposited in the body, will bind to certain immune cells through Fc receptor and down regulate their activity due to over saturation of receptors with Fc binding. This is similar to the development of anergy in T or B cells against self-antigens, where the T and B cell receptors get saturated with self antigens due to their abundance and anergize the cells. Similar to this, immune complexes are known to suppress the immune response in a patient.

Idiotypic regulation

It is mind-boggling to note the diversity generated by the genes of immunoglobulins and T and B cell receptors. It is roughly estimated that an immune system is capable of generating 10^{11} distinct antibodies each with a different specificity. Each antibody contains multiple **idiotopes,** which is nothing but antigenic determinant variable region of an antibody. A sum of the individual idiotope is called the **idiotype.** In some cases, a particular idiotope and the actual antigen-binding site, which is called **paratope**, are identical, in other cases the idiotopes consist of variable region sequences outside the antigen-binding site. To explain this in 1973, Niel Jerne proposed **Network theory**. This theory proposes that antibodies produced against a particular antigen during the earlier response will induce the production of second antibody against the first ones *idiotopes*. The idiotype of the first antibody Ab-1 activated a network of B cells, which recognize the individual idiotope of Ab-1 and then differentiate to produce plasma cells that secrete anti-idiotype antibody Ab-2. Once again individual idiotopes of Ab-2 induce the new set of B cells to produce anti-anti-idiotype Ab-3. At one point, newly formed antibody (anti-anti-idiotype) may resemble the idiotope of the first one (Ab-1), and the network now limits itself and decreased levels of antibody are generated in each successive activation. This type of network may be working within the T cell branch while producing $\alpha\beta$ and $\gamma\delta$ T cell receptor.

Neuroendocrine regulation of immune system

Clinical observations carried out in the past have clearly indicated that psychological factors affect immunity. There are reports implicating stress in immune suppression. Since stress and psychological behaviour of an individual are complicated physiologic processes, the response shown by an individual will be of neurological and endocrinological type. Both these responses interact at various levels and influence the immune response. The interactions appear to be bi-directional, where neuroendocrine system regulates immune response and an active immunity induces changes in both neural and endocrine functions (Fig. 13.6).

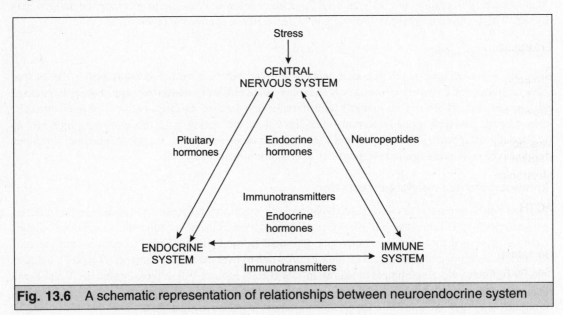

Fig. 13.6   A schematic representation of relationships between neuroendocrine system

There are many neuroendocrine mediators and autonomic nerve innervations into lymphoid organs, which bring in close interaction between central nervous system with immune system. During periods of stress, strong emotions are evoked like depression, anger, fear elicited. In such cases, involvement of sympathetic nervous system predominates. The sympathetic nervous system is known to release two types of neurotransmitters, namely *acetylcholine* from cholinergic nerve fibers and *nor-adrenalin* (nor-epinephrine) from adrenergic nerve fibers.

In periarteriolar sheath intricate anatomic association between T lymphocytes and interdigitating cells with sympathetic nervous system has been observed. In primary and secondary lymphoid organs there is innervation of autonomic nervous system, particularly by adrenergic sympathetic nerve fibers. These fibers often end in regions where lymphocytes are clustered. During periods of stress the hypothalamus acts on the anterior pituitary (adenohypophysis) and stimulates the secretion of adrenocorticotrophic hormone (ACTH), which acts on adrenal cortex and induces the secretion of glucocorticoids and hydrocortisone. In addition to this stress response also stimulates adrenal medulla through sympathetic nerve innervations and causes the secretion of epinephrine from the adrenal medulla. There are other neuroendocrine mediators like growth hormone, prolactin, melatonin, endorphins and enkephalins, which are associated with stress response. These have been shown to either enhance or suppress the immune response (Table 13.1).

Table 13.1 Immunomodulators of neuroendocrine system.

Factors	Action	Immune response affected
Glucocorticoids (hydrocortisone)	Suppression	Antibody production, NK cell activity, cytokine production
Catecholamines (epinephrine)	Suppression	Lymphocyte proliferation in response to mitogens
Acetylcholine	Enhancement	Lymphocytes and macrophages in bone marrow
β- Endorphin	Enhancement/Suppression	Antibody production, activation of macrophages and T cells
Enkephalin	Enhancement/Suppression	T-cell activation (enhanced at low dose and suppressed at high dose)
Prolactin	Enhancement	Macrophage activation and IL-2 production
Growth hormone	Enhancement	Antibody production, macrophage activation, IL-2 production
Vasoactive Intestinal Peptide (VIP)	Enhancement/Suppression	Cytokine production
Melatonin	Enhancement	Mixed lymphocyte reaction (MLR), antibody production
ACTH	Enhancement/Suppression	Cytokine production, NK cell activity, antibody production, macrophage actvation
Somatostatin	Enhancement/Suppression	Response to mitogens
Sex hormones	Enhancement/Suppression	Lymphocyte transformation, MLR

Source: D. N. Khansari et al., 1990, Immunology Today **11**: 170.

The second circuit involves intimate relationship between hormone receptors, hormone, anti-hormone and anti-idiotype response. The cells involved in immune system have receptors for various types of hormones: corticosteroids, insulin, growth hormone, oestradiol, testosterone, β-adrenergic agents, acetylcholine, endorphins and enkephalins. Glucocorticoids, androgens, estrogens and progesterone are known to depress the immune response, whereas growth hormone, thyroxin and insulin enhance the immune response. Spleen, thymus, bone marrow and fetal liver are innervated by autonomic and primary sensorial neurons. These are primary immunological organs. Neonatal sympathectomy with 6-hydroxy dopamine and surgical denervation of the spleen enhances the immune responses.

When there is a peak response to antigen challenge, glucocorticoid levels in the blood are reported to be higher in order to suppress the immune response. Interleukin-1 (IL-1) and other lymphokines, which are not well characterized, are known to stimulate glucocorticoid synthesis, which is achieved through pituitary adrenal axis. There are two network interactions between the immune and the neuroendocrine systems. The first type would involve the increased synthesis of glucocorticoids under the influence of IL-1 and a thymus hormone generated during the immunological response. In turn the glucocorticoids would exert feed back suppression by influencing several processes including production of IL-1 and IL-2 (Fig. 13.7).

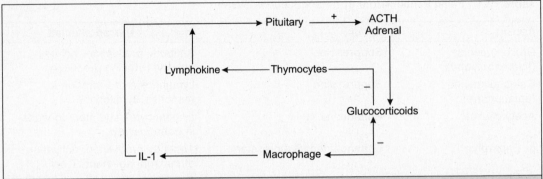

Fig. 13.7 The cycle represents the glucocorticoid feed back through IL-1 and lymphokine production.

Corticosteroids

They are potent anti-inflammatory agents bring about reduction in number and activity of immune system cells, which are cholesterol derivatives, include prednisone, prednisolone and methylprednisolone. In humans, guinea pigs and monkeys, corticosteroids bring about decrease in the number of circulating lymphocytes, whereas in hamster, mouse, rat and rabbit it results in enhanced apoptosis of lymphocytes. Corticosteroids also reduce both the phagocytic and killing ability of macrophages and neutrophils and in addition they reduce chemotaxis, so that fewer inflammatory cells are attached to the site of T_H cell activation. This may contribute to their anti-inflammatory action. In the presence of corticosteroids the production of IL-1 and class II MHC molecule by macrophages is reduced, which would result in failure in activation of T_H cells.

IMMUNOLOGICAL MEMORY

Typical immune response to infectious agents are followed by a state of long term memory during which subsequent contact with antigen leads to a more effective response and rapid rejection of the pathogen concerned, which has been already explained in primary and secondary immune response. Memory is carried by both T and B cells and reflects a combination of an increased precursor frequency of specifically reactive lymphocytes and a heightened sensitivity to the antigen concerned.

Initial generation of memory cells during the primary response

The primary response to pathogens is often intense and cause small numbers of specific T and B cells to undergo marked clonal expansion followed by differentiation into effector cells. It is found that, upregulation of various homing receptors like members of the b1, b2 and b7 integrin families, activated cells acquire the capacity to penetrate the walls of small blood vessels and can therefore disseminate throughout the body to seek and destroy the pathogen concerned. Effector cells have a relatively short lifespan and most of these cells are eliminated at the end of the primary response. At this stage effector cells are no longer useful and these cells get eliminated to preserve the primary repertoire, thus maintaining the responsiveness to new pathogens. It is observed that elimination of all the cells participating in the primary response would lead to development of tolerance rather than immunity. Memory cell generation therefore, appears to be a process where a small fraction of the cells stimulated in the primary response somehow evade death by apoptosis and survives for prolonged periods. Exact mechanism involved in this evasion of death is not understood.

It is now well established that cell survival requires the continuous expression of certain Bcl-2 gene family members, especially Bcl-2 and Bcl-x$_L$, combined with inhibition of the function of pro-apoptotic molecules such as Bad, Bax and Fas. The fate of the cells generated during the primary response is therefore presumably dictated by the relative expression of anti-apoptotic and pro-apoptotic molecules by the responding cells. The reduced expression of anti-apoptotic molecules may be influenced by number of factors, including cytokines such as IL-2 and a failure to engage the CD28 receptor; death effector cells may also reflect hyperstimulation. Concurrently, memory cell generation is presumably contingent upon upregulation/activation of anti-apoptotic molecules like Bcl-2 through cell contact with IL-2 and Bcl-x$_L$ by stimulation via CD28. These molecules, especially BCl-x$_L$, may function by counteracting Fas-mediated cell death, which suggests that the survival of memory cells is more dependent on the upregulation and or continued expression of anti-apoptotic molecules rather than down regulation of pro-apoptotic molecules. Fas-mediated cell death does make a significant contribution to the elimination of activated T cells. In the case of germinal center (GC) reaction leading to memory B cell formation, GC-B cells express a high density of Fas, which raises the probability that elimination of unselected GC-B cells is Fas mediated. Hence the selection of high affinity B cell mutants in the GC reaction may hinge largely on the maintenance and /or upregulation of anti-apoptotic molecules such as Bcl-2 and Bcl-x$_L$ and may be controlled by the CD40 ligand (CD40L)-CD40 interaction which triggers signaling pathways leading to Bcl family regulation.

It is well established that memory B cell generation is restricted to specialized sites in GC. The situation for T cells, however, is not clear. For these cell it appears that prolonged contact with APCs bearing the co-receptor molecule B7 and continuous exposure to appropriate cytokine i.e. IL-2. In addition to this, to prevent hyperstimulation the density of antigens encountering responding cells should not be too high. It is presumed that, memory T cells arise from a subset of late-comer cells, which only arrive at sites of antigen concentration during the later stages of an immune response. These straggling cells will encounter antigen on professional APCs but only at a relatively low concentration, thus avoiding exhaustion. It is thought that, in a protective microenvironment, these cells would then undergo selective expansion and survival, and therefore explaining the affinity maturation of memory cells. This scheme for memory cell generation is largely hypothetical.

Turnover and lifespan

It has long been argued that memory cells have a prolonged lifespan and can often survive for the lifetime of the individual without the need for secondary contact with the infectious organism concerned. This notion is supported by the observation that immunization against smallpox in childhood using vaccinia virus (VV) leads to an elevated precursor frequency of VV specific CD4$^+$ ad CD8$^+$ cells for up to 50 years. It is generally accepted that most late memory cells are resting cells.

Migratory properties

The original notion that memory cells are recirculating cells, has been challenged by reports that memory CD4$^+$ and CD8$^+$ cells eventually cease migrating through the lymphnodes and accumulate preferentially in the blood and spleen. Moreover, it has been found that memory CD8$^+$ cells do reach lymphnodes, at a slightly lower rate than they reach spleen. Another unexpected finding is that the initial route of antigen administration can radically alter the long-term distribution of memory cells. Therefore, intranasal immunization with virus is reported to cause only short-term cytotoxic T lymphocytes memory in spleen but long-term memory in the mesenteric lymphnode. In contrast, opposite distribution of memory cells is seen after intraperitoneal immunization.

Factors Controlling the Long-term Survival of Memory Cells

Over the past 10 years there has been quite a lot of debate on this issue of whether long-term memory cells require some form of chronic stimulation. Recent information on this topic is summarized below.

Role of specific antigen

The notion that memory cells survival requires persistent contact with antigen comes from the observation that T and B cell memory cells can decline rapidly following adoptive transfer unless the primed cells are co-transferred with specific antigen.

Bystander stimulation

It is well established that primary responses to viruses cause intense proliferation of T cells. Although a significant proportion of the dividing cells are antigen specific, the bulk of the proliferative response is thought to reflect a bystander reaction elicited by non-antigenic-specific stimuli. In viral infections in mice bystander proliferation of T cells is largely restricted to the $CD44^{hi}$ subset of $CD8^+$ cells and is probably elicited through production of cytokines, especially type I interferon (IFN-α and IFN-β). Interestingly, after a brief proliferative response, the progeny of these cells differentiate rapidly into long-lived cells expressing the typical semi-naive $-CD44^{hi}CD45RB^{hi}CD62L^{hi}$ phenotype of resting memory $CD8^+$ cells. This finding suggests that the intermittent contact of antigen specific memory $CD8^+$ cells with cytokines released during nonspecific viral infections could provide these cells with a survival boost thus helping to maintain memory.

Requirement for Cell-cell Communication

Under normal physiological conditions immunological memory is apparent in three different cell types, namely $CD4^+$ and $CD8^+$ T cells, and B cells.

Role of B cells in T cell memory

It is well established that deposits of antigen can survive for prolonged periods in the form of antigen-antibody complexes bound to the surface of follicular dendritic cells (FDCs). Hence continuous low-level contact with FDC bound antigen could play a significant role in maintaining the survival of memory cells. In the case of T cells this idea can be assessed by studying the fate of memory cells generated in the absence of B cells, for example μMT mice; in these mice, the lack of antibody production prevents the formation of immune complexes on FDCs.

A number of immunologists have examined the induction of $CD8^+$ T cell memory in μMT mice. The general finding is that the generation and long term survival of memory $CD8^+$ cells is much the same in μMT mice as in normal mice. Therefore, contact with B cells or antigen-antibody complexes seem to be largely irrelevant for $CD8^+$ memory cell survival. In the case of viral infection, however, this conclusion only applies when the primary response is sufficient to cause the complete elimination of live virus.

The role of B cells in controlling $CD4^+$ cell memory is more controversial and the data is fragmentary, therefore until a clear picture does not emerge, it is not going to be presented.

Role of CD4+ cells in CD8+ cell memory

Although primary responses of CD8$^+$ cells require help from CD4$^+$ T$_H$ cells in certain situations, the presence of helper cells is not required for CTL response during viral infection. Nevertheless, CD4$^+$ cells might be required for the generation and /or protracted survival of CD8$^+$ memory cells. This issue has been addressed by studying CD8$^+$ cell memory in MHC class II deficient mice. When such mice were infected with high dose of LCMV, the return in virus titers after the primary response caused the complete disappearance of specific CD8$^+$ cells, presumably as a result of exhaustion. Direct evidence on the role of CD4$^+$ cells in long-term CD8$^+$ cell memory has come from studies with the HY antigen. In this model the presence of CD4$^+$ T$_H$ cells is known to be crucial for the primary CTL response to HY. Therefore, to study the role of CD4$^+$ cells in memory, mice have to be primed with HY antigen in the presence of CD4$^+$ cells and then subsequently depleted of these cells. The key finding in this study is that continuous treatment with anti-CD4$^+$ antibody starting at one month after priming mice with HY failed to cause a detectable decline in HY specific CD8$^+$ memory cells even after several months of antibody treatment. This observation suggests that, once CD8$^+$ memory cells are formed, the long-term survival of these cells does not require help from CD4$^+$ cells.

Role of CD4+ cells in B cell memory

Recent work suggests that contact of B cells with antigen in the absence of CD4$^+$ cells fails to cause long term-memory, thus, when purified populations of hapten-primed B cells were adoptively transferred to nude mice containing pre-localized specific antigen-antibody complexes, the memory B cells survived for only a few weeks. Long-term survival of these cells did occur, after co-injection of specific CD4$^+$ T helper cells. These findings imply that the maintenance of long-term B cell memory requires continuous interaction with antigen specific CD4$^+$ cells.

Nevertheless, the data on this topic are still fragmentary, and much more information will be needed to address certain issues before reaching to any conclusion, which I hope will be available when I come out with the next edition of this book.

Exercise

1. Give detailed account of effector response of cell-mediated immunity (20 marks).
2. Explain how immunological memory is produced (20 marks)
3. Write notes on (10 marks each)
   (a) Humoral effector response
   (b) Cytotoxic T-lymphocytes
   (c) NK-cell mediated cytotoxicity
   (d) Antibody dependent cell mediated cytotoxicity (ADCC)
   (e) Detection of cell mediated and humoral immunity (one of them could be asked for 5 marks)
   (f) Regulation of immune response
   (g) Neuroendocrine regulation of immune system
4. Write notes on (5 marks each)
   (a) Requirement of cell to cell communication in immune memory

Chapter 14

Cytokines

- General Properties of Cytokines
- Cytokines that Stimulate Haematopoiesis
- The Role of Chemokines in Infectious Diseases
- Cytokine Related Diseases
- Functions of Cytokines
- Cytokines that Mediate Innate Immunity
- Cytokines that Regulate Lymphocyte Activation, Growth and Differentiation
- Cytokines that Regulate Immune Mediated Inflammation

Cytokines are a group of chemical messengers of low molecular weight, proteinacious substances, secreted by white blood cells and variety of other cells in the body in response to various kinds of inducing stimuli. Cytokines serve as messengers of immune system just as hormones serve as messengers of endocrine system. Only the difference between the two is that, hormones act far away from their site of production, whereas cytokines act locally. Like hormones, cytokines bind to specific receptor on the target cell membrane and induce signal transduction that ultimately results in triggering gene expression in target cells. A cytokine secreted by a particular cell when it binds to the receptor of the same cell and induces stimulation of that particular cell is called **autocrine**. If the cytokine secreted by a particular cell acts on a target cell in the immediate vicinity, than it is called **paracrine.** The term cytokine encompasses broad category of protein factors, those secreted by lymphocytes are called **lymphokines,** and those secreted by monocytes and macrophages are called **monokines.** Many of the cytokines secreted by leukocytes are called **interleukins** because; they are secreted by some leukocytes and act upon other leukocytes. There are some low molecular weight cytokines, which are specifically called as **chemokines,** which play an important role in inflammation.

The cytokines produced by T_H subsets have distinct functions. In general, T_H1 derived cytokines promote cell-mediated immune functions, whereas T_H2-derived cytokines primarily elicit a humoral immune response. Thus, differential production of cytokine by activated Tcell subsets *in vivo* has profound effect on the character of the immune response and ultimately on the outcome of infection. Members of each cytokine subset have many cross-regulatory effects on both cytokine production and effector function. For ex. IFN-γ, a T_H1 –derived cytokine, inhibits proliferation of T_H2 cells and blocks T_H2-mediated effector functions such as B cell activation. Conversely, IL-10, a T_H-2 derived cytokine, inhibits expansion of T_H1 cell populations; blocks T_H1 cell cytokine synthesis, and interfere with T_H1 effector functions such as macrophage activation. Depending on the type of infection, the predominance of T_H1 or T_H2 type cytokines expressed can have either a protective or deleterious effect. It is not clear whether T_H1 and T_H2 type responses are due to distinct, developmentally fixed subsets *in vivo*.

GENERAL PROPERTIES OF CYTOKINES

Cytokines are often produced by variety of cells and belong to divers group of proteins and bind to receptors present on numerous cell types, but share number of properties:

1. *Cytokines serve to mediate and regulate immune and inflammatory response during natural and specific immunity.* During the effector phase of natural immunity, microbial products, such as lipopolysaccharides (LPS), directly stimulate macrophages to secrete their cytokines. On the contrary T cell derived cytokines are produced only in response to recognition of foreign antigens. These distinctions are only superficial because the cytokine secreted by one cell may act as regulator of synthesis of another cytokine by other cells.
2. *Cytokine secretion is transient and brief:* Cytokine synthesis each time is initiated by new gene transcription and never preformed and stored as inactive molecules waiting for activation. Such transcriptional activation is usually transient and short-lived mRNAs are produced. Once synthesized, the cytokines are rapidly secreted.
3. *Multiple diverse cell types produce many individual cytokines:* Regardless of the source of their production all of them are grouped under cytokines, even though they are produced by leukocytes, lymphocytes, macrophages or fibroblasts. The cellular source of these molecules is not a distinguishing feature.
4. *Cytokines may show pleiotropism:* Some cytokines may act upon many different cell types bringing about different biological effect in each cell type and this function is referred to as **pleiotropic** action.
5. *Same target cell may show multiple different effects when acted upon by cytokine:* The effects that are shown by the target cell may be simultaneous or may occur over different time frame.
6. *The nature of the target cell for a particular cytokine is determined by the specific membrane receptor born by the target cell:* The receptors for cytokines often show very high affinity with dissociation constant ranging from 10^{-10} to 10^{-12} M.
7. *Cytokines have different biological action on different target cells*: Some cytokines show different biological action on different cells. *Some cytokine actions are redundant:* When cytokines mediate similar functions and share the properties, such cytokines are said to be **redundant.**
8. *Cytokine secreted by one cell may influence the synthesis of another cytokine by other cell:* Some cytokines show cascade effect, where it acts as an enhancer or inhibitor of the production of other cytokine by other cells and provide positive or negative regulatory control.
9. *Cytokines influence the action of other cytokines:* Certain cytokines show **synergism,** where the combined effect of two or more cytokines on cellular activity will be greater than the combined effect of individual cytokines. Some cytokines are **antagonistic**, where the effect of one is opposite of the other.
10. *Many target cells, cytokines act as mitogens:* Certain cytokines act as growth factors and stimulate mitosis of target cell.
11. *Most cellular response to cytokines is signal transduction and gene expression:* Majority of cytokines on binding to the target cell membrane receptor induces signal transduction and initiate gene action.

FUNCTIONS OF CYTOKINES

The functions of cytokines may be grouped into four broad categories.

(1) Stimulators of immature leukocyte growth and differentiation.
(2) Mediators of natural immunity.
(3) Regulators of lymphocyte activation, growth and differentiation.
(4) Regulators of immune-mediated inflammation.

CYTOKINES THAT STIMULATE HAEMATOPOIESIS

Cytokines that are produced during natural immunity and antigen induced specific immune response have strong stimulatory effect on bone marrow stem cells. The entire gamut of leukocyte cell population arouses as a result of progressive division and differentiation of progeny of pluripotent stem cells in the bone marrow. This process is completely dependent on cytokines, which bring about maturation of hematopoietic cells and commit them to a particular lineage by losing the ability to develop into other mature cell types. The cytokine that is responsible for the differentiation and proliferation of bone marrow progenitor cells is called **colony-stimulating factor (CSF).** Different types of CSFs act at different stages of development of bone marrow cells and promote development of cells of different lineage (Fig. 14.1).

Some of the actions of CSFs are influenced by other cytokines such as, tumor necrosis factor (TNF), leukotriene (LT), interferon-γ (IFN-γ), and tissue growth factor β (TGF-β). All of these inhibit growth of bone marrow progenitor cells. Interestingly, the gene clusters for many of CSFs are located on human chromosome 5, including IL-3, GM-CSF, IL-4 and IL-5 have been mapped to the same complex.

c-Kit ligand

The cellular oncogene (c-kit) is known to express a tyrosine kinase transmembane receptor in pluripotent stem cells. The cytokine that interacts with the extracellular portion of this receptor is called **c-kit ligand,** which is also referred to as **stem cell factor.** The extracellular portion of the c-kit receptor is made up of five Ig domains. Stromal cells of the bone marrow as well as, adipocytes synthesize the c-kit ligand. Ffibroblasts and endothelial cells also produce it. It is produced in two forms: a transmembrane 27kD protein and a secreted form of 24 kD and both these types are produced by alternative splicing of the same gene.

Interleukin-3 (IL-3)

It is also called as multilineage colony-stimulating factor (multi-CSF), a product of CD4$^+$ T cells of both T_H1 and T_H2 subsets, with a molecular weight of about 20 to 26 kD and acts on the most immature bone marrow progenitor cells and promotes the expansion of all cell types. Its signal transduction unit is shared with IL-5and GM-CSF. IL-3 is made up of 4 α-helix wound around each other. IL-3 is also known to promote the growth of mast cells derived from bone marrow progenitors. It is observed that many of the actions performed by the murine IL-3 are similar to those performed by human GM-CSF.

Granulocyte-macrophage colony-stimulating factor (GM-CSF)

It is a 22 kD glycoprotein secreted by activated T cells and mononuclear phagocytes, vascular endothelial cells, and fibroblasts. Its receptor is similar to the one for IL-3 and the signal trandsducing unit is also

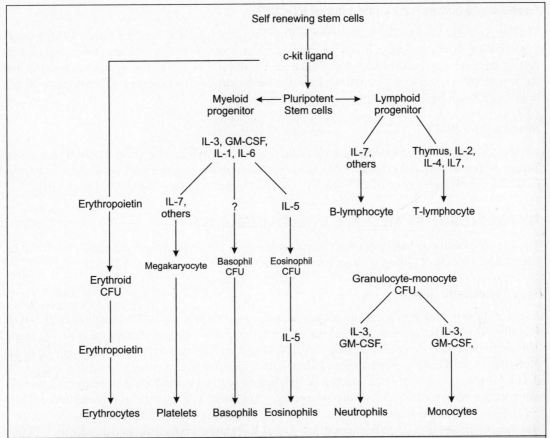

Fig. 14.1   A schematic representation of maturation of blood cells in hematopoietic tissue of bone marrow. CFU = colony forming unit.

similar to the one for IL-3. In mice GM-CSF acts primarily on already committed bone marrow progenitors that develop into leukocytes, therefore presumably acts on more differentiated population of leukocytes as compared to IL-3. In humans, GM-CSF is known to act on non-committed form of leukocytes as well as platelet cells and red blood cells. It mimics the action of IFN-γ and acts as an activator of macrophages. Unlike other cytokines, GM-CSF is not detected in circulation. Therefore, its action is mostly local, i.e. bone marrow or at the site of inflammation by mononuclear phagocytes, vascular endothelial cells and fibroblasts.

Monocyte-macrophage colony-stimulating factor (M-CSF)

It is also called CSF-1, secreted by macrophages, endothelial cells and fibroblasts. The secreted polypeptide is approximately 40 kD and results in a dimer. The receptor of M-CSF resembles that of c-kit and produced by normal cellular counter part of viral oncogene *v*-fms. M-CSF acts on progenitors that are already committed to develop into monocytes, which are mature than those acted upon by GM-CSF. It is not detected in circulation like GM-CSF. Therefore, its action is mostly local in the bone marrow.

Granulocyte colony-stimulating factor (G-CSF)

The same cells that produce GM-CSF secrete it. The secreted polypeptide is approximately 19 kD belongs to 4 α-helical cytokine family. It acts on progenitors of bone marrow, which are mature and already committed to develop into granulocytes. Unlike other CSFs, it is known to circulate and known to bring about neutrophil maturation and release from the bone marrow during severe inflammatory reaction occurring outside the bone marrow.

Interleukin-7 (IL-7)

It is secreted by marrow stromal cells and acts on hematopoietic progenitors committed to the B lymphocyte lineage. Recent *in vitro* studies indicate that IL-7 may also stimulate the growth and maturation of immature $CD4^-CD8^-$ T cell precursors in the thymus but the cellular source of IL-7 in thymus is not known.

CYTOKINES THAT MEDIATE INNATE IMMUNITY

This class of cytokine includes those that protect against viral infection and those that initiate inflammatory reactions as a means of protection from bacterial infection.

Type I Interferon (IFN)

It consists of two serologically distinct groups of proteins named as α and β. The interferon α (IFN-α) is a family of 20 structurally related polypeptides of 18 kD and each encoded by a separate gene. The major cell source of production of IFN-α is mononuclear phagocyte. IFN-β is a single gene product of 20 kD glycoprotein and the cell source is cultured fibroblasts. Other than this, many cells make IFN-α and IFN-β and the most potent signal that induces the production of these interferons is during viral infection. Mononuclear phagocytes on stimulation with antigen stimulated T cells produce both interferons. There is hardly any structural similarity between IFN-α and IFN-β, but both bind to same cell surface receptor and induce similar series of cellular responses. Type I IFN shows 4 principal biologic actions:

1. *Inhibits viral replication:*   IFN induces the cells to produce number of enzymes, one among them is 2'→5' oligoadenylate synthetase. This enzyme interferes with the replication of viral DNA and RNA. IFNs action is paracrine, i.e. virally infected cell produces IFN, which renders protection to neighboring cells not yet infected, and thereby inducing the non infected cells to attain antiviral state.

2. *Inhibits cell proliferation:*   It may prevent certain amino acid synthesis, such as essential amino acids like tryptophan. Since it is known to interfere with DNA synthesis, it is used as antitumor agent in certain tumors like hairy cell leukemia and child hood hemangiomas. IFN-β inhibits normal cell growth.

3. *Increases the lytic potential of natural killer (NK) cells:*   NK cells help in killing virally infected cells (Chapter 13) and this ability is enhanced by IFNs.

4. *It is known to modulate MHC molecular expression:*   In general, IFN increases the expression of class I MHC molecules on virally infected cells and significantly inhibits class II MHC molecule expression. IFN boosts the effector phase of cell-mediated immune response by enhancing the efficiency of cytotoxic T lymphocytes (CTLs). At the same time IFN may also prevent activation of class II MHC-restricted helper T cells, thereby preventing the elaboration of other arm of cell mediated immune response.

Tumor necrosis factor (TNF)

It is the principal mediator of host response to Gram-ve bacterial LPS (lipopolysaccharide) or endotoxin. The major cellular source of TNF is the LPS activated mononuclear phagocytes as well as activated T cells, NK cells and activated mast cells can also secrete TNF. INF-γ produced by activated T cells is known to augment the synthesis of TNF by mononuclear phagocytes. Therefore, TNF is considered to be a mediator of natural and acquired immune response. TNF receptors are present on almost all cell types examined. The biologic action of TNF is concentration dependent. At low concentration (10^{-9} M), TNF acts locally as paracrine and autocrine regulator of leukocytes and endothelial cells. Some of the biological actions, which are critical for inflammatory response to microbes shown by TNF at low concentration are as follows:

1. Expression of adhesion molecules on the vascular endothelial cell surface so that the cell surface becomes adhesive for leukocytes. TNF also acts on neutrophils to enhance their adhesiveness for endothelial cells. This property contributes to accumulation of leukocytes at the site of inflammation.
2. TNF activates neutrophils, eosinophils and mononuclear phagocytes and increases their ability to kill microbes that cause inflammation.
3. Stimulates mononuclear phagocytes to produce cytokines such as, IL-1, IL-6, TNF itself and chemokines.
4. TNF augments expression of class I MHC molecules and exerts protective effect on cells like IFN and potentiates CTL-mediated lysis of virally infected cells.

The systemic action of TNF as means of host responses to infection are as follows:

1. TNF shares the property with IL-1 and acts as pyrogen that acts on hypothalamic thermoregulatory centers and induces fever. Fever production is due to enhanced synthesis of prostaglandins by hypothalamic cells as a result of TNF and IL-1 stimulation. Therefore, prostaglandin inhibitors, such as acetaminophen, paracetamol, aspirin cause reduction in fever.
2. IL-1 and IL-6 secretion as a cascade event by the mononuclear phagocytes is induced by TNF.
3. Serum amyloid A protein by hepatocytes is enhanced by TNF. Acute phase response to inflammatory stimuli is because of IL-6 and IL-1 or TNF induced combination of hepatocyte-derived plasma proteins.
4. The delicate balance between anticoagulant and procoagulant activities of vascular endothelium is altered by TNF.
5. TNF is a strong inhibitor of bone marrow stem cell division. Therefore, chronic administration of TNF may lead to lymphopenia or immunodeficiency. Hence TNF therapy for cancer patients has not become popular.

Lethal effects of TNF at extremely high concentrations can be listed as follows:

1. It causes intravascular thrombosis, due to activation of neutrophils, which plug the vascular passages and altered balance between coagulation and anticoagulation.
2. TNF may act directly or indirectly through prostacyclin and NO produced by endothelial cells on smooth muscles and bring about relaxation of vascular smooth muscle tone thereby reducing the blood pressure.
3. TNF depresses myocardial contractility through the involvement of enzymes such as nitric oxide synthase (NOS) in cardiac myocytes, that produces NO, which inhibits myocardial contractility.
4. TNF causes hypoglycemia by over utilization of blood glucose by muscle cells.

Many of the biologic action of TNF are enhanced by IFN-γ leading to systemic toxicity.

Interleukin-1 (IL-1)

The major source of IL-1 is the activated mononuclear phagocytes and it is the principal mediator of the host inflammatory response in natural immunity. IL-1 is also made by diverse cells types such epithelial and endothelial cells, providing local source of IL-1 in the absence of macrophage infiltrates. During Gram-ve bacterial sepsis, IL-1 can be found in circulation and it acts as endocrine hormone in such situation. There are two different membrane receptors for IL-1, both of which are members of the Ig superfamily. Type I receptor characterized from T cells has higher affinity to IL-1β and the type II receptor characterized from B cells has greater affinity for IL-1α.

The biologic effects of IL-1 are concentration dependent like TNF. At low concentration, IL-1:

1. Induces the synthesis of IL-6 and IL-1 by vascular endothelial cells and mononuclear phagocytes.
2. Acts as mediator of local inflammation.
3. Acts on local endothelial cells to promote coagulation and induces secretion of adhesion molecules on endothelial cell surface to mediate leukocyte adhesion.
4. Causes mononuclear phagocytes and endothelial cells to synthesize chemokines that acts as activators of leukocytes.

The biological effects of IL-1 at high concentration:

1. Exerts endocrine effect and causes fever.
2. Induces synthesis of amyloid A protein by hepatocytes and initiates metabolic wasting or cachexia.
3. Potentiates the tissue injury caused by TNF but by itself it is not lethal.

IL-1 does not share with TNF an ability to increase expression of class I MHC molecules. IL-1 potentiates rather than suppress the action of CSFs on bone marrow.

Interleukin-6 (IL-6)

Mononuclear phagocytes, vascular endothelial cells, fibroblasts and other cells in response to IL-1 synthesize it. IL-6 can be detected in blood circulation following Gram-ve bacterial infection. Some activated T cells also synthesize it. Target cells of IL-6 are hepatocytes and B cells. IL-6 induces hepatocytes to produce certain acute phase proteins like fibrinogen. IL-6 serves as a growth factor for activated B cells late in the sequence of B cell differentiation. It is also secreted by many malignant plasma cells like plasmacytomas or myelomas and act as autocrine growth factor. *In vitro* experiments suggest that IL-6 may serve as co-stimulator of T cells and thymocytes. IL-6 also acts as growth factor of early hematopoietic stem cells of bone marrow.

Chemokines

In recent years, the components of host immunity critical to the early response to infection have been identified and the integration and co-ordination of these components has been worked out in greater detail. Central to the development of an organized host cellular response to infection is the recruitment of immune effector cells such as, neutrophils, monocytes and lymphocytes to the sites of infection. A large number of signaling molecules, which have come to be known as chemokines (chemoattractant cytokines) have been identified as key molecules in recruiting immune cells.

Classification of chemokines

The number and position of the cystein amino-terminal residues have classified Chemokines into three major groups. In general, the chemokines are composed of small protein monomers of 7-10 kD that bind the basic molecule heparin. The CXC family of chemokines has its first two terminal cystein residues separated by a non-conserved amino acid designated as X. The CC family has its two terminal cysteines without separation, and the C family, of which there has been only one member identified to date (lymphotactin), has only single terminal cystein residue. The members of the various chemokine families are shown in Table 14.1.

In general, members of the CXC family are responsible for chemotaxis of neutrophils but nor monocytes, and the CC chemokines are responsible for attracting monocytes and lymphocytes, and to lesser extent basophils and eosinophils, but not neutrophils. The C chemokine, as its name implies, primarily recruits lymphocytes. Interestingly enough, the genes for the CXC chemokines are clustered on chromosome 4, the genes for CC family are found on chromosome 17, and the lymphotactin gene is found on chromosome1. This clustering pattern suggests that the chemokines, within their families, evolved together, whereas the different families evolved separately. There is 20-40% amino acid homology among the various members of the chemokine families.

Table 14.1 Classification of chemokines

Chemokine families	Chemoattractant for
CXC chemokines	**Neutrophils**
IL-8	
Epithelial neutrophil activating protein-78 (ENA-78)	
Growth-related oncogenes α, β, γ (GRO-α,β, γ)	
Granulocyte chemotactic protein-2 (GCP-2)	
Platelet basic protein	
Platelet factor-4	
IFN-γ inducible protein (IP-10)	
Monokine induced by IFN-γ (MIG)	
CC chemokines	**Monocytes, Lymphocytes**
Monocyte chemotactic protein-1, 2, 3, (MCP-1, 2, 3) (basophils, eosinophils)	
Macrophage inflammatory protein 1α, β(MIP-1α, β)	
Regulated on activation normal T cell expressed and secreted (RANTES)	
Eotaxin	
C chemokine	**Lymphotactin**
Lymphocytes	

Source: Schluger, N. W. and Rom, W. N. Curr. Opin. Immunol. 9: 504-508 (1997).

The presence of different cell types in immune response is associated with severe inflammation and tissue destruction and pus formation, usually in a very short period of time. This type of reaction is characteristically associated with bacterial pathogens through the production of CXC chemokines, such as IL-8. IL-8 production is stimulated in response to infection with *Mycobacterium tuberculosis*. The early response to mycobacterial infections such as tuberculosis is also characterized by the recruitment of macrophages. These phagocytic cells engulf the foreign pathogens and become nidus for ganuloma formation, the inflammatory hallmark of mycobacterial disease. These phagocytes also serve as professional antigen presenting cells, which in turn can recruit lymphocytes, which are the other lymphocytes of tissue granulomas. Mycobacterium is capable of stimulating the production of chemokines such as monocyte chemotactic protein (MCP) or macrophage inflammatory protein (MIP).

The Role of Chemokines in Infectious Diseases

Bacterial infections

Several different bacterial pathogens have been shown to be potent inducers of chemokines of various classes, and the level of chemokine produced seem to be affected by the particular strain and species of bacteria and the bacterial component tested as a stimulant. In general acute bacterial infections, such as *Streptococcus pneumoniae*, are characterized by the predominance of neutrophils in the inflammatory reaction, so that the CXC family of chemokines are likely to play a major role in this type of immune response. Other bacterial pathogens which are associated with more sub acute or chronic types of processes involving mononuclear phagocytes and lymphocytes, for ex. *Borrelia burgdorferi*, the pathogen of Lyme disease might be expected to lead to the production of the CC or C classes of chemokines.

Several important bacterial pathogens have been shown to stimulate chemokine production in experimental systems. *Escherichia coli, Pseudomonas aeruginosa and Staphylococcus aureus*, all often associated with severe acute illness and neutrophil recruitment, can stimulate IL-8 production in experimental systems. Peripheral blood mononuclear cells exposed to *Candida albicans, Porphyromonas gingivalis and Actinobacillus actinomycetemcomitans* produced high levels of both MCP-1 and IL-8, whereas *Streptococcus mutans* induced mainly IL-8. In addition, a role of chemokines in the development of the immune response in other organ systems has been shown. Elderly patients with lower respiratory tract bacterial infections demonstrate elevated levels of IL-8 in their sputum and this correlates with both the presence of bacteria in the sputum and also the presence, and amount of neutrophils in the sputum. These bacterial pathogens include *Pseudomonas aeruginosa*. Other chemokines involved in lung inflammation include GRO (growth related oncogene) family. In a rabbit model of lung inflammation, both heat killed *S. aureus* and LPS were able to stimulate the expression of GRO genes as well as the release of GRO from alveolar macrophages in the immune response to these exogenous stimuli. Endogenous stimuli such as tumor necrosis factor-α also caused GRO expression and release.

Many potent pathological bacterial species, such as *Yersinia, Clostridium, Bacteroids* and others are able to cause potent chemokine expression, primarily of the CXC family. In an interesting human study, it has been demonstrated that the gastric levels of IL-8 correlate with the clinical presence and degree of gastritis, which in turn has been strongly associated with infection with *Helicobacter pylori*.

An important aspect of our understanding of the complex nature of the cellular immune response to infections involve the divergence of T helper (T_H) lymphocytes into T_H1 and T_H2 cells. T_H1 cells secrete IFN-γ and IL-2, whereas T_H2 cells predominantly secrete IL-4, IL-5, and IL-10. Various clinical manifestations of disease have been associated with either T_H1 or T_H2 immune response. Lepromatous leprosy lesions, typically necrotic and teeming with bacilli, are composed largely of T_H2 lymphocytes, whereas tuberculoid leprosy lesions, typically more well circumscribed and containing few bacilli, are composed of T_H1 lymphocytes.

Viral infections

A great deal of attention has been focused on the production of chemokines in response to infections both with common respiratory viruses and HIV-1. These CC chemokines are produced both by $CD4^+$ and $CD8^+$ T cells of patients with HIV infection.

CYTOKINES THAT REGULATE LYMPHOCYTE ACTIVATION, GROWTH AND DIFFERENTIATION

The cytokines that act primarily to regulate lymphocytes themselves are IL-2, IL-4 and transforming growth factor-β (TGF-β). The properties of these cytokines are discussed below.

Interleukin-2 (IL-2)

Originally it was called as T cell growth factor (TCGF). It is the major cytokine that stimulates T lymphocyte progression from G1 to s phase of cell cycle. It is produced by $CD4^+$ T cells and to some extent by $CD8^+$ cells also. It acts as an autocrine factor for $CD4^+$ T cells that produce it and on to those nearby, including $CD4^+$ and $CD8^+$ cells, and is also therefore acts as paracrine factor. The gene for IL-2 is situated on chromosome 4 in humans and the secreted IL-2 is 14 to 17 kD glycoprotein. Il-2 is transcribed, synthesized and secreted by T cells only upon activation by antigens and its synthesis is transient, with an early peak of secretion occurring about 4 hours after activation. IL-2 is also known to stimulate the synthesis of other T cell-derived cytokines such as IFN-γ and lymphotoxin (LT). It has been experimentally proved that failure to synthesize adequate quantities of IL-2 results in antigen specific T cell anergy.

IL-2 stimulates the growth of NK cells and enhances their cytolytic function, there by transforming them into lymphokine activated killer (LAK) cells. IL-2 acts as a synergist with IL-12 to induce IFN-γ secretion by NK cells. IL-2 acts as B cell growth factor and stimulates antibody synthesis (Fig. 14.2).

Interleukin-4 (IL-4)

IL-4 has been called the "prototypic immunoregulatory cytokine". Like many cytokines, it can affect a variety of target cells in multiple ways. However, IL-4 has a unique and important role in regulating antibody production, hematopoiesis, inflammation, and development of effector T-cell responses. Dysregulated expression of IL-4 has been implicated in allergy, autocrine growth of tumors, and susceptibility to some infectious diseases. But it also can play a protective role in immunity to some extracellular parasites, in suppressing autoimmune response and in tumor resistance.

IL-4 is a 20 kD glycoprotein and its biological effects are mediated by high affinity IL-4 receptors. This two-chain receptor is found on most cells of hematopoietic lineage as well as some non-hematopoietic cells. The production of IL-4 is tightly regulated. Only a subset of activated T cells, mast cells, and basophils express easily detectable levels, although recent reports demonstrate that human eosinophils are also a source of IL-4. The single copy of IL-4 gene is located on chromosome 5 in humans and found within the clusters of genes encoding other cytokines like IL-3 and IL-5. Based on the different tissue distribution and access to distinct target cells, Tcell, mast cell, or basophil-derived IL-4 may have quite different effects on immunological processes.

Principal functions of IL-4 can be listed as follows:

1. *B cell activation/differentiation factor:* It is called B cell growth factor. IL-4 induces expression of several cell surface molecules, including class II MHC molecules, CD23 (the low affinity Fcε

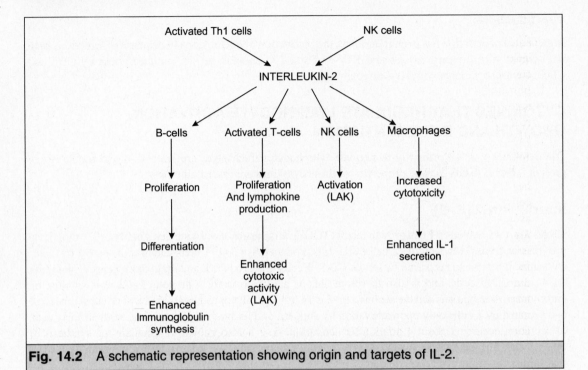

Fig. 14.2 A schematic representation showing origin and targets of IL-2.

receptor). It regulates apoptosis in both normal and transformed B cells. It regulates isotype switching, particularly IgG1 and IgE.

2. *IL-4 influences Cell differentiation:* IL-4 plays a key role in hematopoiesis by stimulating colony formation by precursors of erythroid cells, megakaryocytes, mast cells, and cells of the granulocyte/macrophage lineage. It also has inhibitory effects on progenitor cell growth, suggesting a regulatory function. IL-4 induces myeloid cell progenitor and mast cell expression of c-kit, the receptor for the hematopoietic growth factor, stem cell factor (SCF). IL-4 is critical for the development of a subset of IL-4 producing CD4[+] T helper cells, and can also influence development of CD8[+] effector cells that produce IL-4. IL-4 has co-stimulatory activity for early thymocyte population. Depending on experimental system, IL-4 can enhance, or inhibit T cell cytolytic activity.

3. *IL-4 affects cells that contribute to the inflammatory response:* Many of the activities of IL-4 indicate that it is a major contributor to late phase inflammatory reactions. It induces mitosis in endothelial cells as well as expression of a cell surface VCAM-1 like adhesion molecule. This molecule causes an increase in lymphocyte, eosinophil, and basophil adhesion to the endothelium that results in transendothelial migration to local inflammatory sites. IL-4 also modulates cytokine production by endothelial cells and monocytes as well as the phagocytic activity of neutrophils. It is a chemotactic factor for eosinophils, and induces expression of the low affinity IgE receptor on these cells. Additional effects of IL-4 on immune cells recruited for inflammation include the activation of monocyte and T cell cytotoxicity and an increase in monocyte C2 production.

4. *IL-4 plays a central role in the development of allergic response:* An immediate type hypersensitivity response occurs when mast cells are activated by cross-linking of their high affinity Fcε receptor. Mast cells have long been appreciated as the pivotal effector cell in these types

of responses due to the activation dependent release of number of pharmacological mediators, such as histamine. IL-4 produced by mast cells can signal B cells to induce Cε switching and thus directly influence the activation-state of the cells by promoting IgE production. Mast cells themselves may contribute to this process through their ability to mediate contact-dependent help for B cells. Immunoglobulin isotype switching is thought to occur primarily in the germinal centers of lymph nodes where the contact-dependent interactions between T and B cells can occur. IgE production requires at least two signals: one delivered by IL-4 through interaction with the IL-4 receptor, and another cell contact-dependent signal delivered via interaction of CD40 on B cells with CD40L on the surface of T cells.

In humans, high levels of IL-4 are associated with allergic diseases such as atopic dermatitis and hay fever. In these diseases, which are characterized by high IgE titers and high numbers of mast cells, local IL-4 production may be influenced primarily by resident skin or pulmonary mast cells as well as recruited T cells.

5. *Role of IL-4 in Tumor immunity:* IL-4 is also known to play important role in anti-tumor immunity. It influences the activity of lymphokine activated killer (LAK) cells and natural killer (NK) cells and increase the tumoricidal activity of macrophages. In a study direct injection of IL-4 into region of draining lymph nodes in tumor bearing mice induced a potent anti-tumor response. At present, human clinical trials to test the efficacy of IL-4 immunotherapy in a variety of human tumors such as melanoma have yielded encouraging results. In contrast to its effect IL-4 has been implicated as an autocrine growth factor for mast cell and B cell tumors in mice and in human T cell leukemia's. These cells exhibit dysregulated, high constitutive production of IL-4 and, in some cases, proliferate in response to this cytokine. IL-4 also influences the growth of endothelial cells that are involved in angiogenesis, a process essential for the establishment of some tumors. This provides another mechanism by which IL-4 can indirectly influence tumor survival.

6. *Regulation of immune response to infectious and autoimmune diseases by IL-4:* It has been proposed that IL-4 and other cytokine, such as IL-10, provide an anti-inflammatory function and limit tissue damage in immune responses to microbes and autoimmunity by inhibiting prolonged T cell activation. The ability of IL-4 to convert cytotoxic T cells to IL-4 producing, noncytolytic cells and to inhibit IFN-γ, a cytokine that activates macrophage function, supports this idea. *In vivo* studies have confirmed that IL-4 has both positive and negative effects on infectious diseases outcome. Fr. Ex. IL-4 induces protective IgE response to *Nippostrongylus brasiliensis* infection. In contrast, in progressive leishmaniasis, IL-4 inhibits the protective T cell response. IL-4 has clearly been shown to inhibit the monocyte production of inflammatory mediators such as IL-1, TNF-α and PGE2.

The progression of acquired immunodeficiency syndrome (AIDS) is associated with an increase in the ability of stimulated T cells to produce IL-4. IL-4 can induce a switch of the CD8$^+$ effector cells to noncytotoxic cytokine producing cells that are thus unable to carry out elimination of virally infected cells (Fig.14.3).

Cells that produce IL-4

CD4$^+$ T cells: IL-4 is considered the hallmark of the cytokines selectively produced in a TH2 type immune response and plays a central role in the regulation of the type of TH response that develops. It has been demonstrated both *in vitro* and *in vivo* that exposure of naïve CD4$^+$ cells to IL-4 during initial exposure to antigen directs the development of the TH2 cell population. Thus IL-4 plays an important role, either directly or indirectly, in regulating its own synthesis.

A population of IL-4 producing CD4$^+$ γδ$^+$ T cells were identified in mice infected with either *Listeria monocytogenes or Nippostrongylus brasiliensis.* These cells produce a polarized cytokine response similar to a conventional protective CD4$^+$ αβ$^+$ TH response. The nature of the response was dependent on the infectious agent: IL-4 response predominated in *Nippostrongylus* infected mice, and IFN-γ response prevailed in *Listeria* infections, where a cell mediated response is more beneficial. During the first 13 days after primary infection, the synthesis of IL-4 by these cells was essentially limited to this γδ$^+$ population. Thus, γδ$^+$ T cells may also be classified into distinct subsets based on cytokine production, and can be a source of IL-4 early in infection that helps to amplify a TH2 response (Fig. 14.3).

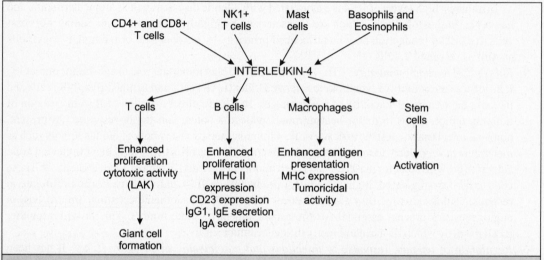

Fig. 14.3   A schematic representation showing origin and targets of interleukin-4 (IL-4).

CD8$^+$ T cells: IL-4 production by CD8$^+$ cells appears to be dependent on the differentiation state of the cells and the stimulation conditions used to activate the cells. Some activated human CD8$^+$ T cell clones express both IL-4 and IFN-γ, suggests a THO like cytokine profile. Included among these are T cell clones derived from leprosy patients with Lepromatous but not the tuberculoid form of the disease.

NK1$^+$ T cells: Recently, subset of T cells was described that may play a role in the initiation of IL-4 production by TH and TC subsets. They are distinguished by the cell surface expression of receptors first identified on NK cells and are referred to as NK1$^+$ T cells. NK1$^+$ cells are often CD8$^-$ and CD4$^-$, but a CD4 single positive population of cells has also been described. This population was first identified in experiments showing that spleen cells from mice primed with α-CD3 antibody injection produced significant levels of IL-4 without subsequent priming or a source of exogenous IL-4. NK1.1$^+$ CD4$^+$ cells also appear to be responsible for IL-4 independent IL-4 production in the thymus and bone marrow. Injection of staphylococcus enterotoxin B induces IL-4 production by these cells, indicating that superantigens can initiate this prompt response.

It has been proposed that IL-4 production by NK1.1$^+$T cells plays a crucial role in the initiation of TH2 response as well as IgE production. The NK1$^+$ T cell population, via stimulation through the TCR, is the only T cell type that has been shown to produce high levels of IL-4 without prior antigen priming and is most likely an initial front line producer of IL-4 (Fig. 14.3).

FcεRI⁺ cells: Mast cells and basophils are best known for their role as the critical effector cells in IgE-dependent immediate-type hypersensitivity reactions. However, it is now clear that these cells are an important source of several cytokines. Interestingly, the profile of cytokine produced by both types of cells resembles that of TH2 cells. This discovery has broadened the view of the role these cells in regulating the inflammatory response. Both mast cells and basophils are stimulated to produce IL-4 via cross-linkage of the high affinity IgE receptor, an event that also induces release of a number of other mediators, including histamine.

Mast cells

Mast cells constitutively produce IL-4 at low levels and store it in secretory granules. FcεRI-mediated activation of cells results in increased production as well as release of preformed stores of IL-4. The released IL-4 may be associated with cell membrane in some cells, protecting it from digestion by chymase released from the granules. Membrane-associated IL-4 may also limit the access of functional IL-4 to cells that are in close contact with the mast cell, resulting in highly localized response (Fig. 14.3).

Basophils

The expression of IL-4 in basophils was first described in a population of non-B non-T cells from spleen and bone marrow. These cells were found to be FcεRI⁺ and have the morphological characteristics of basophils. In addition, they produce very large amounts of IL-4 when compared with the mast cell lines studied, and express IL-4 when stimulated through FcγRII as well as FcεRI.

IL-4 has also been detected in peripheral blood basophils. Although mast cells have fixed tissue localization, basophils circulate, are recruited to sites of active inflammatory reactions, and are involved in the late phase inflammatory responses. Therefore, in addition to their other inflammatory functions, basophils are likely to be involved in maintaining the TH2 type response in late phase reaction (Fig. 14.3).

Eosinophils

Eosinophils are recruited to sites of allergic and inflammatory reactions and are critical mediators of these responses. Eosinophils appear subsequent to the appearance of basophils but are a dominant polymorphic leukocyte in these reactions. Recently it was discovered that eosinophils have the capability to produce, store, and secrete IL-4. As in mast cells IL-4 is stored in cytoplasmic granules. It has previously been demonstrated that eosinophils express FcεRIIb, the low affinity IgE receptor and Fcγ receptors. Analogous to basophils, eosinophils are implicated in the support of inflammatory responses, and may do so by maintaining a TH2 like cytokine environment by providing an additional source of IL-4 (Fig. 14.3).

Transforming growth factor-β (TGF-β)

It is a 25 kD disulfide linked glycoprotein homodimer that plays a crucial role in embryonic development, tumorigenesis, wound healing, fibrosis and immuneregulation. It was first identified as a product of virally transformed malignant cells. At present it is well known that TGF-β is produced by platelets, activated macrophages, B cells and T cells. TGF-β is synthesized in an inactive form and is activated by proteases before it binds to the receptor. TGF-β exists in many isoforms and each form has its own receptor, with varied biological potency. TGF-β acts as both stimulatory as well as inhibitory molecule. It is stimulatory to fibroblast, monocyte and neutrophil chemotaxis; it stimulates monocyte IL-1 and

TNF-α secretion and enhances helper T cell function. It has inhibitory effects on IL-1R expression, respiratory burst, and cytotoxic effects of activated macrophages. It also inhibits monocyte and T cell, and B cell differentiation. It inhibits immune function in chronic inflammatory reactions. Other inhibitory effects of TGF-β include IFN-γ production by T cells, cmyc and GM-CSF gene transcription, IL-2R, class II MHC expression, cytotoxic T cell development, LAK production, NK cell production and TNF-α production (Fig. 14.4).

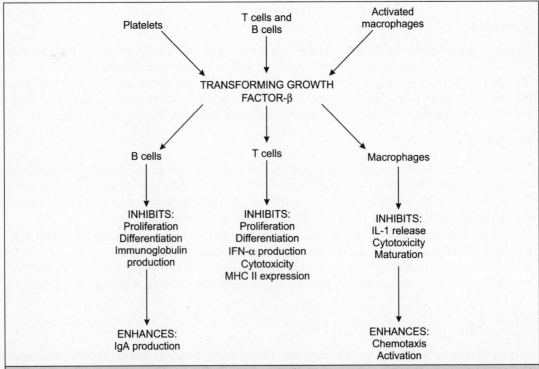

Fig. 14.4 A schematic representation showing the origin and targets of transforming growth factor-β.

B cells stimulated by IL-2 are inhibited by TGF-β. Therefore, it blocks light chain IgG1 and IgM production as well as terminal differentiation of B cells. It causes lipopolysaccharide-stimulated lymphocytes to express IgA and enhances the heavy chain switching to IgA. IL-5 is known to act as synergist of TGF-β and promote IgA response. Although TGF-β is largely a negative regulator, it may promote some positive reactions in the host to prevent chronic inflammation and promote healing. It is a chemoattractant of fibroblasts, regulates their growth, and upregulates the production of collagen as well as fibronectin. It acts on neutrophils to inhibit adherence to endothelial cells, thereby decreasing the intensity of inflammatory reaction.

CYTOKINES THAT REGULATE IMMUNE MEDIATED INFLAMMATION

In this category, cytokines derived from antigen activated CD4$^+$ and CD8$^+$ T cells. They primarily serve to activate the functions of nonspecific effector cells hence they play key role in the effector phase of cell-mediated immune response. Cytokines involved in this section are described below:

Interferon-γ (IFN-γ)

It is referred to as type II interferon, a homodimeric glycoprotein of 21 to 24 kD subunits. Each subunit is made up of 18 kD polypeptide of identical nature but due to glycosylation, size variation occurs. Production of IFN-γ is initiated by the antigen and is enhanced by IL-2 and IL-12. It is produced by both naïve (T_H0) and T_H1 CD4$^+$ helper T cells and nearly all CD8$^+$ T cells. It is also produced in large quantity by NK cells in T cells deficient mice (nude mice) (Fig. 14.5).

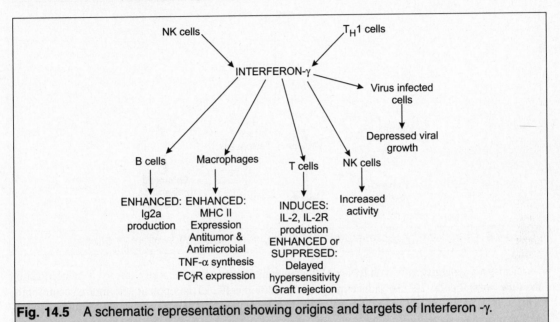

Fig. 14.5   A schematic representation showing origins and targets of Interferon -γ.

IFN-γ is antiproliferative and antiviral. It induces antiviral state in healthy cells like type I IFN. It differs from Type I IFN in several properties, because it mainly serves in immunoregulation. Some of the properties of IFN-γ are listed below.

1. It is potent activator of macrophages. It facilitates killing of microbes in phagosomes of macrophages by enhancing respiratory burst. It is also known to induce macrophages to kill tumor cells. Therefore, IFN-γ is also called macrophage activation factor (MAF)

2. IFN-γ increases class I MHC molecule expression. It is also known to enhance class II MHC expression by wide variety of cells.

3. It promotes differentiation of naive CD4$^+$ T cells to T_H1 subset and inhibits the proliferation of T_H1 cells. Maturation of CD8$^+$ T cells (CTLs) is also facilitated by IFN-γ. By acting on B cells, it inhibits class switching to IgG1 and IgE.

4. It enhances the cytolytic activity of NK cells.

5. Promoted CD4$^+$ T cell lymphocyte adhesion and morphologic alteration in the blood vessels, thereby promoting extravasation.

6. It activated neutrophils and enhances respiratory burst in them to facilitate killing of microbes in phagosomes.

Lymphotoxin (LT)

It has 30% homology to TNF-β and competes with it for binding to the same cell surface receptors. It is a glycoprotein of approximately 21 to 25 kD produced by activated CD4$^+$ and CD8$^+$ T cells. In humans LT and TNF genes are located on chromosome 6 in tandem. Normal B cells do not produce it but cultures B cell lines are known to produce it. It is found in both free and cell membrane bound form (Fig. 14.6).

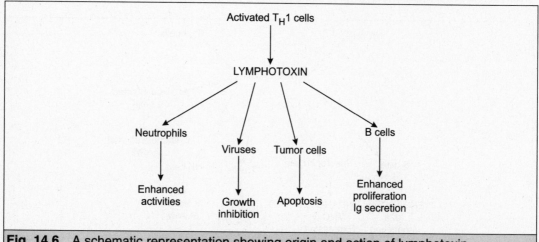

Fig. 14.6   A schematic representation showing origin and action of lymphotoxin.

LT may act synergistically with IFN-γ. Malignant transformed cells are more prone to LT induced killing than the normal cells. LT can induce apoptosis in certain cells. LT is a potent activator of neutrophils, which gives added advantage to them for inflammatory reaction. LT activates vascular endothelial cells, which promotes secretion of adhesion molecules and vascular adhesion of cells and extravasation of cells.

Interleukin-5 (IL-5)

It is a 45 kD homodimeric glycoprotein produced by T$_H$2 subset of CD4+ T cells and by activated mast cells. It enhances IgA production by B cells precommitted to IgA synthesis and makes them differentiate into IgA producing plasma cells. It also induces the appearance of the homing receptor CD44 on the surface of activated B cells, suggesting that it has a role in lymphocyte trafficking (Fig. 14.7).

IL-5 acts synergistically with IL-2 to induce cytotoxic T cell activity. It acts as an eosipnophil chemotactic factor and promotes differentiation of precursors of eosinophils in bone marrow.

Interleukin-10 (IL-10)

It is an immunosuppressive glycoprotein of 19 to 21 kD, secreted by TH2 subset of CD4$^+$ T cells, some B cells, as well as by activated macrophages. IL-10 acts on activated macrophages to suppress their secretion of IL-1, IL-12, TNF-α and free radicals of oxygen. It stimulates the production of IL-1RA by macrophages and down regulates the production of MHC class II thereby affecting their antigen presenting ability. IL-10 supports mast cell proliferation by acting synergistically with IL-3 and IL-4. It has a inhibitory effect on

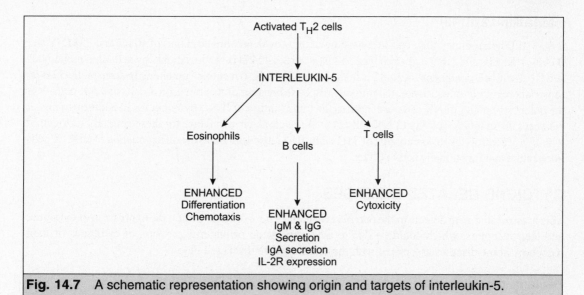

Fig. 14.7   A schematic representation showing origin and targets of interleukin-5.

the production of IL-2 and IFN-γ by T_H2 cells. It also acts as potent stimulator of activated B cells, inducing MHC class II expression and promoting growth (Fig. 14.8).

In humans IL-10 is produced by both TH1 and TH2 cells and downregulates both cell types. As a result it inhibits, IL-4-induced IgE synthesis.

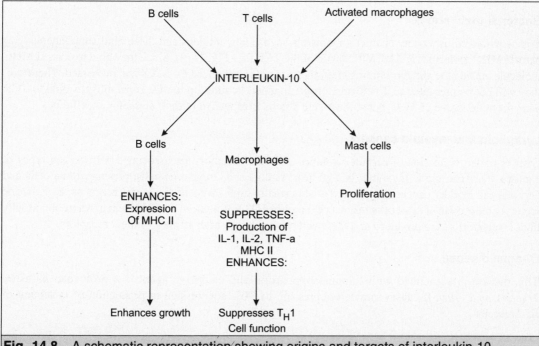

Fig. 14.8   A schematic representation showing origins and targets of interleukin-10.

Interleukin-12 (IL-12)

It is a 70 kD heterodimer polypeptide consisting of two covalently linked chains of 40 kD and 35 kD. T and B cells, NK cells and monocytes produce 35 kD, whereas 40 kD is produced only by activated monocytes and B cells. 40 kD component of IL-12 is homologous to the IL-6 receptor containing Ig domain. IL-12 is an important regulator of cell-mediated immune response because of its effects on T cells and NK cells. It is the potent stimulator of NK cells and induces the transcription of IFN-γ by NK cells. In addition to this, it enhances the cytolytic activity of NK cells as well as acts as growth factor for these cells. IL-12 together with IFN-g controls the differentiation of TH1 cells. IL-12 also stimulates the differentiation of CD8$^+$ T cells into mature and functionally active CTLs.

CYTOKINE RELATED DISEASES

This is associated with defects in the complex regulatory networks governing the expression of cytokines and their receptors, which could be due to over expression or under expression of cytokines or their receptors. Some diseases associated with these features are discussed below.

Bacterial septic shock

This occurs due to overproduction of cytokine during bacterial infection. This condition may develop within few hours following infection by certain gram-negative bacteria such as *E. coli, Klebsiella pneumoniae, Nesseria meningitidis, Pseudomonas aeruginosa and Enterobacter aerogenes.* The symptoms of septic shock include drop in blood pressure, diarrhea, fever and hemorrhagic blood clotting in various organs. The reason for septic shock is bacterial endotoxins stimulate macrophage to over produce IL-1 and TNF-α.

Bacterial toxic shock

Toxins produced by variety of microorganism's act as superantigens and these bind simultaneously to class II MHC molecules and the Vβ domain of the TCR (see Fig. 11. 9). Since they bind to class II MHC molecule outside the antigen-binding cleft, they are not internalized by APCs and processed. Therefore, they will not be presented to T cells in a proper manner. In addition to this, superantigens bind to TCR away from the grove of TCR, but still activate T cells irrespective of their antigenic specificity.

Lymphoid and myeloid cancers

Over or under expression of certain cytokines and their receptors are associated with certain types of cancers. For ex. Cardiac myxoma (benign heart tumor) cells, myeloma cells, plasmacytoma cells and cervical and bladder cancer cells produces abnormally high levels of IL-6, which acts as an autocrine factor for the growth of these cells. Another example is HTLV-1 induced T cell leukemia, where abnormally high levels of IL-2 are produced and these cells also produce high affinity trimeric receptors.

Chagas disease

This disease is associated with immunosuppression and causative agent is a protozoan parasite-*Trypanosoma cruzi*. It causes immunosuppression by 90% suppression in production of α subunit of IL-2 receptor.

Exercise

1. Give an account of: (5 marks each)

    (a) Cytokine that regulate haematopoieisis
    (b) General properties of cytokines
    (c) Cytokine related diseases
    (d) Type I interferon
    (e) Tumor necrosis factor
    (f) Interleukin –1
    (g) Interleukin – 2
    (h) *Transforming growth factor-*β
    (i) *Interferon - *γ

2. Give a descriptive account of: (20 marks each)

    (a) Cytokines that regulate innate immunity
    (b) Cytokines that regulate lymphocyte activation, growth and differentiation
    (c) Cytokines that regulate immune mediated inflammation

3. Describe the functions and properties of interleukin – 4 (10 marks)

Chapter 15

Complement System

- The Complement Components
- Classical Complement Pathway
- Alternative Complement Pathway
- Lectin Pathway of Complement
- Consequences of Complement Activation
- Evasion of Complement-Mediated Damage by Microbes
- Complement Deficiencies

The complement system plays a critical role in the defense of the body in association with antibodies and the cells of the immune system. In other words, it is the major effector of the humoral and cellular immune system. It consists of 30 serum and membrane proteins. The complement system consists of various enzymes and proteins, which on activation interact with one another in a regulated manner called as **cascade reaction**, which ultimately results in antigen clearance and inflammatory response. Uncontrolled activation of complement can lead to massive cell destruction. The Belgian scientist Jules Bordet, who coined the term "alexine", discovered the complement system in 1893. Paul Ehrlich later introduced the term "complement" because they facilitate removal of antigen-antibody complex from the body.

There are two pathways of complement activation: the classical pathway and the alternative pathway. The alternative pathway has been already dealt in innate immune response (Chapter 2). Both the pathways share a common terminal reaction sequence that results in macromolecular membrane attack complex (MAC), which causes lysis of variety of cells that includes bacterial, infected host cells and viruses. When the complements are activated, variety of diffusible chemokines are released into circulation, which cause localized vasodilation and attract phagocytic cells, leading to inflammatory reaction. Some of the complement products are known to activate B lymphocytes. The phagocytes that possess receptors for these complement products readily phagocytose antigens coated with complements.

The Complement Components

The complement system consists of proteins that are labeled numerically with the prefix C- for ex. C1, C2, C3 etc., or designated by the alphabet-B, D, P etc. There are 19 of these components found in the serum of an individual and constitute about 10% of the globulin fraction of serum. They circulate in the serum in inactive form and many of them proenzymes and have their active site masked. When the complement is activated the active site is exposed by proteolytic cleavage of the proenzyme and the active site is exposed. The activation step of complement involves a sequential enzyme cascade reaction in which proenzyme product of one step becomes the enzyme catalyst of another step. Half-life of each activated complement component is very short. Complement components are synthesized at various sites throughout the body. Most C3, C6, C8, and B are made in the liver, and C2, C3, C4, C5, B, D, P and I are synthesized by macrophages. In addition to this complement components are also produced by blood monocytes, epithelial cells of gastrointestinal and genitourinary tracts. As a result, these components are readily available for defense at sites of inflammation where macrophages accumulate. Small letters of alphabets denotes the peptide fragments formed by the activation of complement. The smaller fragment designated by letter "a" and larger fragment by "b". The smaller fragment diffuses in the surrounding area and acts as chemokine and the larger fragment attaches itself to the target near the site of activation. The complement fragments interact with one another to form functional complexes, mainly enzymes. Bold Italics in this text designate those complexes, which have enzymatic role.

Classical Complement Pathway

This pathway is initiated by the formation of soluble antigen-antibody complexes or by the antibody bound to the antigen on a suitable target, such a bacterial cell. The complexing of antibody with antigen results in conformational changes in Fc region of the antibody, which exposes the receptor of the complement component C1. The C1 complement component consists of three separate proteins, C1q, C1r and C1s. They are held together in a complex-$C1qr_2s_2$ by Ca^{2+} ions. C1q looks like a six-stranded whip when viewed by electron microscopy (Fig. 15.1).

It is the globular heads that bind to the heavy chains of antigen-bound IgG and IgM. It is observed that, when pentameric IgM is bound to antigen on a target surface, at least three binding sites for C1q are exposed. Therefore, IgM can readily activate C1 complement. On the other hand, IgG molecule contains only one C1q site in the CH_2 domain of the Fc, so that firm C1q binding is achieved only when two IgG

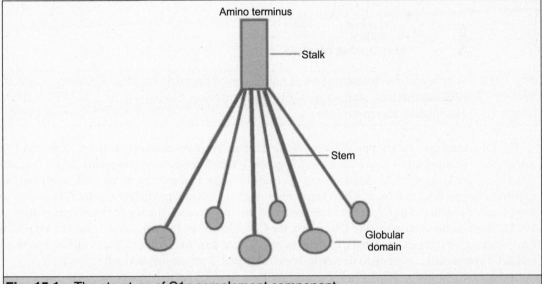

Fig. 15.1   The structure of C1q complement component.

molecules are bound within 30 to 40 nm of each other on a target surface, providing two attachment sites for C1q. Once C1q is bound, the tetrameric $C1r_2$-$C1s_2$ protease complex can bind tightly enough to become sequentially activated; The *C1r* autoactivates and subsequently cleaves C1s subunits. It is the activated *C1s* that cleaves C4 and C2 (Fig. 15.2).

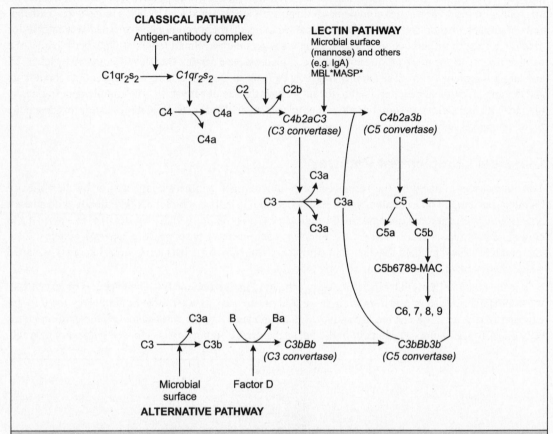

Fig. 15.2 A schematic representation of complement cascade reaction showing classical and alternative pathway. MBL* = mannose binding lectin; MASP*= MBL associated serine proteases.

The C4 component is a glycoprotein containing three polypeptide chains-α, β, and γ. Activated *C1s* acts on the α chain of C4 to cleave off a small fragment (9kD) from the amino terminus, called C4a and leave the major fragment C4b. Removal of C4a causes change in the shape of the C4b, as a result an exposed thioester bond is broken, which generates a reactive carbonyl group that enables C4b to bind to nearby cell membrane. The C2, second component of the complement, is a single chain glycoprotein of 102 kD, binds to the exposed part of C4b, where the C2 is cleaved by the activated *C1s* into C2a and C2b components. C2b diffuses away and C2a remains with C4b to form a complex *C4b2a*, which is a protease called **C3 convertase**, referring to its role in converting the C3 proenzyme into active form.

The third complement component is C3, which is most important of the complement components. It is a heterodimer of 190kD, consists of β chain of 70kD and α chain of 120kD linked by two disulfide bonds. Hydrolysis of short fragment-C3a (6kD) from the amino terminus of the α chain by the C3 convertase results in the formation of many molecules of C3b. Some of the C3b binds to *C4b2a* to form a trimolecular complex-*C4b2a3b* called **C5 convertase.** The C3b part of this complex binds to C5 and alters its structure, so that the *C4b2a* can cleave the C5 into C5a and C5b components. C3a and C5a constitute anaphylatoxic components and diffuse away, whereas C5b binds to the antigenic surface. C5b initiates the formation of membrane attack complex. Some of the C3b component does not bind to *C4b2a*; instead it diffuses away and binds to particulate antigens and immune complexes (antigen antibody complexes) functioning as opsonin and facilitates phagocytosis of the bound substance or opsonized substance (Fig. 15.3).

Alternative Complement Pathway

This pathway involves four serum proteins C3, factor, H, factor B, Factor D and properdin. Unlike the classical pathway, which is activated by antigen antibody complex, this pathway is activated by the antigenic property of gram-negative or gram-positive bacteria. C3 complement is spontaneously broken down in the serum and it binds to bacterial surface or cell surface.

Depending on the type of cell surface the alternative pathway either gets activated or suppressed. Under normal circumstances the C3b bound to normal cells will be bound by another factor called H factor to form C3bH. This complex is susceptible to digestion by another enzyme like factor called I. Factor H and I destroy C3b as fast as it is generated and as a result alternative pathway of C3 convertase action remains inactive. On the other hand, if C3b binds to activating surface such as gram-positive and gram-negative bacterial cells then it is not destroyed. The mammalian cell membrane consist of high level of sialic acid, which contributes to rapid inactivation of bound C3b molecules on host cells, whereas bacterial cell surfaces have low levels of this molecules. Sialic acid enhances binding of H factor to the C3b bound cell surface thereby initiating the decay of C3b. When C3b remains bound to the cell surface for long time, it initiates alternative pathway of complement. Bound C3b can bind to another serum factor B and expose a site on the surface of B factor that acts as substrate for another enzyme called factor D. Factor D breaks down factor B into smaller fragment Ba, which diffuses away and a larger fragment Bb, which remains with C3 to form a complex *C3bBb*. This complex has C3 convertase activity and it is analogous to *C4b2a* complex in the classical pathway. *C3bBb* has a very short half-life of only 5 min unless serum protein properdin binds to it. On binding to properdin, its half-life gets extended to 30 min (Fig. 15.4)

More C3b component will be generated in an amplified manner by the action of *C3bBb* on the C3, thereby 2×10^6 molecules of C3b can be deposited on an antigenic surface in less than 5 min. Furthermore, another complex *C3bBb3b* generated by the action of *C3bBb* on C3 will act as **C5 convertase** analogous to *C4b2a3b* complex in the classical pathway. C5 is bound by the nonenzymatic C3b component and subsequently is hydrolyzed by *C3bBb* to generate C5a and C5b. The C5a diffuses into the surrounding and acts as anaphylactic substance and C5b binds to the antigenic surface.

C3b may be also generated by other methods. For. ex. Enzymes of phagocytic cells or those generated by thrombin action on platelets. As a result, C3b is generated at the site of thrombosis and inflammation.

Lectin Pathway of Complement

Activation of the lectin pathway is initiated by mannose binding lectin (MBL) recognizing mannose on bacteria, by IgA and probably, by structures exposed on damaged endothelium. MBL is homologous to

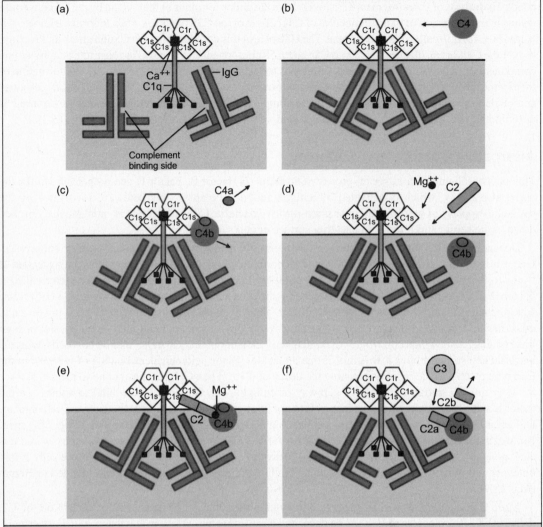

Fig. 15.3   A diagrammatic representation of classical complement pathway on the cell membrane. Antibodies recognize antigens and form complexes with them. When two IgG molecules are bound to same antigens and lie adjacent to each other , they activate complement C1. C1 is made up of 3 subunits C1q, C1r, and C1s held together by clacium. C1q binds to complement binding site or antibody.

(a) C1q bound to antibody is activated and becomes enzymatic *C1q* which becomes *C1qr2s2*.

(b) **and (c)** *C1qr2s2* enzyme is activated and acts on complement C4 that comes in contact with C1s which breaks into C4a and C4b. C4b binds to cell membrane and C4a is released.

(d) C2 comes in contact with the activated C1s.

(e) C2 is split into C2a and C2b

(f) C2a combines with C4b and C2b is released . C4b2a forms an enzyme whose substrate is C3

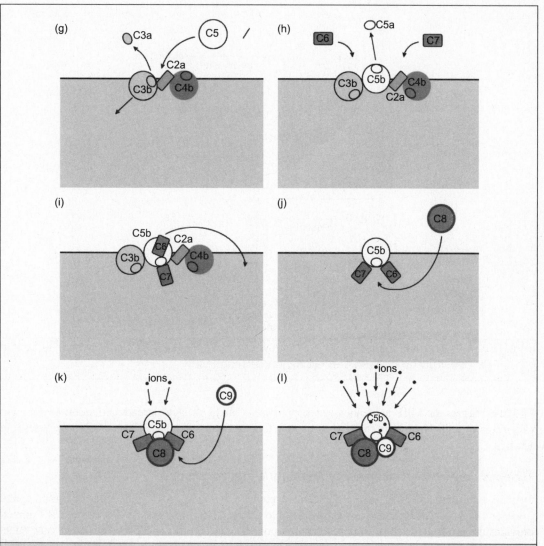

Fig. 15.3 Contd.

   (g) C3 is split into C3a and C3b by C4b2a. C3a is realeased and C3b combines with *C4b2a* to form *C4b2a3b* enzyme complex.

   (h) *C4b2a3b* acts on complement C5 and splits it into C5a and C5b. C5b is bound to *C4b2a3b* to form another enzyme. C5a is realeased. Complement 6 and 7 bind to C5b to form another complex.

   (i) C5b bound to C6 and C7 acts as enzyme *C5b67*.

   (j) C5b67 binds to C8 on the cell surface at a new site.

   (k) Cell bound by C5b678 now develops leaky pore.

   (l) Addition of C9 to these pores greatly enlarges the pore size and speeds up the inflow of water and ions causing the cell to swell and burst.

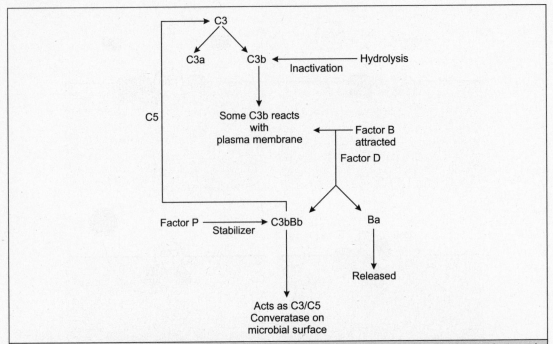

Fig. 15.4   A schematic representation of involvement of alternative pathway of complement in destruction of bacterium as an innate response.

C1q and triggers the MBL associated serine proteases (MASPs). Downstream activation of the lectin pathway is virtually identical to classical pathway activation forming the same C3 and C5 convertases (Fig. 15.2).

Terminal complement pathway or Membrane attack complex

C3b acts as the initiator of the terminal complement pathway by binding to C5 and rendering C5 susceptible to either *C4b2a or C3bBb* attack and splitting it into C5a and C5b components. The large C5b fragment provides the binding site for the subsequent components C6, C7, C8, and C9 of the membrane attack complex (MAC). C5b is highly labile component and gets inactivated within 2 min if it does not bind to C6. Up to this point whatever complement reaction took place are on the hydrophilic surface of the membrane or in the liquid phase (serum or plasma). Soon after the formation of C5b6 complex it binds to C7 on the membrane surface resulting in hydrophilic-amphiphilic structural changes to expose hydrophobic regions, which serve as binding site for membrane phospholipids. C5b67 complex, if occurs on the membrane surface it will insert the complex into the membrane and if the complex occurs in the fluid medium on the antigen antibody complex, it will dissociate from the immune complex and binds to the neighboring cell membrane and initiate **"innocent bystander lysis"**. This innocent bystander lysis is highly harmful to normal cells and in various types of diseases associated with immune complex mediated reaction tissue damage results from this process.

Membrane bound C5b67 attracts C8 complement and binds to it resulting in its structural change, so that it too undergoes a hydrophilic-amphiphilic structural change exposing a hydrophobic region, which helps in interaction with plasma membrane. By this time C5b678 creates a small pore of 10 A° diameter on the membrane, which may lead to lysis of the red blood cells but not of nucleated cells. The final step in the generation of membrane attack complex would be the binding of C9 complement to C5b678 complex. As many as 10 to 16 molecules of C9 (**poly-C9**) can bind to C5b678 and undergo hydrophilic-amphiphilic structural change so that they also can insert into the membrane. Completed MAC assumes a cylindrical form and increases the diameter of the pore to 70 to 100 A° initially formed by C5b678 (Fig. 15.5). From such a large pore, ions and cellular contents can easily leak, the cell cannot maintain osmotic balance, hence leads to lysis by the influx of water and loss of electrolytes.

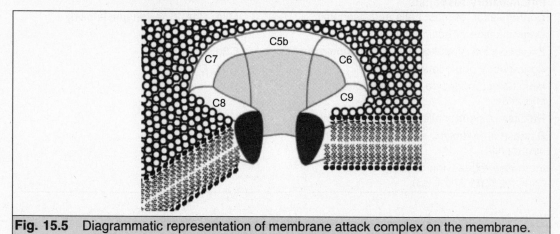

Fig. 15.5 Diagrammatic representation of membrane attack complex on the membrane.

Recently some proteins have been discovered, which are capable of activating the complement in a different manner, they are called mannose-binding proteins. Certain cytokines released by phagocytes, like IL-1, IL-6 and TNF-α of which IL-6 is known to stimulate hepatocytes to produce several new proteins. One of the proteins secreted by liver cells in response to IL-6 is mannose-binding protein. It is observed that majority of bacteria have mannose as major component in their cell wall. The mannose-binding protein, thus attaches to any bacteria found in the free circulation. When the protein binds to mannose residue in the bacterial cell wall, it forms a potent opsonin. This also significantly enhances the complement deposition by the alternative pathway. Mannose-binding protein is structurally similar to C1q complement component, but it cannot activate classical complement pathway.

CONSEQUENCES OF COMPLEMENT ACTIVATION

Complement serves as major effector of defense mechanism to destroy invading microorganisms and viruses. It is an important mediator of the humoral immune response and helps in amplification of humoral arm of defense system. Many of the biological activities of the complement are dependent on receptor binding, which are expressed on different type cells. Some complement receptors play regulatory role by facilitating their binding and degrading them to inactive products. In addition to MAC mediated cell lysis, other complement components participate in the inflammatory response, opsonization of antigen, viral neutralization and clearance of immune complex (Table 15.1).

Opsonization

Phagocytic cells possess Fc receptor for immunoglobulins and the Cr1 receptor for C3b. Therefore, both antibody and complement coated antigens bind to the phagocytes through these receptors and get

Table 15.1 Biological effects mediated by complement components

Effects	Complement components
Opsonization of particulate antigens and enhancing their phagocytosis	C3b, C4b, C3bi
Viral neutralization	C3b, C5b-9 (MAC)
Clearance of antibody-antigen complex	C3b (through pahgocytosis)
Inflammatory response:	
Degranulation of mast cells and basophils	C3a, C4a, C5a (anaphylatoxin)
Degranulation of eosinophil	C3a, C5a
Extravasation of leukocytes and chemotaxis	C3a, C5a, C5b67
Aggregation of platlets	C3a, C5a
Inhibition of monocyte and macrophage migration	Bb
Release of neutrophils from bone marrow	C3c
Release of hydrolytic enzymes from neutrophils	C5a
Increased expression of complement receptor (CR1 and CR3)	C5a

phagocytosed. Neutrophils on activation may secrete their lysosomal enzymes, which cause inflammation and tissue damage as well as activate C3 and C5 complement.

Removal of immune complexes

It is very crucial for the body to get rid off the antigen-antibody complexes. Otherwise the immune complexes may get deposited in vital organs and cause tissue damage. Complements facilitate in getting rid of immune complexes through phagocytosis or by CR1 receptor on RBCs. Deposition of immune complexes in kidney due to absence of certain complement components leads to kidney damage.

Immune regulation

C3 plays a dominant role in enhancing the B cell response as well as increases the uptake of antigen-C3 complexes by APCs. C3a is found to be inhibitor of NK cells and T cell activity, but C5a is found to be both T and B cell stimulator. C5a enhances the production of IL-1 by macrophages. Stimulation of macrophages by C5a results in enhanced expression of CR1, CD11a/CD18, CD11c/CD18, CD16 and CD45.

Cytolysis

Cell lysis brought about by complement as an end product of activation of complement through MAC formation is an essential step in getting rid of infected cells and bacterial cells. C9 component of the complement belongs to the class of proteins called perforins that are implicated in cell lysis mediated by cytotoxic T cells and NK cells and eosinophils. Bacterial cell lysis involves two hit process because initial hole driven by C9 component destroys outer cell wall. Once the outer cell wall is destroyed, second hit by the complement on the membrane occurs, which ultimately results in bacteriolysis. Among the pathogenic viruses shown to be lysed by complement-mediated lysis are herpes virus, myxovirus, retrovirus and paramyxovirus.

Chemotaxis

Certain byproducts C5a, C5b67, C3c and Bb of the complement cascade act as chemotactic factors for different types of cells. For ex. C5b67 acts as chemotactic factor for Neutrophils and eosinophils, whereas C5a acts as chemotactic factor for not only neutrophils and eosinophils but also for macrophages and basophils. C3c promotes leukocyte proliferation and migration of leukocytes from bone marrow.

Inflammation

The complement components C3a and C5a promote anaphylaxis by promoting degranulation of mast cells and also on their own act as anaphylatoxic substance because they can bring about smooth muscle contraction of bronchial and intestinal wall. They promote vascular permeability and induce lysosomal enzyme release from neutrophils, histamine and serotonin release from platelets, and thromboxane release from macrophages.

EVASION OF COMPLEMENT—MEDIATED DAMAGE BY MICROBES

Gram positive bacteria are generally resistant to complement-mediated lysis because of their thick peptidoglycan cell wall, which prevents insertion of MAC into the inner membrane. Some bacteria possess elastase that inactivates C3a and C5a, which are the key components of inflammatory reaction. Certain resistant strains of gram negative bacteria produce increased amount of lipopolysaccharide in their cell wall, which results in the formation of smooth variety and prevents the insertion of MAC into the bacterial membrane so that complex is released from the bacterial cell rather than forming a pore. In *Neisseria gonorrhoea,* the resistant strain shows noncovalent interaction with MAC thereby preventing insertion into the outer membrane of the bacterial cell. Some other species of bacteria *Candida albicans,* protozoan *Trypanosoma cruzi,* and virusus *vaccinia, Herpes simplex, and Epstein-Barr virus* mimic certain complement regulatory proteins thereby inhibiting the complement cascade.

COMPLEMENT DEFICIENCIES

Genetic deficiencies of complement components result in increased susceptibility of an individual to infections and immune complex diseases (Table 15.2).

Table 15.2 Diseases associated with complement deficiencies

Deficient complement component	Diseases
C1q	Systemic lupus erythematosus (SLE), bacterial Infections, glomerulonephritis, Hypogammaglobulinemia
C1r	SLE, Rheumatoid disease, recurrent infections Renal disease
C1s	SLE
C2	Glomerulonephritis, rheumatoid arthritis SLE, Recurrent infections

Contd.

Table 15.2 Contd.

Deficient complement component	Diseases
C3	Glomerulonephritis, recurrent infections
C4	SLE
C5	Recurrent infections, SLE
C6	Gonorrhoea, meningococcal infection
C7	Recurrent Neisserial infections
C8	SLE, Neisserial infections
C9	Neisserial infections
I	Recurrent infections
H	Hemolytic uremia
P	Nesseirial infection

Exercise

1. Give a detailed account of classical complement pathway (20 marks).
2. Write notes on alternative complement pathway (15 marks).
3. Write short notes on: (5 marks each)

   (a) Membrane attack complex
   (b) Consequences of complement activation
   (c) Evasion of complement mediated damage by microbes
   (d) Complement deficient diseases

Chapter 16

Vaccines

- Active Immunization through Designing Vaccines
- Vaccines from Whole Organisms
- Polysaccharide Vaccines
- Outer Membrane Protein Vaccines
- Vaccines in the form of Toxoids
- Vaccines from Recombinant Vectors
- DNA as Vaccines
- Vaccines from Synthetic Peptides

Edward Jenner and Louis Pasteur made the first attempt of vaccination for human diseases. Since then many vaccines have been developed for major afflictions of human beings. The disease such as diphtheria, measles, mumps, poliomyelitis, whooping cough (pertussis), rubella (German measles) and tetanus has declined sufficiently due to WHO policy of vaccination of children on war footing. Vaccination is a cost-effective process for disease prevention. One of the best examples of vaccination is complete eradication of small pox, a deadly disease, which afflicted mankind many year's back. Since 1977 not a single case of small pox has been reported anywhere in the world.

Recent advances in immunology through understanding of molecular aspect of T cell and B cell receptors and their interactions with epitopes has enabled the immunologist to design vaccines to maximize humoral and cellular immune response. Understanding of antigen processing and presentation of antigenic determinants by antigen presenting cells (APC) has enabled molecular immunologists to design vaccines to maximize antigen presentation by class I or II MHC molecules. Genetic engineering techniques have been used to improve the vaccines to maximize the immune response to selected antigenic determinants. Active immunization can be achieved through natural infection by a microorganism or it can be acquired artificially through the administration of vaccines.

As the name implies, active immunization through vaccination plays an active role in proliferation of antigen sensitive T and B-lymphocytes resulting in the formation of immune memory cells. Active immunization by artificial means can be achieved by following strategies:

1. Attenuated organisms (avirulent)
2. Inactivated organisms (Killed)
3. Purified microbial macromolecules
4. Cloned (genetically engineered) microbial antigens

5. Synthetic peptides
6. Anti-idiotype antibodies
7. Multivalent complexes

Active immunization by vaccination has resulted in the reduction in number of deaths by infectious diseases in infants. Vaccination schedule can begin at 2 months of age and should be over by 15 years. A 1995 update schedule for vaccination recommended by Center for Disease Control (CDC), Atlanta, U. S. A is listed in Table 16.1.

To achieve life long immunity as indicated in Table 16.1, child hood immunization requires multiple boosters at appropriately timed intervals. Multiple immunization with oral polio vaccine is necessary to ensure a sufficient immune response to be generated against each of the three strains of poliovirus that make up the Sabin vaccine.

Table 16.1   CDC recommended (1995) vaccination schedule for infants and children.

Age	Vaccination
Birth to 2 months	Hepatitis B
2 months	Diphtheria-Pertussis-Tetanus (DPT), Poliomyletis (OPV)
Hemophilius influenzae (Hib)	Type b
4 months	DPT, OPV, Hib
6-18 months	Hepatitis B, OPV
12-15 months	DTP, Varicella zoster (VZV), Measels, Mumps, Rubella (MMR)
4-6 years	DPT, OPV, MMR
11-12 years	Diphtheria-Tetanus, VZV

*Sabin vaccine consists of 3 attenuated strains of poliovirus.

One of the reasons for multiple immunization schedules is because of presence of maternal antibodies in the infants, which were gained passively through placenta or mothers milk. For example, passively acquired maternal antibodies bind to epitopes on the DPT vaccines, thereby blocking adequate immune activation. Therefore, this vaccine must be given several times to achieve adequate immunity. Passively acquired maternal antibodies also interfere with MMR vaccine, because it is not given before 12-15 months of age. In the developing countries, measles vaccine is given at 9 months of age, because 30-50% of children in these countries contract the disease before 15 months of age.

Vaccination of the adult's varies, depending on the severity of the disease. Vaccination for meningitis, pneumonia and influenza if given to individuals living in larger groups (Military camps, pilgrimage and excursion groups) or individuals with reduced immunity (elderly). Generally international travelers are also routinely vaccinated against yellow fever, cholera, plague, typhoid, typhus etc. Some countries insist on these vaccinations before giving entry permit to the visitors into their country.

Active Immunization through Designing Vaccines

First and the foremost thing before designing any vaccine, is to study the activation of humoral and cell mediated immune response shown by a particular antigen. Secondly, the potentiality of development of immunologic memory by the particular antigen needs to be considered. For example, vaccines may produce a protective primary response but may fail to produce immune memory cells. In such cases, individual becomes susceptible to second infection by same pathogen.

Memory cell production plays an important role in immunity and partly it is dependent on incubation period of the pathogen. For example, influenza virus has a very short incubation period, i.e. less than 3 days. Individuals infected with influenza readily show disease symptoms by the time immune memory cells are activated. Therefore, maintaining high levels of neutralizing antibodies in free circulation by repeated immunization is necessary for effective protection against influenza. For pathogens with a longer incubation period, for example, poliovirus does not need higher levels of circulating neutralizing antibodies at the time of infection because, poliovirus requires more than 3 days to start infection of central nervous system. Due to this longer incubation period, sufficient time is provided for memory B cells to respond with production of high levels of serum antibodies. Thus, the polio vaccine is also designed to induce production of high levels of immune memory cells. If an immunized individual is later exposed to the poliovirus, these memory cells will respond immediately and within 2 weeks of time produce high levels of serum antibody, which protects the individual from infection.

Vaccines from Whole Organisms

Many of the commonly used vaccines to date consist of inactivated (Killed) or live but attenuated (avirulent) bacterial cells or viral particles (Table 16.2). The important primary characteristics of these two vaccines are given in Table 16.2.

Table 16.2 Types of vaccines commonly used for human immunization

Whole Organism	
Pathogens or disease	*Types of vaccines*
Bacterial cells	
Plague	Inactivated
Pertussis	Inactivated
Cholera	Inactivated
Tuberculosis	Attenuated BCG
Viral particles	
Influenza virus	Inactivated
Rubella virus	Inactivated
Polio (Salk)	Inactivated
Polio (Sabin)	Attenuated
Yellow fever	Attenuated
Measles	Attenuated
Mumps	Attenuated
Varicella zoster (Chicken Pox)	Attenuated
Purified Macromolecules	
Toxoids	
Tetanus	Inactivated exotoxin
Diptheria	Inactivated exotoxin
Capsular polysaccharides	
Nesseria meningitis	Polysaccharide
Streptococcus pneumonia	23 distinct capsular polysaccharides
Hemophilius influenzae type b	Polysaccharide + Protein carrier
Surface antigen	
Hepatitis B	Recombinant surface antigens (HbsAg)

Attenuated Bacterial or Viral Vaccines

Pathogenicity of certain microorganisms can be attenuated so that they lose their ability to cause disease. At the same time attenuated organisms retain the capacity to undergo transient growth in an inoculated host. Generally, attenuation of a bacteria or virus is achieved by growing them for a prolonged periods under abnormal culture conditions or in unnatural host. By this procedure mutants are selected that are better suited to growth in the abnormal culture conditions but fail to grow to such an extent in original host. The development of vaccine for tuberculosis was achieved through growing *Mycobacterium bovis* on a medium containing excessive bile for 13 years. The vaccine developed from the attenuated strain of *M. bovis* is called Bacillus Calmette Guerin (BCG). Sabin vaccine for polio was obtained by growing poliovirus in monkey kidney epithelial cells. The vaccine for measles contains a strain of rubella virus that was attenuated by growing in duck embryo cells and later in human diploid cell lines.

There are some disadvantages and advantages from the attenuated vaccines. The ability of many attenuated vaccines to replicate within the host cells makes them particularly suitable for inducing cell-mediated immune response. Attenuated vaccines show transient growth thereby, providing prolonged immune system exposure to the individual epitopes on the attenuated organisms. This results in increased immunogenicity and memory cell production. Therefore, these vaccines often require only a single dose of administration (Table 16.3).

Table 16.3 Comparison of primary characteristics of attenuated (live) and inactivated killed vaccines

Characters	Attenuated	Inactivated
Method of production	Virulent strain grown under adverse culture conditions or prolonged growth in unnatural host or passage through different unnatural hosts	Virulence is inactivated by chemical treatment or by γ radiation
Requirement of booster dose	Generally single booster dose is required	Mulitple booster doses are required
Stability	Less stable	More stable and resistant to natural temperature fluctuations. Does not need refrigeration
Typr of host immune responses	Produce both cell mediated and humoral immune response	Mainly produces humoral response
Tendency to revert	May revert to original virulent strain by recombination with wild type strain or reverse mutation	Does not revert to virulent form

The Sabin oral polio vaccine consists of three strains of attenuated polioviruses. These viruses colonize intestinal area and induce protective immunity against all the three virulent strains of poliovirus. Sabin vaccine induces production of secretory IgA, IgM and IgG class of antibodies. Unlike other vaccines, Sabin vaccine requires three times administration at definite intervals. Because, the three strains of attenuated viruses interfere with each other's replication in the intestine. Generally with first time immunization, one strain will predominate in its growth, thereby inducing immunity against that strain. In the second immunization, immunity generated by the previous strain will limit the growth of the previous predominant strain. This results in one of the remaining two strains to predominate and induce immunity. Finally, with the third immunization, immunity to all the three strains is obtained.

Some of the disadvantages of attenuated vaccines are the possibility of their reversion into virulent forms. The rate of reversion in Sabin polio vaccine is 1 in 4 million doses of vaccine. In some cases, post-vaccine complications may develop in individuals. For example, in some cases, measles vaccine consisting of attenuated strain of Edmonston-Zagreb virus is known to cause immunosuppression thereby placing the vaccinated infant at a greater risk of infection with other disease causing pathogens.

Inactivated Bacterial or Viral Vaccines

This is another common method in vaccine production. The pathogen is inactivated by heat or by chemical hence it is no longer capable of replicating in the host. During inactivation process, it is critically important to maintain the structures of epitopes on surface antigens. Heat inactivation generally leads to protein denaturation, which may lead to alteration in epitope structure and failure in immune recognition. Chemical inactivation with formaldehyde has met with success. Sabin vaccine and pertussis (Whooping cough) vaccines are produced by formaldehyde treatment. In the case of killed vaccines repeated booster doses are often needed to maintain the immune status of the host, where as attenuated vaccines generally require only one dose to induce long lasting immunity. Killed vaccines predominantly induce humoral immune response, whereas attenuated vaccines induce cell mediated as well as humoral immune response (Table 16.3).

In rare instances, where quality control procedures were not properly followed while producing killed vaccines led to complications in the host. For example, due to inadequate treatment of pathogens by formaldehyde paralytic polio from Salk vaccine and pertussis from pertussis vaccine were caused in the host. Otherwise, killed vaccines are very safe and cause less complication.

Vaccine from Purified Macromolecules

The risks associated with attenuated or killed whole organism vaccines can be overcome by preparing vaccines from purified macromolecules of pathogens. There are three general forms of such vaccines in current use. Capsular polysaccharides, inactivated exotoxins and recombinant surface antigens.

Polysaccharide Vaccines

It was early in the twentieth century that the ability of pneumococcal capsular polysaccharides has potential as vaccines were recognized. Meningococcal, pneumococcal and *Hemophilus influenzae* type b (Hib) polysaccharide vaccines have been found to be protective in the field trials. In the field trials it has been observed that infants mount poor immune response to polysaccharide vaccines. The age at which the vaccine administered is found to play an important role for capsular polysaccharides and Meningococcal group A polysaccharides being an example of early responsiveness as low as 3 months of age. With respect to Hib polysaccharide vaccine, significant immune response and clinical protection can be induced only in the age group 18 months and above. Another issue of major concern is the poor response in the infants and lack of immunological memory, have prevented the use of polysaccharide vaccines on a large scale.

The mechanism and immunological properties of polysaccharide vaccines can be listed as follows:

- Polysaccharides contain repeating units of epitopes within one molecule, which can result in cross-linking of antigen receptors on the surface of B-lymphocytes.
- Polysaccharide capsules of certain bacteria are known to possess antiphagocytic properties therefore they show virulence. Coating of the capsule by antibody or complement greatly increases the ability of neutrophils and macrophages to phagocytize such virulent pathogens. These findings have enabled immunologists to develop vaccines from purified polysaccharides. The vaccine against *Streptococcus pneumoniae* (causes pneumonia), consists of 23 different antigenic capsular polysaccharide components. This vaccine induces opsonizing antibodies and it is administered to high-risk groups, such as infants and spleenectomized patients. *Neisseria meningitidis* is known for bacterial meningitis is also controlled by vaccine against its purified capsular polysaccharides.
- Many bacterial polysaccharides are known to activate alternative pathway of complements leading to deposition of C3b on to polysaccharides. C3b can bind to complement receptor 2 (CD21 or CR2) on the surface of B-lymphocytes. Co activation of CR2 and mIgM receptor on the surface of B lymphocyte will lead to induction of antibody production. In the neonatal B lymphocytes CR2 expression is very low, therefore the poor responsiveness of infants to polysaccharides.

Both $CD4^+$ $\alpha\beta$ as well as $\gamma\delta$ T cell receptor can affect the B cell response in non MHC-restricted manner. Polysaccharide specific B cells are known to be present at birth. It has been possible to induce T cell immune response by using carrier protein and the T cells specific for the carrier protein become involved in the activation of B-lymphocytes specific for the polysaccharide. Such conjugate vaccines can induce clinically relevant immune response as well as immunological memory in infants.

Hib Polysaccharide Vaccine

The Hib polysaccharide vaccine poly-ribose-ribitol-phosphate (PRP) has been found to be 90% efficacious at the age of 18-24 months or older in preventing Hib infection. Because of the immunological shortcomings of the polysaccharide vaccines, conjugate vaccines are produced. For example PRP-diphtheria (PRP-D) toxoid vaccine was found to be 90% efficacious after a primary immunization series of three doses at the age of 3, 4 and 6 months. Infants and children vaccinated with Hib conjugates have been shown to possess IgG and IgA in their saliva.

Vaccine against *Hemophilus influenzae* type b (Hib) consists of type b capsular polysaccharide antigen covalently linked to protein carrier-tetanus toxoid. This polysaccharide-protein conjugate is more immunogenic than the polysaccharide alone. The conjugate is capable of stimulating T_H cells, it enables class switching from IgM to IgG. It is also capable of inducing memory B cells but not memory T cells specific for pathogen.

Salmonella O-antigen specific conjugates

As early as 1977, preparation of *Salmonella* serotype BO specific O-antigen-protein conjugate was described. This conjugate was based on oligosaccharide of the O-polysaccharide chain obtained by the use of specific bacteriophage associated endo-a-rhamnosidase. The resulting conjugate was shown to yield substantial quantity of BO antibody upon injection in rabbits. Using coupling procedure based on the principles of conversion of oligosaccharide into its corresponding aldonic acid and conjugating with the carrier protein by a water-soluble carbodiimide produced the first conjugate vaccine. The newer approach is by using 2-(4-isothiocyanotophenyl)-ethylamine derivatives for covalent conjugation, which allows the preparation of non-cross-linked conjugates as opposed to aldonate method. These conjugates were found to be highly immunogenic in rabbits with a titer of 20 to 50 thousand.

Recently, *Salmonella typhi* O-polysaccharide conjugated to tetanus toxoid was used as vaccine by introducing reducing groups into the O-antigenic polysaccharide side chain through periodate oxidation, after which it was conjugated to tetanus toxoid by reductive amination. The immunogenicity of cross-linked conjugate was checked in mice using microgram dose of *S. typhi* antigen in Alhydrogel adjuvant. The antibodies showed complement-mediated lysis of *S. typhi*. Immunized mice were fully protected against challenge with 10 LD_{50} of *S. typhi* Ty2.

S. typhi: Vi-antigen specific conjugates

S. typhi in contrast to other *Salmonella sp.* Carries a special type of antigen called Vi-polysaccharide (Vi for virulence). Vi-polysaccharide was conjugated to the B subunit of the heat labile toxin of *E. coli* and also to a recombinant exoprotein A from *Pseudomonas aeruginosa*. Both the conjugates elicited higher antibody titers against Vi in mice and guinea pigs than the non-conjugate type of Vi-polysaccharide vaccines.

Shigella: O-antigen specific conjugates

O-specific polysaccharide of *Shigella sonnei and S. Flexneri* type 2a covalently bound to *Pseudomonas aeruginosa* recombinant exoprotein A, were evaluated in 192 Israeli soldiers. As early as 14 days after immunization up to 90% of those given *S. sonnei* vaccine and over 70% of those receiving the *S. flexneri* type 2a vaccine showed a four fold or greater increase in serum IgG and IgA titers. The predominant subclass was IgG1. Follow-up after two years of the same individuals showed significantly higher titers, indicating long-lasting immune response towards both the *Shigella* vaccines.

E. coli: O-antigen specific conjugates

By using different O-antigens from *E. coli,* several groups have prepared different types of vaccines, one of them being from the detoxified serotype O111 lipopolysaccharide conjugate with tetanus toxoid as carrier protein. A spacer arm (adipic acid dihydrazide) was used as linker for the conjugate. Serotype O157 conjugate prepared in the similar manner evoked much better response than the O-111 and the conjugates were able to evoke IgG response with bactericidal activity.

Outer Membrane Protein Vaccines

Bacterial vaccines that are in use at present in large scale are composed of killed or attenuated whole cells, toxoids and polysaccharide-protein conjugate vaccines. For ex. Diphtheria, pertussis, tetanus, bacille Calmette-Guerin, *Hemophilus influenzae* type b conjugates, cholera and typhoid are used for human immunization. Recently new subunit pertussis vaccines containing pertussis toxoid with surface protein such as **filamentous hemagglutinin (FHA)** and **pertactin** are the first two surface proteins to become part of widely accepted vaccines for human immunization. At present vaccine research and development for the pathogenic strains such as *Neisseria gonorrhoea, N. meningitidis, H. influenzae and Moraxella catarrhalis* are under way. Since these bacteria share many of the surface characteristics, vaccine development efforts against these species are dealt here.

Neisseria gonorrhoea

(a) Pili   The abundance, easy accessibility of pili and the critical adhesion function to eukaryotic cells led to the development of parenteral pilus vaccine. In human volunteers, the vaccine induced high titer antibody production, which showed opsonic and adhesion-blocking activities with broad cross-reactivity. Although high titer antibodies were produced in subjects, they were still susceptible for gonococcal infection. It became evident that gonococcal pili show remarkable polymorphism among intra and interstrain. The intrastrain antigenic variability is due to the reciprocal recombination of gene pilE with intrastrain silent copies of pilin genes, pilS. Recent findings show that PilC is located close to the outer membrane and neisserial fibers are covered with O-linked trisaccharides on one side are the prime candidates in vaccine production.

(b) Outer membrane protein PI or Por   This is the most abundant protein from the gonococcal outer membrane is available for vaccine production and it is called PI or Por, the gonococcal porin. Unlike the pilin, Por has limited variability in its serotype determinants. Anti-Por antibodies induced in humans are known to show bactericidal activity. The Por vaccines designed to cover almost all serotypes were found to be ineffective due to other impurities like PIII or reduction modifiable protein (Rmp) and lipopolysaccharide (LPS). It was observed that antibody induction to Rmp block antibody activity directed against porin. Similarly, LPS sialylation prevents Por-mediated bactericidal antibody killing.

(c) Opacity associated proteins or PII   The presence of PII gives rise to the formation of opaque colonies due to interbacterial association. A strain of *N. gonorrhoea* can express many of PIIs. PIIs help in adhesion properties of gonococci in addition to pili. There are 12 different (opa) genes associated with the expression of opacity protein. These genes are regulated in response to addition or deletion of CTCTT pentanucleotide coding repeating units. This leads to total repertoir of antigenic variation and hindrance in vaccine development. At present a model for opa has been proposed assuming four-cell surface exposed, variable regions for the vaccine development.

Vaccines in the form of Toxoids

Some pathogenic strains of bacteria produce exotoxins, which produce many of the disease symptoms resulting from infection. For example, by purifying the bacterial exotoxin of diphtheria and tetanus vaccines are produced by neutralizing the exotoxins with formaldehyde to harmless toxoid. Vaccination with toxoid results in development of antitoxoid antibodies, which are also capable of binding to toxin. On binding to toxin, the antibodies neutralize the toxic effects of toxin. One of the problems encountered with vaccines produced from purified macromolecules is the difficulty involved in obtaining sufficient quantity of purified molecules. At present this problem has been overcome by cloning the gene for toxin of diphtheria and tetanus in a suitable host so as to produce enough quantity of toxin molecules for the production of vaccine.

Vaccines from Recombinant Vectors

Genes encoding major antigens of virulent pathogens can be introduced into attenuated viruses or bacteria, which serve as vectors. The vectors replicate in the host cell, expressing the genes encoding major antigens of pathogens. Wide range of organisms have been used as vectors for vaccines, which include, vaccinia virus, attenuated poliovirus, canary pox virus, adenoviruses, BCG strain of *Mycobacterium bovis* and the attenuated strain of *Salmonella*.

Attenuated vaccinia virus used for eradication of small pox has been widely employed as vector for vaccine production. The genome of this virus can be engineered to carry several dozen foreign genes without impairing its capacity to infect host cells and replicate. The procedure involved in producing vaccinia vector for carrying the gene of a pathogen is given in Fig. 16.1.

The degree of expression of inserted foreign pathogenic gene is quite high in vaccinia virus, which serves as a potent immunogen in an inoculated host. At present, gene for hepatitis B surface antigen, *Herpes simplex* and influenza have been successfully inserted into vaccinia genome. Laboratory trials of this vector vaccinia have shown that it induces production of antibodies and cell mediated immune response against the engineered products.

Vaccines produced from other attenuated vectors may prove safer than the vaccinia vaccines, because vaccinia may become virulent in individuals suffering from severe immune suppression. Therefore, Canary

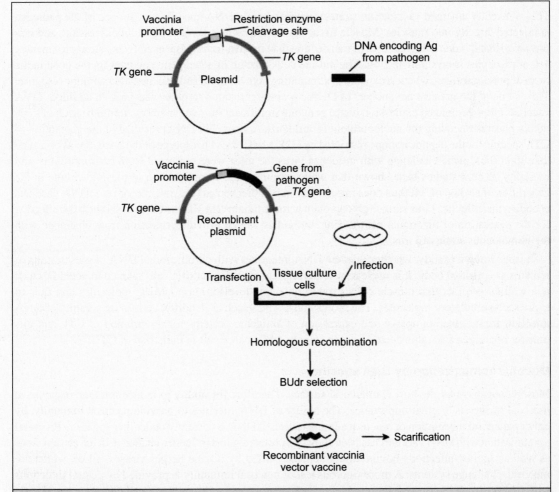

Fig. 16.1 Creating vaccinia virus vector through genetic engineering for Hemophilus influenzae.

poxvirus has been recently tried as a vector for vaccines, since it does not appear to be virulent in individuals with severe immune suppression. It is similar to vaccinia and has the ability to carry multiple genes.

Another possible attenuated bacterial vector, which has been genetically engineered to carry genes from cholera bacterium is *Salmonella typhimurium*. The main advantage is that salmonella is capable of infecting muscle cell lining of intestine. Hence it is capable of inducing secretory IgA production. It has been possible to induce increased production of secretory IgA at mucosal lining of intestine, which has enabled to achieve effective immunity against cholera, gonorrhea. One of the poliovirus strains from Sabin vaccine is an effective candidate for safe vector vaccine. In this case, out side capsid protein of the poliovirus is replaced by gene encoding the epitope of choice. Resulting chimera vector is capable of expressing the desired epitope in a highly accessible manner on the poliovirus nuclear capsid.

DNA as Vaccines

This is recently emerged vaccination strategy where plasmid DNA encoding an antigen of the pathogen is injected directly into muscles. Muscle tissue shows the highest levels of protein expression, and it is presumed that it is due to higher level of transfection than in other tissues. But even in muscle approximately 1% of myocytes shows transfection. The muscle cells take up injected gene and express the gene in the form of protein antigen, which is capable of stimulating both humoral and cell mediated immune response. This is one of the greatest advantages of DNA vaccines compared to other vaccines. In addition, DNA vaccines allow prolonged expression hence generate significant immune memory. Immunization of mice with a plasmid encoding the nucleoprotein of influenza A virus (NP DNA) resulted in the generation of CTL specific for the peptide epitope restricted by H2K MHC class I haplotype of the mice. It was observed that upon subsequent challenge with influenza virus the mice were protected from both morbidity and mortality. Recent studies have shown that while intramuscular immunization of plasmid results in the generation of stronger CMI than does immunization by other routes (i.v., i.d., s.c. or i.p.). DNA vaccines encoding the influenza virus surface glycoprotein hemagglutinin (HA) have also been shown to be effective for the generation of functional neutralizing antibodies, which provide protection from challenge with the homologous strain of virus.

It is not known exactly, whether injected DNA integrates with chromosomal DNA of muscle cells or remains as episomal body. It is unclear, whether muscle cells or dendritic cells take up injected DNA. It is a well-known fact that muscle cells express only low level of class I MHC molecules and fails to express co-stimulatory molecules. The professional APCs such as dendritic cells in the vicinity of DNA injection are involved in uptake and expression of antigenic proteins for the priming of CTL and this transfer of antigen from transfected muscle cells to APCs can result in induction of CTL.

Mucosal immunization by DNA vaccine

Most pathogens enter the host via mucosal surface. Therefore the ability to induce immune response at mucosal surface is of great importance. The ability of DNA vaccines to provide mucosal immunity, by either parenteral inoculation or mucosal administration of DNA is currently under investigation. Prenteral immunization with DNA vaccines has been shown to protect against influenza challenge in ferrets, chickens as well as against infectious bovine thinotracheitis caused by bovine herpes viruses, all of, which are mucosal, challenge systems. A more rigorous test of mucosal immunity is provided by genital infections with herpes simplex virus and human immunoefficiency virus and by enteric pathogens such as *Vibrio* and *Shigella* sp. against which parenteral immunization is generally only marginally effective.

Herpes virus applied vaginally in guinea pigs is a well-developed model for human genital herpes infection and provides an opportunity to study mucosal lesions caused by the infection. Immunization with DNA, encoding HSV-2 envelope glycoproteins are also known to produce serum antibodies similar to those resulting from vaginal infection with HSV-2. Vaginal secretions obtained prior to viral challenge contained gD and gB specific antibodies of the IgG subclass. Rouse and his team have shown that a DNA vaccine encoding HSV-1 gB induces $CD4^+$ cytotoxic T lymphocytes, which are protective against murine zoster infection model. DNA vaccines designed to be administered mucosally by direct application of saline formulated plasmids intranasally or intravaginally. Administration by these routes has resulted in generation of local antibodies against HIV antigens and HSV antigens, while intranasal inoculation with influenza HA DNA resulted in protection from challenge with virus. Addition of mucosal adjuvant, such as cholera toxin or incorporation of plasmid into cationic liposomes is in the offing for the delivery of DNA vaccines mucosally.

DNA delivery through live vectors

In this approach the DNA is delivered through a live vector, such as bacteria, in which the plasmid to be delivered is present and it is delivered only after the infection of the cell. An example of this approach is to use an attenuated bacterium, such as an auxotrophic mutant of *Shigella* containing a mammalian DNA expression plasmid into cells in vivo. The bacterial strain was a mutant unable to replicate in the absence of diaminopimelic acid (DAP) into which plasmid encoding reporter protein β-galactosidase was introduced. Such a mutant was able to invade the cell, but since it lacks DAP, which is a critical component of the cell wall, and because mammalian tissue does not contain DAP, such mutants lyse upon cell division, releasing the plasmid into the cytoplasm of the infected cell. Antibody responses against the antigens were observed in the sera following two administration of this recombinant vector. In addition antigen specific spleenocyte proliferation was also observed and the results are favourable.

DNA as adjuvant

It has been known for some years that bacterial DNA is mitogenic for lymphocytes, and that these stimulatory effects may be related to the sequence of nitrogenous bases and the methylation pattern. It is only recently, the evidence for a role for these effects on the immunogenicity of DNA vaccine has emerged. In general, DNA vaccines administered intramuscularly result in the induction of T_H1-type responses as indicated by antigen-specific stimulated secretion of IL-2 and interferon-γ by spleenocytes from animals immunized with various DNA vaccines. It is observed that repeated immunization with various DNA coated onto gold beads into the skin by a biolistic device (gene gun) gradually raises a T_H2-type response. Some DNAs have immune enhancing effect due to specific sequence of nitrogenous bases and methylation pattern in the plasmid. The particular sequence in stimulatory to NK cells and lymphocytes in vitro, inducing them to secrete cytokines. A specific sequence AACGTT when inserted in a DNA vaccine encoding β-galactosidase, has been shown to enhance immune response against the encoded protein.

Recently an improved method for delivery of DNA vaccine has been discovered, which is called **gene gun or biolistic approach.** This method involves coating microscopic gold particles with plasmid DNA and delivering it through the skin into underlying muscle layer with an airgun or electric gun. Helium gas under high pressure is used for delivering the particles or current of 15 to 20 Kv is used. At present the method is being tested for its efficacy in animal models. So far, the results are encouraging and vaccines delivered in this manner have been able to induce protective immunity against different strains of pathogenic antigens.

It is still not clear about the consequences of long term antigen expression in a host. Persistent expression of antigen may eventually lead to a state of autoimmunity or immunologic non-responsiveness due to tolerance.

Vaccines from Synthetic Peptides

Synthetic peptide vaccines for HIV, influenza, diphtheria toxin, hepatitis B virus and malaria parasite are currently being evaluated for their efficacy. To prepare synthetic peptides vaccines, it is necessary to understand the nature of B cell and T cell epitopes. Synthetic peptides are designed in such a way that they strongly bind to hydrophilic region of the B cell epitope. Ideally, vaccines designed for inducing humoral immunity should contain immunodominant B cell epitopes in their peptides.

For an effective memory response for both humoral and cell mediated immunity, good number of memory T_H cells are necessary. In order to achieve this, a successful vaccine must therefore have an immunodominant T cell epitopes. Since T cell epitopes interact with MHC molecule, which differ in their ability to present peptides or antigens to T cells. MHC polymorphism within a species influences the level of T cell responsiveness by different individuals to different antigens. Probably, different sub-population of T cells recognizes different epitopes. Some synthetic peptides generate helper T cell response and some suppressor T cell response. Those that show suppressor response are of immense use in treating autoimmune disease.

Multivalent sub-unit Vaccines

Recombinant protein vaccines and synthetic peptide vaccines have limitations in their applications, because they tend to be poorly immunogenic. More often they tend to induce humoral immune response and less likely cell mediated immune response. At present new innovative techniques have been designed to develop multivalent vaccines that can present multiple copies of antigenic epitope or a mixture of peptides to immune system.

One of the approaches to produce multivalent vaccines is to attach monoclonal antibodies to a solid support (matrix) and then react it with antigen to produce solid matrix-antibody-antigen (SMAA) complex. The resulting complex is used as vaccine. By attaching heterogeneous monoclonal antibodies to the solid support, it is possible to bond different peptides or antigens composing immunodominant epitopes of T and B cells to the solid matrix as shown in Fig. 16. 2a. Particulate nature of this complex contributes to increased immunogenicity by facilitating phagocytosis by macrophages and neutrophils. The complex is also capable of inducing humoral and cellular immune response.

Other methods of obtaining multivalent vaccines are by utilizing detergents, liposomes or immunostimulating complexes (ISCOMs). Detergents are used for preparing micelles from proteins. On mixing protein with detergent and later removal of detergent leads to formation of micelles, where individual proteins will orient in such a way that hydrophobic ends get turned in and hydrophilic ends get turned out to form spherical bodies. Liposomes are prepared by mixing protein antigens with phospholipids. They form bilayered vesicles by enclosing within them protein antigen. ISCOMs are lipid carriers prepared by mixing protein antigen with detergent and a glycoside called Quil A. Liposomes and ISCOMs appear to fuse with plasma membrane thereby delivering the antigen in intracellular area, where it can be processed through cytosolic pathway and induce cell mediated immune response (Fig. 16. 2b and 16.2 c).

At present, protein components of influenza virus, measles virus, HIV and hepatitis B are incorporated into ISCOMs, liposomes and micelles and are being assessed for their vaccine property.

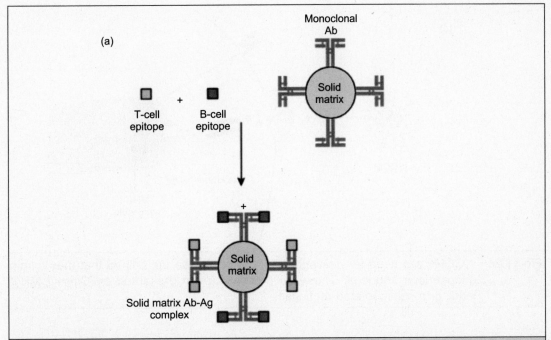

Fig 16.2a Solid matrix antigen-antibody complex is designed so as to contain synthetic peptides representing T-cell epitopes (gray) and B-cell epitopes (dark gray).

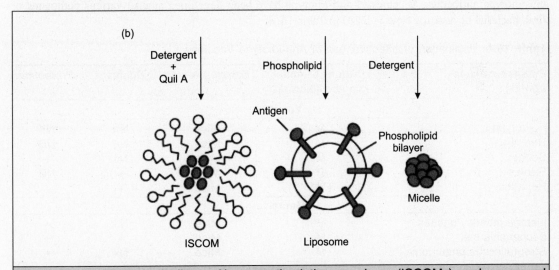

Fig 16.2b Liposomes, micelles and immunostimulating complexes (ISCOMs) can be prepared by mixing extracted antigens with respective substances as indicated

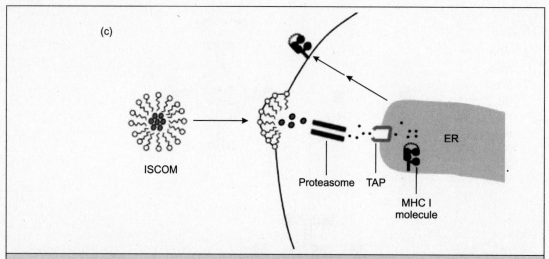

Fig 16.2c ISCOMs are used for delivering the antigen inside the cell so that they mimic endogenous antigens. These on processing are presented on Class I MHC leading to cell-mediated response.

Anti-Idiotype Vaccines

Generation of an effective immune response to a dangerous pathogen without exposing the individual to the killed or attenuated pathogen as vaccine has opened a new doorway in vaccine therapy. It is called anti-idiotype antibodies. Vaccines of anti-idiotype have been developed against various pathogens of viral, bacterial or parasitic type as listed in Table 16. 4.

Table 16.4 Evaluation of effectiveness of Anti-idiotype Vaccines.

Disease causing agents	Nature of Anti-idiotype vaccines	Species tested	Adjuvant	Protection
Viruses				
Polio type I	M	Mice	Nil	Nil
Reo virus	M	Mice	Nil	ND
Sendai	M	Mice	Nil	+
Rabies	P	Mice	+	ND
Hepatitis	P/M	Mice	+	+
Bacteria				
Listeria monocytogenes	M	Mice	Nil	+
Escherichia coli	M	Mice	+	+
Streptococcus pneumonia	M	Mice	Nil	+
Parasites				
Schistosoma mansoni	M	Rat	Nil	+
Trypanosoma cruzi	P	Mice	+	ND
Trypanosoma rhodesiense	M	Mice	Nil	+

Key: P=polyclonal, M=monoclonal, ND=not determined
Source: ZANETTI, M. ET AL., *Immunol. Today* **8:** 18-25. 1987.

Exercise

1. What are Vaccines? Give detailed account types of vaccines and their role in active immunity (20 marks).
2. Write briefly on: (10 marks)
   (a) Attenuated and killed vaccines
   (b) Polysaccharide vaccines
   (c) Protein and toxoid vaccines
   (d) Vaccines from recombinant vectors
   (e) DNA vaccines
   (f) Subunit and synthetic peptide vaccines

Chapter 17

Immune Response to Infectious Diseases

- Viral Infection And Immunity
- Cell-Mediated Immune Response Against Virus
- Viral Strategies Of Immune Evasion
- Immune Response Against Bacterial Infection
- Immune Response Against Protozoan Parasites
- Immune Response Against Helminthine Parasites
- B Cell Effector Mechanisms Against Chronic Infections

Generally, pathogens use variety of strategies to escape immune detection in a host. Many of them have the ability to change their antigenic markers on the membrane, some are able to grow within the host cell, thereby reducing their antigenicity and protected from immune attack. Some parasites are able to shed their antigens from the membrane to avoid immune detection. There are pathogens, which can mimic host cell membrane antigens, either by producing it by them self or by acquiring it from the host cell membrane. Some pathogens have further evolved their own complex system to suppress the host immune response.

Throughout the human history, infectious diseases are the major cause of millions of deaths every year. Although wide spread use of vaccines and drugs have reduced the death rate from infectious diseases in developed countries, infectious diseases are the leading cause of mortality in developing countries. It is estimated that over 600 million people are infected with tropical diseases and 20million die each year. It is not only a tragedy for these countries; some diseases are re-emerging with drug resistance such as malaria and tuberculosis.

Viral Infection and Immunity

When the viral infection occurs, a number of specific immune effector mechanisms are called in to destroy and eliminate the virus from the body. Both innate and adaptive immune responses play an important role in containing the invading pathogen.

The innate response involves the rapid recognition of general molecular patterns of pathogens or post-translational modifications initiated in the infected host cells. Eosinophils, monocytes, macrophages, natural killer cells and soluble mediators such as components of the complement system and acute phase reactions are either bactericidal or activate cellular functions that eradicate pathogens. Viral infections also induce potent antiviral response mediated by interferons. Confrontation of the innate immune system with pathogens leads to its activation and prepares the adaptive immune system to respond approximately. Adaptive immunity is conveyed by both humoral and cellular elements.

Neutralization of viral antigens by humoral antibodies

Antibodies produced as a result of humoral immune response against specific viral antigens are responsible for prevention of spread of virus during acute infection and against re-infection. Most viruses have the ability to express surface protein molecules that are capable of binding specifically to host cell membrane molecules. Epstein-Barr virus binds to type 2 complement receptor on B cells, influenza virus binds to sialic acid residues in membrane glycoproteins and glycolipids; rhinovirus binds to intracellular adhesion molecules (ICAM).

Humoral antibodies when bind to viral antigenic determinants or receptors, will prevent the binding of virus to the host cells, which results in blockade of infection by the virus. Secretory IgA blocks binding of virus to host cells, thus preventing infection or re-infection. IgG and IgM and IgA antibodies block fusion of viral envelope with host cell plasma membrane. IgG and IgM also enhance phagocytosis of viral particles (opsonization). Moreover, IgM antibody agglutinates viral particles. Complements activated by IgG and IgM antibodies mediate opsonization by C3b and lysis of enveloped viral particles by membrane-attack complex.

Cell-mediated Immune Response against Virus

Although antibodies play a key role in preventing the spread of viral infection, they are not able to completely eliminate the virus once the infection has occurred-particularly when virus has entered latent phase by incorporating its DNA into host genome. Once the infection is established, it is only cell-mediated mechanism, which includes $CD4^+$ T_H cells, $CD8^+$ T_C cells are the main components. In the process, T_H1 cells, which come in contact with the viral antigens, undergo activation and produce certain cytokines as immune-mediators, which includes, IL-2, IFN-γ and TNF. IFN-γ induces antiviral state in a cell by acting directly on it and IL-2 acts indirectly by activation of CTL precursors into effector cells. IL-2 and IFN-γ, which plays an important role in defense during the first days of viral infections until a specific CTL response develops, also, activate NK cells. CTL activity arises within 3-4 days after viral infection peaks by 7-10 days and then declines. Within 7-10 days of primary infection most virions are eliminated.

The role of B cells in primary viral infection

The importance of B cells during primary infections varies for different viruses. In fact, the multitude of distinct viruses covers the whole spectrum of effector mechanisms critically involved in protection. The spectrum ranges from viruses controlled exclusively by antibodies, to those controlled by antibodies together with T cells and to those controlled exclusively by T cells (Table 17.1).

Vesicular stomatitis virus (VSV), polyoma virus and rotavirus are impressive examples of viruses that are exclusively controlled by B cells-apparently in the complete absence of T cell help. These viruses exhibit highly repetitive surface antigens and therefore induce specific virus neutralizing IgM antibodies

Table 17.1   Effector mechanisms involved in protection from primary and secondary infections by viruses.

Virus Family/ Group	Virus/ Disease	Critical Effector Mechanism	
		Primary Infection	Secondary Infection
Reoviridae	Rotavirus	Ab	Ab
Papovaviridae	Polyoma	Ab	Ab
Rhabdoviridae	VSV	Ab (T$_H$)	Ab
Togaviridae	Sindbis	Ab (T$_H$)	Ab
Flaviviridae	Flavavirus	Ab (T$_H$)	Ab
Orhtomyxoviridae	Influenza	Ab, T$_H$, CTL	Ab
Picornaviridae	Polio	Ab, T$_H$	Ab
Encephalomyocarditis		Ab, T$_H$, CTL	Ab
Poxviridae	Ectromelia	CTL (Ab)	Ab
Hepadnaviridae	Hepatitis B	CTL (Ab)	Ab
Arenaviridae	LCMV	CTL	Ab (CTL)
Retroviridae	SIV	CTL	Ab (CTL)
Retroviridae	HIV	CTL	Ab (CTL)

Ab=antibody, CTL=cytotoxic T lymphocyte, T$_H$=T helper cell
Source: BACHMANN, M. F. AND KOPF, M. *Curr. Opin. Immunol.* 1999. **11:** 332-339.

in the absence of T$_H$ cells. Although the isotype switch from IgM to IgG or IgA is usually inefficient in the absence of T cell help, the high titer IgM antibodies and/or the relatively low IgG/IgA antibody levels are apparently sufficient to control the viral infection in the acute phase.

Sindbis virus and flavivirus are additional examples in which mainly antibodies and not T cells protect from primary infection; however, it appears that long-lived T cell dependent B cell response may sometimes be required for long-term control of infection. In fact, although T cell independent IgM antibodies can control VSV early, long-term survival of the host is enhanced by the presence of T$_H$ cells that mediate isotype switching.

Influenza virus may be placed next in the spectrum as an example where both B and T cells are critical for protection, since both B cell deficient and T cell deficient mice have been found to be highly susceptible to influenza virus infection. Interestingly, not only CD8$^+$ T cells but also T$_H$ cells are known to be involved in antiviral protection; however, the latter do not directly exhibit antiviral activity. Specifically, viral clearance is only increased in the presence of B cells, indicating that T$_H$ cells protect by increasing the production of specific antibodies. Thus, although influenza virus induces efficient IgM responses in the absence of T cell help, this is apparently not sufficient to confer full protection. Other examples of viruses for which both B and T cells are involved in protection from primary infection are poliovirus and encephalomyocarditis virus. For poliovirus, T$_H$ cells were shown to mediate antiviral protection by enhancing B cell responses. T cells are involved in protection against encephalomyocarditis virus infection, since mice deficient in either MHC class II or MHC class I are hypersusceptible to infection.

On the T cell side of the spectrum lie ectromelia and hepatitis B virus, for which CD8$^+$ T cells play a predominant role while CD4$^+$ T cells and B cells seem dispensable for control of primary infections. The best examples of exclusively T cell controlled viruses are lymphocytic choriomeningitis virus (LCMV), simian immunodeficiency virus (SIV) and HIV. B cells are not required to resolve primary LCMV infections since B cells deficient mice are fully competent to control the virus during the first weeks after inoculation; moreover, protection has been shown to be exclusively mediated by CD8$^+$ T cells. For SIV, it has been recently demonstrated by depletion experiments that CD8$^+$ T cells are critical for control of virus during acute infections. For HIV, no direct experimental evidence is available; however, frequencies of HIV specific CTLs inversely correlate with levels of plasma load of viral RNA, indicating that CD8$^+$ T cells play a critical role in controlling the virus. B cells seem to be of limited importance for the outcome of SIV and HIV infections.

It is interesting to note that the structure of the virions and the repetitiveness of the neutralizing viral epitopes correlates with importance of B cell responses for the control of primary viral infections. B cells are pivotal for elimination of viruses that are structurally highly organized; such viruses induce B cell responses in the absence of T cell help and often form serotypes. The impact of T cell independent B cell responses may be two fold: first, the T cell independent antibodies may directly mediate antiviral protection; secondly, specific B cells are activated and expanded early-facilitating subsequent cognate collaboration between T cells and B cells.

The role of B cells in secondary viral infections

All viruses can be exclusively controlled by antibody if the antibody is present in the organism before infection. Most, if not all, successful antiviral vaccines are based on the induction of neutralizing antibodies. Under these circumstances, viral diseases may be completely inhibited by neutralization of viruses before any cellular infection occurred-as has been shown by VSV. The most interesting example of protection mediated by preexisting antibodies in complete absence of T cells is exhibited by nearly all in early life. Antibody is transferred from the mother to the immunocompetent fetus via blood and/or milk. This antibody is able to protect the newborn child from a variety of viral infections including hepatitis B, rubella virus, influenza virus, respiratory syncytial virus, poliovirus and herpes virus. In addition, preexisting neutralizing antibodies are able to protect from viral infections that are otherwise exclusively controlled by CTLs during primary infections. Such viruses include hepatitis B virus, LCMV and intravenously administered SIV and primary isolates of HIV.

The observation that antibody-mediated protective memory is long-lived, as exemplified by life long protection against re-infection with viruses mediating childhood diseases, is readily explained by the notion that elevated levels of antibodies are present in the serum for decades in humans. In contrast, protective T cell memory is usually more short lived, most probably because memory T cells are known to lose some-although not all-effector functions in the absence of continuous re-stimulation by antigen.

The role of B cells in persistent viral infections

It is observed that, the dynamic virus-host interactions can typically have three different outcomes: first-and most commonly-viruses replicate, induce and immune response and are either eliminated by the immune system or kill the host (acute infection); second, some viruses are able to subvert the immune system and establish a carrier status with high virus load present in the serum, as may be the case after LCMV or hepatitis B virus infection (persistent infection); third, some viruses are able to hide from the immune system and to replicate at very low, undetectable levels as has been shown for herpes virus, LCMV and some retroviruses that integrate into host genome (latent phase). HIV may behave exceptionally, since relatively high viral titers are maintained for extended time periods in the face of a strong and ongoing immune response. Such a situation may differ from the persistent infection as observed after infection with high dose of LCMV, where the virus has overwhelmed the immune system and specific T cells have been exhausted. Thus, early symptom free phase of HIV may be characterized best as an extended primary infection and the same effector mechanisms are probably involved in inhibition of viral replication both early and late after HIV infection.

Interestingly the situation is different for latent infection by LCMV. Acute infection with LCMV are resolved by CD8+ T cells even in the complete absence of B cells; however, several months after the acute infection and long after clearance of the virus to undetectable levels-LCMV is found to flare up again in B cell deficient mice. These data indicate that viruses that are controlled by CTLs during acute infection phase may be held in check by specific antibodies during the latent infection phase. These considerations are supported by the observation that neutralizing antibodies specific for herpes virus are of help in keeping the viral load low in neuronal cells; however, application of exogenous antibodies may be needed to reduce or even eliminate viral load in persistent viral infections.

Viral Strategies of Immune Evasion

1. Blocking the proteins

Many viruses are known to produce proteins that interfere at various levels with specific and non-specific host defenses. Many cells in response to viral infection produce IFN-α and β. These cytokines induce antiviral protein production in nearby non-infected cells called DAI. Viruses such as Epstein-Barr virus and adenovirus are capable of overcoming the antiviral effect of the interferons by blocking or inhibiting the action of DAI.

2. Complement inhibition

Viruses reacted upon by antibodies require complement activation resulting in direct lysis of viral particles or opsonization and elimination of virus through phagocytosis. Many viruses have evolved strategies to evade complement-mediated destruction. For ex. Vaccinia virus induces the production of proteins that bind to the C4b complement component, inhibiting the classical pathway. Similarly, Herpes simplex virus has a glycoprotein component that binds to the C3b component of the complement, thereby inhibiting both classical as well as alternative pathway of complement.

3. Antigen variation

A good number of viruses escape immune attack by constantly changing their antigens. For ex. Influenza virus continuously changes antigens resulting in frequent infection with new strain. Due to the absence of protective immunity against these newly emerging strains, repeated infections occur. Similarly antigenic variation among rhinoviruses has affected vaccine production against common cold. The degree of antigenic variation is highest in HIV (AIDS) virus, which accumulate mutations at a rate of 65 times faster than influenza virus.

4. Evasion of MHC class I antigen presentation

Activity of class I restricted CD8[+] cytotoxic T lymphocytes (CTLs) is responsible for eradication of virus infected cells. Pathogens that attenuate class I expression would have selective advantage through elimination of class I molecules from the cell surface. This makes the virally infected cells become temporarily invisible to CTLs and allows the virus to proliferate. Elimination of surface class I expression as a strategy for deceiving the immune system is not without risk to the virus. NK cells can recognize cell deficient in self-MHC products. Every step in the assembly and trafficking of the class I complex presents a suitable target for this strategy (Figs. 12.3 and 12.4). Quite a number of viruses can down regulate the transcription of class I genes, and in doing so, prevent expression of class I products. Other components of class I presentation pathway such as TAP and the LMPs are also targets for transcriptional control. Even their partial down regulation could frustrate T cell recognition of the infected cell.

5. Proteolysis

The first step in the generation of an antigenic peptide is proteolysis of cellular proteins. There are two examples of interference with cytosolic proteolysis. In human cytomegalovirus (HCMV)-infected cell's expression of viral phosphoprotein, pp65 inhibits the generation of HCMV specific T cell epitopes. The second example is the Epstein-Barr virus (EBV)-encoded EBNA-1 protein, which contains a Gly-Ala repeat that interferes with its proteasomal proteolysis. A single amino acid substitution can eliminate the protective cleavage site required for the generation of a mouse leukemia virus-derived epitope and thus avoid CTL recognition. Most probably, the polymorphism of the MHC evolved in part to accommodate these types of escape strategies, maximizing the likelihood that for a pathogen in question at least some peptides can be presented by the MHC alleles present in the population. MHC products are exploited in a fundamentally different way by HIV virus. In HIV infected individuals, HIV variants evolve in which peptide epitopes recognized by HIV specific T cells have sustained exactly the type of mutation that transforms these peptide ligands into antagonists, thus actively silencing HIV specific T lymphocytes.

6. Retention and destruction of class I MHC molecule

Even if assembly and peptide loading of class I molecules are completed successfully, the final complex must be delivered to the cell surface, if T cells have to recognize them. Some viruses are capable of detaining properly assembled class I molecule at the site of synthesis. Eg. HCMV. Murine CMV (MCMV) is subtly different: its m152 gene product, gp40, likewise causes intracellular retention, but does so in cisternae of Golgi complex. In HIV infected cells, the action of the Vpu product abolishes expression of class I molecules before their egress from the ER. Vpu is also capable of down regulation of CD4.

7. Internalization of class I MHC molecule

MHC class I molecules may be retained in or purged out from ER, but even when they reach the cell surface, they are not safe from viral proteins that modify their function. The HIV Nef protein, modifies the endocytic machinery so that the co-receptor CD4 is cleared from the cell surface and down modulates surface expression of class I molecules. Nef may interact with the adaptor complex AP-2, a set of proteins that link cargo molecules such as receptors to the coat proteins of the vesicles that transport them. Nef is thought to modify the AP-2 complex to facilitate endocytosis of CD4 and class I molecule.

8. NK cells

They destroy variety of virus infected cells early during infection. NK cells are normally prevented from killing their targets by inhibitory signals provided through interaction of receptor on NK cells with self-MHC products. Human CMV encodes its own UL18, which acts as decoy for NK cells. CD94 on NK cells acts as a receptor for UL18.

9. Interference with trafficking along the endocytic pathway

Pathogens can rearrange the intracellular trafficking machinery without causing overt cytoplasmic effect. They could modify endocytic pathway either directly or through control of cytokine production. IL-10 is capable of preventing the surface display of MHC class II molecules by inhibiting their recruitment from intracellular compartments to the cell surface. The IL-10 homologue encoded by EBV is known to impede the display of peptide loaded class II molecules, therefore delay the process of T cell recognition. The E_6 protein of the BPV is known to interact with components of AP-1 adaptor complex, which affects intracellular distribution of class II products or the antigens destined for presentation by them. The adaptor complex AP-3 may be essential for orchestrating traffic involving endocytic components and may allow further splitting of steps targeted by E_6 products of BPV or HIV Nef. Vacuolar acidification is brought about by H+ adenosine triphosphatase, whose subunit may be replaced by E5 product of BPV, thereby preventing acidification of endosome and lysosome. Even a slight elevation of endosomal pH might spare certain antigens from proteolysis and thus prevent their presentation. Helicobacter pylori VacA toxin inhibits acildification of the endosomal system in a very similar manner, thus preventing li-dependent antigen presentation.

10. Negative cytokine regulation

Cytokines are proteins secreted by activated immune cells that regulate immune and inflammatory responses. It is observed that, many viruses benefit from antagonism of cytokine activity. Cytokines can be positive or negative regulators of the immune response and for this reason some viruses encode their own cytokines. EBV encodes a protein homologous to the cellular cytokine IL-10, which is a negative regulator of IL-12. IL-12 itself a cytokine that promotes IFN-γ production and have a profound impact on the development of T_H1 and T_H2 like cytokine producing cells. EBV-encoded IL-10 is also known to down regulate TAP expression as its cellular counter part does.

Viruses may also neutralize cytokine activities. Adenoviruses encode four such genes that antagonize the effect of tumor necrosis factor (TNF). The products of these genes are found at different location in the infected cells, suggesting that they may act independently to interrupt different stages of TNF induced biological activities. The effort exerted by the adenoviruses for neutralizing TNF strongly suggests its importance in the control of adenovirus infection.

In contrast to the adenovirus, pox viruses and herpes viruses modulate cytokine differently. Both encode functional cytokine receptors. EBV encodes a soluble neutralizing receptor for CSF-1 (macrophage colony stimulating factor), four other herpes viruses carry membrane bound receptors for chemokines.

Members of the pox virus family, collectively encode an impressive array of soluble cytokine receptors that bind and block the activity of IFN-γ, the α and β IFNs, TNF and IL-1. These later cytokines are among the most potent regulators of inflammatory reaction and immune function.

A, different form of cytokine regulation is manifested by measles virus. The virus binds specifically to CD46, a cellular complement regulatory protein found on monocytes, which are a prime target for measles virus infection *in vivo*. When measles virus binds and cross-links CD46, the production of IL-12 by monocytes is inhibited, hence generalized immunosuppression of cell-mediated response.

11. Inhibition of apoptosis

It functions as a protective mechanism, in that parasite-infected cells killed by CTL and NK cells undergo apoptotic death. Virus infection can also induce apoptosis more directly and may restrict virus infection by killing off the host cell before the release of progeny virions. One of the best examples of apoptotic interference involves a pox virus protein termed crmA, which resembles serine protease inhibitor (serpin) but functionally inhibits Asp-specific cystein protease (caspases), such as the IL-1β conversion enzyme (ICE). This caspase inhibition is probably how crmA blocks apoptosis induced by CTL, TNF or Fas. The exact mechanism of crmA-mediated inhibition are still unclear, but may be involved in inhibition of granzyme-B, as Asp-Xaa-Specific serine protease released by CTLs that proteolytically activate apoptosis inducing protein. Inactivation of FLICE, a caspase that is part of the death inducing signal complex (DISC) associated with the cytoplasmic tail of Fas. Several members of herpes virus family encode FLICE inhibitory proteins or V-FLIPs that interfere with recruitment and activation of FLICE. In this manner, V-FLIPS protects against cell death induced by activation of members of the TNF-receptor family.

IMMUNE RESPONSE AGAINST BACTERIAL INFECTION

Bacteria enter the body through a number of natural entry routes such as respiratory tract, GI tract and genitourinary tract or through unnatural routes, such as damaged or broken mucous membrane or the skin. Immune response to bacterial infection is mainly through humoral antibodies except in the case of intracellular infection, in which case delayed type hypersensitivity plays an important role. If the virulence and the infection caused by the bacteria are very low, then localized tissue phagocytosis may be able to mount a non-specific defense and eliminate the bacteria. If the strain is virulent and high scale infection occurs than strong immune response will be evoked.

Immune response against extracellular and intracellular bacteria

Extracellular infection by bacteria is known to induce production of humoral antibodies, which are generally secreted by the plasma cells in the lymph node and the submucosa of the respiratory and GI tracts. The reaction of the antibody at several levels is illustrated in the Fig.17.1.

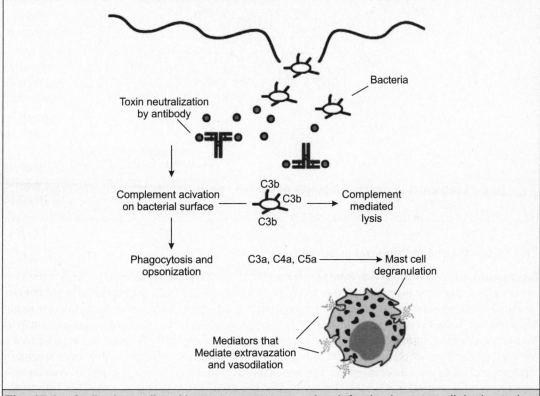

Fig. 17.1   Antibody-mediated immune response against infection by extracellular bacteria

The antibody that readily recognizes and binds to antigen on bacterial cell membrane will invite C3b complement component. These two complexes cause opsonization, which increases the possibility of phagocytosis and thus clearance of the bacterium. Localized inflammatory reaction may also develop as a result of antibody-mediated activation of complement system. For ex. Complement split products, such as C3a, C4b and C5a act as anaphylatoxins, which cause degranulation of mast cells and thus vasodilation and extravasation of lymphocytes and neutrophils from the blood into the tissue spaces. These are the main components of the inflammatory response. Some other complement split products also act as chemotactic factors, which attract neutrophils to the site of infection, thereby increase the phagocytic activity. In the case of Gram-ve bacteria, complement activation leads to direct lysis of the organisms. Specific antibodies (antitoxins) neutralize the exotoxins and phagocytes remove endotoxins of the bacteria and the toxin-antibody complexes.

Cell-mediated immune response is generated against intracellular bacteria and this infection does not even spare immune cells. Generally delayed type hypersensitive reaction occurs in these types of infections, where cytokines secreted by T_{DTH} play an important role, which includes IFN-γ. This cytokine is known to activate macrophages, which will succeed in killing of intracellular pathogen (Fig. 17.2).

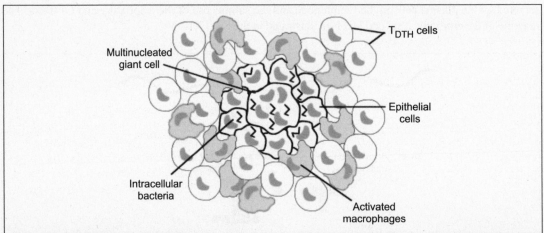

Fig. 17.2   Diagrammatic representation of granuloma formation due to prolonged T_{DTH} response

The role of B cells in bacterial infections

Mechanisms involved in protection from primary bacterial infections are quite complex, while antibodies usually play a major role in protection from secondary infection (Table 17.2). In general the innate immune system is very important for the control of primary bacterial infections, as has been directly demonstrated for protection from streptococcal infection or lipopolysaccharide (LPS) mediated endotoxic shock. In both cases, complement-together with natural antibodies in the case of LPS- has been shown to be critical for host survival; however, specific antibodies are mainly responsible for protection from secondary streptococcal infection. The detailed mechanisms involved in protection from primary *Salmonella typhi* infection remain unclear, it is evident that antibodies can efficiently protect from secondary infections.

Mechanisms involved in protection against *Bordatella pertussis,* the causative agent of whooping cough, have been studied in various gene deficient mice. During primary infections, B cells were observed to be essential for bacterial clearance. Additionally, production of IFN-γ by T_H1 cells was essential to prevent an atypical, disseminated disease. Similarly, during secondary infections, both B and T_H cells were found to be involved in protection.

Table 17.2 Effector mechanisms involved in protection from primary and secondary infections by bacteria.

Bacterial family/ group	Bacteria/ disease	Critical effector mechanisms	
		Primary Infection	Secondary Infection
Gram +	Streptococcus	C	Ab (C)
Gram +	Listeria	Innate, T_H1	T_H1, CTL
Gram +	Bordatella	Ab, T_H1	Ab, T_H1
Gram -	Chlamydia	T_H (B)	Ab
Gram -	Salmonella	Complex	Ab (T)

C=complement, T_H=T helper cell, Ab=antibody, CTL=cytotoxic T lymphocyte, B=B cell
Source: BACHMANN, M. F. AND KOPF, M. *Curr. Opin. Immunol.* 1999. **11**: 332-339.

Antibodies have been implicated in control of variety of secondary infections-including *Streptococcus, Bordatella, Brucella, Chlamydia, Coxiella, Ehrlichia, Francisella, Legionella, Ricketsia and Shigella,* with the exception of *Listeria*.

Evasion of host immune response by bacteria

There are four primary steps in bacterial infection and at each step a host defense mechanism acts and prevents it from spreading. Many bacteria have evolved a strategy to evade these defenses. Some bacteria have the ability to produce surface molecules, which enhance their ability to attach to host cell membrane. A number of Gram-ve bacteria produce hair-like protoplasmic projections on their body called pili, which enable them to attach to the cells of the genitourinary and intestinal tract. Some bacteria like *Bordatella pertussis,* produce sticky adhesion molecules that help them to attach to ciliated epithelial cells of upper respiratory tract.

It is well known that secretory IgA antibody can block bacterial attachment to mucosal epithelial cells, which is the first line of defense against infection in the host. However, some bacteria, such as *Neisseria gonorrhea, Hemophilus influenzae* and *Neisseria meningitidis* have the ability to cleave the secretory IgA molecule at the hinge region by their protease secretion. Due to this half-life of the IgA is shortened; hence it is unable to agglutinate microorganisms at the mucosal surface. Some bacteria have the ability to change the surface antigens, thereby preventing recognition by IgA. For this purpose bacteria adopts a method called gene conversion, where one or more gene segments or mini-cassettes of silent genes replace the gene sequences of the coding region. This has been observed in *N. gonorrhoea*, which attaches itself to the epithelial lining of urethra and cervix through pili. In this organism pili consists of a special protein called pilin, which undergoes tremendous variation due to gene conversion and produce antigenically different pilin protein in *N. gonorrhoea,* which gives the bacteria an added advantage of avoidance of reaction with antibodies.

In some bacteria, such as *Streptococcus pneumoniae,* produce polysaccharide capsule on their surface, which is effective in inhibition of phagocytosis. There are 84 different serotypes in *S. pneumoniae*, which produce different types of polysaccharide molecules; hence antibody produced against one serotype will not react with the other serotype. Therefore, *S. pneumoniae* can cause disease in the same host with different serotypes. Some *Staphylococci* secrete an enzyme *coagulase*, which produces fibrin coat around the organism, thereby protecting it from phagocytosis.

As in the case of viruses, some bacteria have the ability to interfere with complement system. For ex. *Pseudomonas* secretes an enzyme-*elastase*, which is capable of inactivating both C3a and C5a complement components. They are anaphylatoxic and responsible for inflammation. Due to their inhibition by elastase, localized inflammation fails to occur at the site of infection. Some Gram-ve bacteria produce long side chains on lipid A moiety of the cell wall-core polysaccharide, which helps to resist lysis mediated by complement reaction.

Mycobacterium tuberculosis and Mycobacterium leprae survive in the intracellular environment of the phagocytes and escape from the host defense mechanism. Other bacteria like, *Mycobacterium avium and Chlamydia* have the ability to inhibit lysosomal fusion with phagosomes, thereby preventing lysis.

IMMUNE RESPONSE AGAINST PROTOZOAN PARASITES

Protozoan parasites are unicellular, intracellular or extracellular pathogens that cause plethora of diseases in humans, such as amoebiasis, African sleeping sickness, malaria, leishmaniasis and toxoplasmosis. Depending on the location of the parasite within the host body, type of immune response shown also varies. In most instances, the host responds to these unicellular parasites and limits parasitic replication, which would otherwise result in chronic infection. Disease usually develops either from immunopathological side effects, from unchecked parasitic growth due to immunosuppression, or due to parasitic resistance. Generally control of chronic infection is maintained by cell-mediated and humoral immune mechanisms.

Many protozoans have been shown to induce remarkably enhanced NK cell activity in chicken, fish, human and mouse hosts following infection with the genuses: *Babesia, Cryptosporidium, Eimeria, Ichthyopthirius, Leishmania, Plasmodium, Theileria, Toxoplasma and Trypanosoma*. The rapid elevation in cytotoxic response induced by *Leishmania, Toxoplasma and Trypanosoma* suggests that NK cells may participate in the innate phase of host resistance against protozoa.

The Effector function of NK cells during Protozoan infection

The two major effector functions of NK cells include Lysis of target cells and the production of cytokines involved in the stimulation of other immune cells. Recent reports indicate that, the latter function is the primary resistance mechanism of these cells in protozoan infection. The destruction of protozoa by NK cells is known to occur by the lysis of extracellular organisms or by the destruction of infected cells. In an experiment, NK cells from mice treated with the NK cell inducer poly (IC) or infected with *Trypanosoma cruzii* exhibited lytic activity against extracellular trypomastigotes, a blood stage of the parasite, and epimastigotes an invertebrate form of the parasite. Similarly, NK cell-mediated extracellular parasite destruction has been observed using extracellular tachyzoites of *Toxoplasma gondii and Tetrahymena pyriformis*, which are opportunistic human protozoan pathogens. NK cells have also been shown to destroy host cells (e.g. macrophages) infected with *Plasmodium falciparum, Trypanosoma gondii or Leishmania major.*

Cytokine dependent effector functions of NK cells

NK cells are known to be an important source of IFN-γ and TNF-α, two cytokines, which play a major role in activating macrophages, to kill both intracellular and extracellular microorganisms. In an experiment, addition of heat killed bacteria to spleen cells from T-cell deficient sever combined immunodeficient (SCID) mice resulted in the production of high levels of NK cell-derived IFN-γ. This response was shown not be a consequence of direct interaction between the pathogen and NK cells but rather a secondary effect of IL-12 and TNF-α induced from activated macrophages in the cultures. Similar studies carried out with the intracellular protozoan pathogen such as *T. gondi* revealed the same pattern of IL-12 and

TNF-α dependent pathway of NK cell IFN-γ synthesis, stimulated by both live tachizoites as well as parasite extracts. IFN-γ is known to be a crucial mediator of innate resistance to protozoan infection. NK cells also produce number of other important mediators, which may influence host resistance to protozoan infections. These include chemotactic proteins-IL-8 and macrophage inflammatory protein (MIP-1a), GM-CSF, macrophage colony stimulating factor (M-CSF) and IL-3.

Mechanism of NK cell activation by Protozoa

At present it is believed that protozoans activate murine NK cells, which includes both cytokine production and lytic activity, primarily through an indirect mechanism involving stimulation of monokines such as IL-12 from APCs. *L. major* and *T. gondi* are also known to indirectly stimulate NK cells in humans. In the murine model, protozoan stimulated spleen and peritoneal cell populations are known to synthesize high levels of IL-12 and TNF-α and these cytokines in the absence of parasite act synergistically to induce IFN-γ production by purified NK cells. These observations indicate that monokine induction is the primary mechanism by which protozoan parasites stimulate NK cell activation. A number of structurally distinct molecules have been implicated in the induction of IL-12. For ex, a protein highly homologous to a eukaryotic ribosomal protein has been implicated in the induction of IL-12 by *L. braziliensis*. In contrast, recent work on *Plasmodium sp., T. cruzi, T. brucci and T. gondi* indicate that, glycolipids as inducers of IL-12 and TNF-α. In all four protozoan species, glycolipid anchors have been postulated to be the major structures triggering the production of these cytokines, which are important for stimulating the activity of NK cells. In addition to these cytokines, other cytokines like IL-1β, IL-2, IL-7 and IL-15 as well IFN-γ has also been implicated in stimulation of NK cells by certain protozoan parasites. It is presumed that, in addition to IL-1β, IL-2, IL-7, IL-12, IL-15 and TNF-α other cytokines may act as positive regulators of NK cell function in protozoan infection.

Regulation of protozoan-triggered NK cell activity

Since NK cells show a transient response against protozoan infection, it is suggested that the activity of these cells may be tightly regulated. The cytokine IL-10, TGF-β and to a lesser extent IL-4, have been shown to inhibit parasite-induced IFN-γ production and NK cell induced lysis. For ex, *L. major* is known to stimulate increased synthesis of IL-10 and TGF-β within 1 day after infection and addition of monoclonal antibody (mAb) against both of these cytokines are known to cause increased NK cell associated IFN-γ production by cells from infected mice. It is observed that IL-10 deficient mice rapidly succumbs to infection with an avirulent parasite strain, a phenomenon found to be associated with the overproduction of type I cytokines (IL-12, TNF-α and IFN-γ) as well as enhanced NK cell lytic activity. The exact mechanism by which IL-10 and TNF-β specifically inhibit protozoan mediated NK cell activation is not clear. It is suggested that both IL-10 and TNF-β inhibit the synthesis of IFN-γ similar to the inhibition observed with IL-12 and TNF-α synthesis by macrophages. The relevance of existence of this indirect pathway is supported from the experimental evidences documented from *T. gondi* infected IL-10 deficient mice. Direct inhibition of NK cell function, i.e., IFN-γ synthesis and lysis also seems to be likely because of the stimulatory effects of exogenously administered IL-12 are greatly reduced in the presence of either IL-10 or TGF-β. The exact nature of such direct regulation is not clear but it is presumed that modulation of receptors for either IL-12 or other cytokines involved in amplifying the IL-12 response (ex. IL-1β, IL-2R, IL-15R, TNF-αR) or down modulating the costimulatory molecules (ex. CD28) on the NK cells.

Immune response against Plasmodium infection

Malaria is caused by various species of Plasmodium, of which *P. falciparum* is the most virulent and responsible for brain malaria and maximum casualties. Rest other species *P. vivax, p. malariae* cause malarial fever. The pathogens are transmitted through *Anopheles* mosquito. Malarial disease occurs in 600 million people all over the world and annually it causes 1-2 million deaths. At present eradication of malaria programme has got tangled into another problem of drug resistance of parasites, in addition to pesticide resistance of vector-mosquito. Hence, vaccine development against the pathogen is on priority and various laboratories in the world are trying various strategies of development of vaccine by modern biotechnology.

In many parts of the world malaria is endemic to the region, where immune response to the pathogen is very poor. It is observed that children with less than 14 years of age show very low immune response against the Plasmodium infection and it accounts for more than 50% mortality in the children in these endemic areas. Most people living in endemic regions have life long low level infection by plasmodium and they have detectable level of antibodies in their serum against *sporozoite* stage of the plasmodium. Even then the degree of immunity is far from complete and there are number of factors which contribute to low level of immune response to Plasmodium. First and the foremost are changing of surface antigens at different stages of parasitic life cycle. Intracellular phases of the life cycle in the liver and erythrocytes reduce the chances of immune activation. Furthermore, the most accessible stage, the sporozoite lasts only for 30 min in the blood is not sufficient enough to activate the immune response. Even if antibody is developed, the parasite has evolved a strategy of sloughing off the surface antigen coat, thus antibodies fail to bind to their body.

The role of B cells in plasmodium infection

Mouse models of the erythrocyte stage of various species of malarial parasite showed that control of acute and chronic infection is primarily dependent on both $CD4^+$ T cells and B cells, with some contribution of CTLs and $\gamma\delta$ cells. While B cell deficient (μMT) mice infected with *Plasmodium chabaudi chabaudi* were able to limit the acute early parasitemia, they failed to eliminate the parasite and instead developed chronic, relapsing parasitemia with high peak numbers. Transfer of immune serum into infected μMT mice partially suppressed recrudescent parasitemia, indicating that antibodies are important in control of chronic infection; furthermore μMT mice also failed to control secondary infection with *P.c. chabaudi*, demonstrating that B cells are crucial for protective memory responses.

Design of vaccines against Malaria

At present vaccines have been tried against sporozoite stage. In one strategy of vaccine development, the *P. falciparum* sporozoites are irradiated by X-rays and injected into nine volunteers. Later these volunteers were challenged with virulent *P. falciparum* through mosquito bite. It was revealed that six of the nine volunteers were completely protected. Even though, the results are encouraging, greatest problem of this immunization strategy is breeding of mosquitoes to obtain plasmodium sporozoites, which is impractical for immunization of millions of people living in endemic areas.

Current biotechnological approach to produce vaccine is aimed at producing subunit vaccines consisting of epitopes that can be recognized by T cells and B cells. One such vaccine designed consists of 3 epitopes from merozoite proteins together with a conserved domain from the sporozoite protein called SPf66. Clinical trials have shown that the vaccine has 75% efficiency. Presently this vaccine is being tested in Africa and in Latin America.

Immune response against Trypanosoma

It is flagellated protozoan and two species of Trypanosoma are known to cause sleeping sickness in Africa. The disease progresses through several stages, beginning with blood, where the parasites undergo multiplication every 4-6 hrs. From there the disease spreads to the nervous system causing meningoencephalitis leading to loss of consciousness. Trypanosomal surface is covered by variant surface glycoprotein (VSG) antigen, which stimulates effective humoral antibody response. The antibodies against VSG successfully eliminate most of the parasite from the blood stream both by opsonization and subsequent phagocytosis as well as complement-mediated lysis. Some organisms show 1% variation in VSG and will escape antibody attack. These variant organisms begin to proliferate in the blood stream and cause new wave of infection in the individual. The successive wave of infection is due to antigenic shift by which trypanosomes can evade the immune response to their glycoprotein antigens. In this way single infection is able to escape the humoral antibodies generated in response to the preceding variant, so that waves of parasitic forms of the same variant parasite keeps occurring repeatedly.

An individual trypanosoma carries a large repertoire of VSG genes, which are clustered at multiple chromosomal sites. A trypanosome expresses only one VSG gene at a time. Activation of VSG gene results in duplication of the gene and its transposition to a transcriptionally active site at the telomeric end of a specific chromosome. Activation of another VSG gene displaces the previous one from the telomeric expression site. It is because of this property of continuous shift in epitopes of VSG, makes it difficult to develop a vaccine against African sleeping sickness.

The role of B cells in Trypanosoma infections

Trypanosoma cruzi is a parasitic protozoan that causes Chagas disease, which is the major cause of heart disease within endemic areas. The importance of B cells and antibodies in both acute and chronic stages of Chagas disease is well documented in humans and led to the conclusion that antibodies are the major immune effector mechanisms controlling *T. cruzi* infection, in particular after secondary infections. Additionally studies in mice lacking CD4$^+$ T cells or CD8$^+$ T cells suggests that both T cells subsets are involved in control of *T. cruzi* infection. By using μMT mice it has been demonstrated that B cells or antibodies are not required for the protective mechanisms that lead to survival and reduction of parasitemia of mice vaccinated with paraflagellar rod proteins, an efficacious immunogen, before infection with an otherwise lethal dose; however, before the idea of an important role for B cells during *T. cruzi* infection is discarded, studies are under way in B cell deficient mice on the BALB/c background, which is a strain that exhibits high parasitemia.

IMMUNE RESPONSE AGAINST HELMINTHINE PARASITES

Helminths are large multicellular organisms that do not multiply in large numbers in humans and they are not intracellular pathogens. They are more accessible to the immune system. Even then, immune response developed against them in an infected individual is very poor, because helminthes are generally few in numbers in a host. Hence the immune system is not strongly engaged.

In the world more than a billion people are infected with *Ascaris,* which is a roundworm that infects the small intestine. About 300 million people are infected with *Schistosoma haematobium*, a trematode worm, which is a blood parasite of intestinal wall, liver and bladder. Several nematodes and platyhelminths are parasites of domestic animals like pig, sheep etc. They enter the human body through improperly cooked meat. The important helminths are: *Taenia,* a tapeworm found in cattle or pigs and liver fluke found in sheep liver, *Trichinella* spiral roundworm found in pork.

In the case of *Schistosomiasis*, although an immune response does develop, it is insufficient to eliminate the adult worms even though the adults are confined to intramuscular sites. Since the adult worms are motile, they move from one area to other, hence evade localized buildup of immune and inflammatory cells. Schistosomes live up to 20 years in a host and the adult Schistosomes are known to have a unique property of decreasing the antigen expression on its outer membrane and also they are known to enclose themselves in host derived glycolipids and glycoprotein coat. These strategies help in masking the antigens. Among the frequently observed host glycolipid-glycoprotein coatings are ABO blood group antigens, which are recognized by the body as self-components contributing to life long persistence of these organisms.

There are three species of Schistosomes, which infect humans in different regions of the world. They are *Schistosoma mansoni*, *S. japonicum* and *S. haematobium*. It is observed that, when S. mansoni infection occurs, IgE titer in the blood goes up and shows localized increase in mast cell degranulation and increased number of eosinophils (Fig. 17.3). Degranulation of mast cells release pharmacological mediators that increase the infiltration of cells like macrophages and eosinophils. The eosinophils have Fc receptor for IgE and IgG and they bind to antibody-coated parasite. Once bound to the parasite, eosinophils undergo

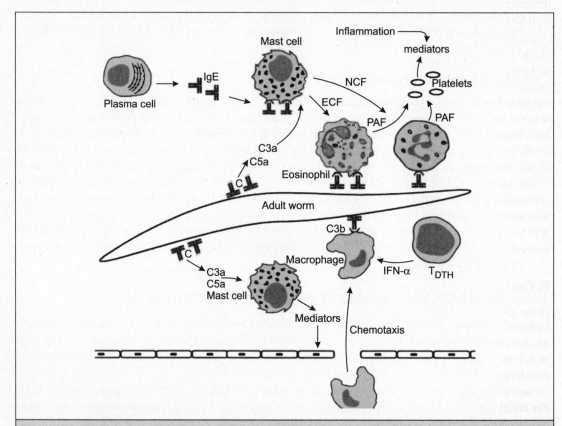

Fig. 17.3 Diagrammatic representation of IgE mediated immune response against helminth parasite (*Schistosoma mansoni*). Key: ECR = Eosinophil chemotactic factor, NCF = Chemotactic factor, PAF = Platelet activation factor.

degranulation to release basic proteins and sulfotransferase. This results in antibody dependent cell-mediated cytotoxicity (ADCC). Basic proteins released by eosinophils are toxic to helminths.

At present various strategies to develop vaccines against young schistosomules or cercariae antigens is underway because they are most susceptible to immune attack. Schistosome cDNA libraries are ready and various antigen markers from this library have been identified and cloned. Experiments using cloned cercariae or schistosomule antigens are presently underway to assess their ability to induce protective immunity in animal models.

The role of B cells in helminth infections

Infections with tissue dwelling filarial nematodes are usually persistent and may cause elephantiasis, chronic skin lesions and blindness. Mechanisms for acquired immunity remain elusive. Mouse model of infection with *Onchocerca lienalis* and *Brugia malayi* clearly demonstrated that B cells are dispensable for the control of both primary and challenge infection; however, vaccine derived from tropomyosin of *Onchocerca* can confer protective immunity, which is at least part antibody-mediated. Additionally, it has been shown that filaria can interfere with B cell activation by secretion of a glycoprotein that differentially modulates the expression and activation of isoforms or protein kinase C and disrupts the coupling of surface immunoglobulin to the mitogen-activated protein kinase pathway in B cells.

Several species of schistosome worms, which are a distinct group of helminths, are responsible for the chronic parasitic disease bilharizis. The formation of granulomas around eggs in the liver is the main pathogenic event. In a murine model of acute and chronic *Schistosoma mansoni* infection, formation of hepatic egg granulomas and hepatic fibrosis are dependent on T_H2 type cytokine responses. Recently it has been convincingly demonstrated that B cells downmodulate the hepatic pathology during acute and in particular, during chronic infection; however, B cell deficient mice did not exhibit increased parasitic load. B cells appear to inhibit liver pathology through mechanisms dependent on a functional Fc receptor (FcR) γ chain, indicating that antibody mediated stimulation of FcRs on macrophages triggers the release of anti-inflammatory mediators such as transforming growth factor (TGF)-β and prostaglandins.

Efficient protection to schistosome infection by vaccination with irradiated cercaria requires both a cell-dependent and humoral immune component. Immunity induced by vaccination was reduced by less than 50% in both IFN-$\gamma^{-/-}$ mice and in B cell deficient mice whereas it was almost nil in mice lacking both IFN-γ and B cells. Thus, although specific antibodies can mediate some protection, presence of both antibodies and T_H1 cells is required to prevent disease upon secondary infection.

B Cell Effector Mechanisms against Chronic Infections

In the great majority of cases, antibodies are the relevant effector mediators for protection against viral, bacterial or parasitic infections; nevertheless, it is interesting to note that B cell deficient mice fail to resolve chlamydial infections because they are unable to generate protective T cell response in the absence of B cells. An important effector mechanism of antibodies is neutralization of pathogens by blocking infectivity. Viruses neutralizing antibodies usually inhibit cellular infection by blocking the interaction of viruses with the cellular receptor or by inhibiting fusion of the virus with cellular endosomal membranes. For rabies virus and vesicular stomatitis virus, it was shown that neutralizing antibodies block infection by covering up the viral surface. In addition, induction of conformation changes in the viral envelope has also been suggested to inhibit viral infectivity.

The role of antibody-dependent complement activation in antiviral protection is relatively ill defined. Complement decorated bacteria are more efficiently phagocytosed by macrophages and neutrophils and may also stimulate innate immunity. Indeed, complement deficient mice have been found to be hypersusceptible to primary and secondary streptococcal infection; moreover the classical pathway of complement activation, together with natural antibodies, is crucial for LPS clearance from the serum. Local and systemic C3 complement component responses have been shown to be regulated by IL-6, a proinflammatory cytokine triggered early during infection. This cytokine possibly link impaired antibody responses and the susceptibility to a variety of pathogens that is observed in IL-6 deficient mice. Antibodies may also directly inhibit bacteria by inhibition of bacterial motility and by prevention of bacterial attachment to target cells. A further well-known mechanism of action of antibodies that is beneficial to the host is toxin neutralization. The efficiency of the latter mechanism is demonstrated by the success of tetanus and pertussis vaccines, which are based on immunization with inactivated toxins.

Plasmodium may serve as a good example where direct inhibition of a parasite by antibodies has been observed. Specific antibodies against either the circumsporozoite antigen or the *P. falciparum* erythrocyte membrane protein 1 (PfEMP1)-a family of highly polymorphic parasite proteins expressed on the infected erythrocyte-may interfere with the attachment of sporozoite to hepatocytes or with the attachment of merozoites to endothelial cells, respectively, and so provide immunity to malaria.

Exercise

1. Give a detailed account of mode of viral infection and explain how immune response develops against viral infection (20 marks).
2. Describe the strategy of viral immune evasion (20 marks).
3. Explain the mode of immune response against bacteria and add a note on immune evasion by bacteria (20 marks).
4. Give a descriptive account of immune response against protozoan parasites (20 marks).
5. Write an account on immune response against helminth parasite (20 marks)
6. Write notes on role of B cells against: (10 marks each)
    (a) Viral infection
    (b) Protozoan infection
    (c) Helminth infection

Chapter 18

Hypersensitivity

- Type I-IgE-Mediated Hypersensitivity
- Basophils and Mast Cells
- Mediators of Type I Reactions
- Passive Transfer Anaphylaxis
- Localized Anaphylaxis
- Late Phase Reaction
- Detection of Type I Hypersensitivity
- Allergens
- Mechanism of IgE-Mediated Degranulation
- Consequences of Type I Reactions
- Cutaneous Anaphylaxis
- Infantile Eczema or Atopic Dermatitis or Allergic Eczema
- Treatment of Type I Hypersensitivity

- Type II Hypersensitivity or Antibody Mediated Cytotoxic Hypersensitivity
- Type IV Delayed Type Hypersensitivity or Tdth Mediated Hypersensitivity
- Type III-Immune Complex Mediated or Antibody-Antigen Complex Mediated Hypersensitivity
- Type V-Stimulatory Hypersensitivity

When an immunologically sensitized individual comes in contact with same antigen second time, it leads to secondary boosting of the immune response. The secondary response may be excessive leading to tissue damage if the antigen is present in large dose or the cellular and humoral immune response is at a heightened level. Heightened immune response evokes a battery of effector molecules. Generally, those effector molecules induce mild subclinical, localized inflammatory reaction, which help in removal of antigens without causing excessive damage to the tissue in the host. In rare instances, this inflammatory response may be more severe and cause tissue damage. Such a reaction is called *hypersensitivity or allergy*. There are several types of hypersensitive reactions, which can be distinguished on the basis of effector molecules generated during the course of reaction. IgE antibodies are found attached to mast cell membrane. On reacting with antigen, they cause degranulation of mast cells, thereby releasing histamine and other biologically active substances. IgG and IgM antibodies on reacting with antigens, stimulate complement system, whose effector molecules in this reaction are membrane attack complexes, such as C3a, C4a, and C5a. Antibody involved hypersensitive reactions are immediate type. In delayed type hypersensitive (DTH) reaction, the effector molecules are various cytokines secreted by separate population of T cells, called T_{DTH}. As it became apparent that different types of immune mechanisms give rise to different types of hypersensitivity, Comb's and Gel defined four types of hypersensitivity and at present fifth one viz. *Stimulatory* has been added (Table 18.1). Type I, II, III, and V and depend on the interaction of antigen with humoral antibody and it is called immediate hypersensitivity. Type IV is called delayed

Table 18.1 Comb's and Gell classification of hypersensitive reactions

Type	Descriptive name	Initiation time	Mechanism	Type of manifestation
Immediate Type				
I	IgE- mediated, anaphylactic and atopic hypersensitivity	20-30 min	IgE bound to mast cells and basophils reacts with Ag and induces cross-linkage thereby releasing vasoactive mediators	Systemic or generalized anaphylaxis: hay fever, asthma, Hives (anigiodema or urticaria), food allergies, eczema
II	IgG, IgM- mediated cytotoxic	5-8 hrs	Ab directed against surface antigens, causes cell destruction via complement activation or ADCC reaction	Blood transfusion reactions, autoimmune hemolytic anemia, Rh factor (erythroblastosis foetalis)
III	Immune complex- mediated hypersensitivity	2-8 hrs	Ag-Ab complex deposited in different areas of body induce complement activation and inflammatory response	Localized: Arthus reaction Generalized reaction: Rheumatoid arthritis, glomerular nephritis, serum sickness *lupus erythematosus*
V	Stimulatory hypersensitivity			
Delayed Type				
VI	Cell mediated hypersensitivity	24-72 hrs	Sensitized T_{DTH} (delayed type hypersensitivity) cells release cytokines that activate macrophages and T-cytotoxic cells	Graft rejection, contact dermatitis, tubercular lesions

type hypersensitivity because of its longer time course and it involves receptors bound to the lymphocyte surface.

The detailed classification of hypersensitivity is as follows:

Type I- Anaphylactic, Atopic hypersensitivity

Type II- Antibody dependent cytotoxic hypersensitivity

Type III- Immune complex mediated hypersensitivity

Type IV- Cell mediated (delayed type) hypersensitivity

Type V- Stimulatory hypersensitivity

TYPE I-IgE-MEDIATED HYPERSENSITIVITY

Certain class of antigens referred, as *allergens* are responsible for type I hypersensitive reaction. In this case like all other antigens, these allergens stimulate humoral immune response through the same mechanism as described in Chapter 10 and 12, resulting in production of antibody secreting plasma cells and memory cells. Only the difference in this case from the conventional humoral response is that, the plasma cells secrete excessive quality of IgE.

This antibody has its Fc receptors on mast cells and basophilic membrane. IgE on binding to Fc receptors on the basophilic and mast cell membrane, **sensitize** them. Such sensitized cells when react with allergens through IgE molecules, bring about degranulation of these cells (Fig. 18.1). Degranulation of these cells results in release of pharmacologically active mediators, which exert biological effect on smooth muscle linings. Thereby, inducing vasodilation or constriction of smooth muscles, which may be systemic or localized depending on the amount of mediators released.

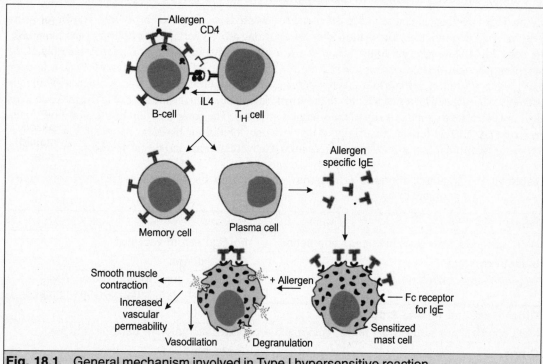

Fig. 18.1 General mechanism involved in Type I hypersensitive reaction

Components Involved in Type I Reaction

Before dealing with the mechanism of degranulation, it is felt necessary to give the details of components involved in type I reaction, which are dealt here with.

ALLERGENS

Generally, majority of humans mount an immune reaction against different parasitic infection by producing IgE. Hence, IgE levels in the serum of patients with parasitic infection will be higher compared to normal individuals. These levels come to normal only when the parasite is successfully cleared from the body. The term allergen refers to antigens specifically of stimulatory type I hypersensitivity in allergic as well as **atopic** (hereditary) individuals.

Most of the allergens enter the body through the oral or nasal route and bring about allergic reaction on mucous membrane surface, where IgE is available. Some of the common allergens encountered by humans in their day-to-day life are listed in Table 18.2.

Most of the allergens are small proteins or protein bound substances having a molecular weight of 15,000 to 40,000. Some of them are haptens capable of reacting with body proteins and form a stable complex. This hapten-protein complex is capable of stimulating immune response, where IgE, IgG and IgM antibodies may be involved.

The major antibody involved in anaphylactic reaction is IgE or reagenic antibody

In the human antibodies that sensitize the tissue for anaphylactic reactions have been known for many years as reaginic antibodies. These antibodies have a strong affinity for tissue (cytotropic) and can readily be detected 24 to 48 hrs later in the serum of a sensitized individual by injecting small quantity of the serum into the skin of a normal recipient into the injection site. The IgE is present in vary low concentration (10-130 µg/100 ml of serum) in a healthy person. The concentration of IgE in patients with allergic asthma has been found to be much higher than normal individuals although the level of IgE in the circulation does not correlate with the severity of the allergic symptoms. The comparatively low levels of IgE found in serum presumably reflect the affinity of this immunoglobulin for tissue so that freshly made IgE is very soon removed from serum when it comes in contact with the appropriate cell receptors on mast cells.

Table 18.2 Common antigens (allergens) encountered by humans associated with type I hypersensitivity.

Foods	Proteins
Nuts, sea food , egg and milk, peas and beans	Foreign serum vaccines
Insect Products	**Plant Pollens**
Venom of ants, bees and wasps, mosquito saliva	Rag weed, poke weed, timothy, hay, Parthenium, rye, birch, conifers, subabul
Other Plant and Animal Products	
Mold spores, house dust, dust mites, cockroach droppings, animal hair, danders and wool.	
Drugs	**Toxicants**
Penicillin, sulfonamides, anesthetics, salicylates, benzoates	PVC fumes, dioxins, aromatic hydrocarbons (petroleum products) natural and artificial perfumes

IgE appears to have four main activities, namely

(1) Capacity to bind via F_C fragment to mast cells and basophils
(2) Subsequent interaction with antigen that takes place on the cell membrane of the mast cell
(3) Resultant trigger of the release of pharmacological mediators
(4) Attraction of other cell types-eosinophils.

Human atopy and Prausnitz-Kustner (PK) reaction

A significant proportion of humans are susceptible to natural sensitization by a variety of environmental antigens, including pollens, spores, animal danders, house dusts, drugs and foods. These individuals appear to be genetically predisposed or susceptible. This susceptibility is known as atopy; however, the term allergy is often used synonymously. These hyperactive reactions in humans can also be passively transferred to non-reactive subjects by the injection of serum antibodies. In order to avoid generalized reaction and sensitization, a completely localized transfer may be performed. This procedure is referred to as the Prausnitz-Kustner (PK) reaction. Serum from a sensitized individual is injected intradermally into a normal recipient. After a latent period of one or more days, antigen is injected into the same site and a localized wheel and flare reaction occurs within minutes.

BASOPHILS AND MAST CELLS

Basophils are a type of leukocytes, which belong to granulocyte category that circulate in the blood and they account for mere 0.5 to 1.0% in normal human blood. They have a granulated cytoplasm, which stains with basic dyes, hence the name basophils. Electron microscopy of basophil reveals that, it has a multilobed nucleus, few mitochondria, numerous glycogen granules and electron dense membrane bound granules scattered throughout the cytoplasm. (Fig.18.2).

Precursors of mast cells are formed in the bone marrow during hematopoiesis. From there, they are carried to virtually all vascularized areas of the body, where they differentiate and become mast cells. They are abundant in connective tissue, particularly blood vessel lining and lymphatics. Some tissue such as mucous membrane lining of respiratory and gastrointestinal tract and the skin contain large number of mast cells. For ex. Mucous lining of GI tract is known to contain 10,000 mast cells per mm^3. Electron micrograph of mast cells reveal, numerous membrane bound granules distributed throughout the cytoplasm. These granules are known to contain pharmacologically active substances (Fig. 18.3). On activation, mast cells release these mediators from their granules, which bring about type I hypersensitive reaction. Mast cells are also known to secrete certain cytokines, like IL-1, IL-3, IL-4, IL-5, IL-6, GM-CSF, TGF-β and TNF-α. Since these cytokines exert diverse biological effects, mast cells contribute to a broad spectrum of physiologic, immunologic and pathologic processes.

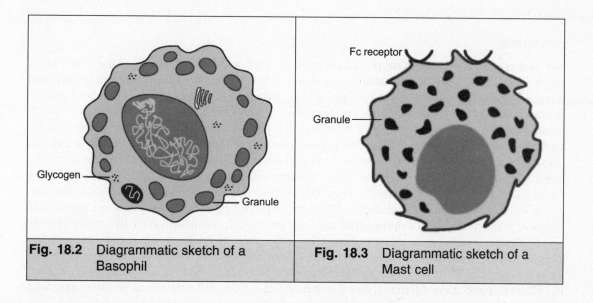

Fig. 18.2　Diagrammatic sketch of a Basophil

Fig. 18.3　Diagrammatic sketch of a Mast cell

MECHANISM OF IgE-MEDIATED DEGRANULATION

IgE is brings about degranulation of mast cells by cross-linking with the receptors. The explosive degranulation and the release of pharmacological mediators are shown in Fig. 18.4. The exact mechanism of activation of mast cells is as follows.

On bridging the receptors by cross linking of IgE molecules on the mast cells, it is rapidly followed by the breakdown of phosphatidyl inositol to inositol triphosphate (IP_3), the generation of diacyl glycerol and an increase in intracytoplasmic free calcium. As in the case of B cell activation phospholipase C activation generates both IP_3 which mobilizes intracellular Ca^{2+} and diacyl glycerol which in turn activate protein kinase C. The biochemical activation of membrane produces membrane active *fusogens* such as lysophosphotidic acid, which may facilitate granular membrane fusion and degranulation, and the series of arachidonic acid metabolites formed by the cyclo-oxygenase and lipoxygenase pathways.

MEDIATORS OF TYPE I REACTIONS

Mediators are pharmacologically active substances that are released after degranulation of basophils and mast cells. They act as an amplifying terminal effector mechanism of type I hypersensitive reaction. Mediator release induced by allergens, results in unnecessary increase in vascular permeability and inflammatory response, whose detrimental effects far outweigh any beneficial effects. Mediators can be classified as primary and secondary.

The primary mediators are produced before degranulation and are stored in the form of granules. The most important primary mediators are histamine, protease, eosinophil chemotactic factor (ECF), neutrophil chemotactic factor (NCF) and heparin.

The secondary mediators are synthesized after target-cell activation or released by the breakdown of membrane phospholipids during degranulation process. The important second mediators are leukotrienes, platelet activating factor, prostaglandins, bradykinin and various other cytokines. The differences in manifestation of type I hypersensitive reaction in different tissues is indicative of variation in involvement of primary and secondary mediators.

Histamine

The most predominant amongst the pharmacological mediator responsible for many of the symptoms of anaphylactic shock is histamine, which can be shown to be liberated *in vitro* when antibody sensitized pieces of various tissues including uterine muscle, lung and intestine are exposed to contact with antigen. Sensitization may be produced by prior injection of antigen into the animal supplying the tissue, which makes antibody as mentioned earlier or the tissue may be sensitized passively by the addition of the antibody produced in another animal. The typical contractions induced in this way in the uterus and intestine are called Schultze-Dale reactions. The histamine is derived from the granules of the mast cells where it exists as its precursor histidine, in combination with heparin; these substances are released by the interaction of antigen with antibody via another pharmacologically active substance, anaphylatoxin, acting together with serum complements. Histamine is formed by decarboxylation of the amino acid histidine, which is the major component of mast cell granules. It constitutes about 10% of the granule weight. Since it is stored in the preformed condition in the granules, its effects are observed immediately after the activation and degranulation of mast cells. Once it is released, it binds to specific receptors on various target cells. There are three types of receptors for histamine, which are designated as H_1, H_2, and H_3. These receptors have different tissue distribution hence show different effects on interacting with histamine. Most of the biologic effects brought about by histamine during anaphylaxis are mediated by

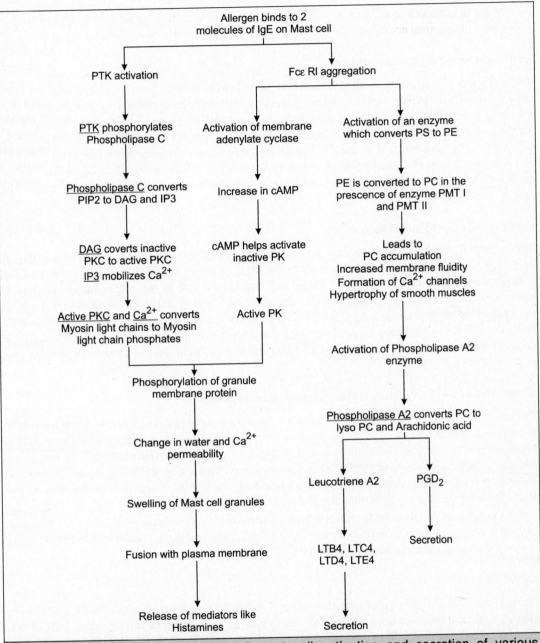

Fig. 18.4 Schematic representation of mast cell activation and secretion of various pharmacological mediators. (PE- phosphatidyl ethanolamine, PS- phosphatidyl serine, LT- leukotriene, PG- prostaglandin, PTK- proteintyrosine kinase, PKC- protein kinase C, PMT- phospholipid methyltransferase, DAG- Diacylglycerol, PC- phosphatidyl choline, PIP_2- phosphotidyl inositol-4,5-biphosphate, IP_3- Inositol triphosphate).

the binding of histamine to H1 receptors. This binding induces increased permeability in blood vessels, contraction of intestinal and bronchial smooth muscles and increased mucous secretion by goblet cells.

Leukotrienes and prostaglandins

The leukocyte-derived group of substances called the leukotrienes, belong to secondary mediators. They are not formed until the degranulation and break down of the mast cells. Together with them prostaglandins are also produced through a series of enzymatic reactions and the plasma membrane is broken down. Therefore it takes longer time for these mediators to show the biological effects. Their effects are more pronounced and long lasting than those of histamine. Leukotrienes are likely to be important in allergy, and appear to account for the activity of slow reacting substance A (SRS-A). The leukotrienes mediate bronchial constriction, increased mucous production and vascular constriction. Prostaglandin D2 also causes bronchial constriction.

Eosinophil chemotactic factor

The eosinophil is thought to play an important part in anaphylaxis by getting them self attracted to the site of the reaction by an eosinophil chemotactic factor (ECF) that is released following the interaction of antibody and antigen on the surface of a mast cell. The precise role of the eosinophil in anaphylactic reactions is not yet clear. It is suggested that the activities of the eosinophil include the release of an inhibitor of histamine after having phagocytosed complexes of antibody and antigen and the repair of the tissue damage brought about in the hypersensitivity reaction. Eosinophil granules contain arylsulphatase, and enzyme that splits SRS-A into two inactive fragments and thus can control the smooth muscle spasm induced by SRS-A.

Serotonin or 5-HT (hydroxy tryptamine) and bradykinin

The other pharmacological mediators of immediate hypersensitivity reactions are 5-hydroxy-tryptamine or serotonin, which causes contraction of plain muscle and increased capillary permeability. It is of uncertain role in anaphylaxis although it is probably involved in local intestinal food allergies; slow reacting substances (SRS-A) has a plain muscle contracting effect acting, unlike histamine, on the larger rather than smaller blood vessels. SRS-A has a particularly marked bronchial constricting effect in man and is probably predominant pharmacological agent in human asthma.

Bradykinins are simple peptides formed from a plasma α globulin (kininogen). They have histamine like effect on smooth muscle and capillaries, and studies have shown that it is present in the blood stream in many species in the early stages of an anaphylactic reaction.

Cytokines

Human mast cells are known to secrete IL-4, IL-5, IL-6 and TNF-α. These cytokines are responsible for alteration of local microenvironment, thereby leading to the recruitment of inflammatory cells such as neutrophils and eosinophils. IL-4 causes increase in IgE production by B cells and IL-5 is responsible for recruitment and activation of eosinophils. The shock in systemic anaphylaxis is due to increased production of TNF-α.

CONSEQUENCES OF TYPE I REACTIONS

The consequences of type I reactions may range from life threatening systemic or generalized anaphylaxis and asthma to mild allergic reactions such as hay fever, eczema, urticaria, etc.

Systemic or generalized anaphylaxis

It is shock like, often fatal, whose onset takes place within minutes of a type I hypersensitive reaction. Magendie first reported it in 1839. He noted that dogs repeatedly injected with egg albumin died. It remained unnoticed till 1902, when two French scientists, P. J. Portier and C. R. Richet observed a similar phenomenon in dogs when they were immunized with extracts obtained from the Portuguese-man-of war, jelly fish and sea anemone.

With the first injection of this extract, there were no adverse symptoms observed, but on challenging the animals after a week with the second dose, severe anaphylactic symptoms developed. The symptoms were, vomiting, bloody diarrhea, asphyxia, unconsciousness and death. They called this *anaphylaxis* (GK: ana = against and phylaxis = protection) to denote that this is an inappropriate reaction, which is against the principle of host protection. For this work, Richet was awarded Nobel Prize in Medicine in 1913.

Systemic anaphylaxis can be induced in a variety of experimental animal models. In the laboratory, injecting a small dose of antigen (sensitizing) into an animal, followed within several days by an intravenous dose of antigen (challenging dose) usually produces generalized anaphylaxis. The manifestation of generalized anaphylaxis varies with different species, in which different shock organs may be affected. The guinea pig, a few minutes after challenge with antigen, will scratch, sneeze, cough and may convulse and can collapse and die. This is primarily the result of respiratory impairment due to constriction of smooth muscles in the bronchioles and leading to bronchial edema. A sharp drop in blood pressure and a generalized increase in vascular permeability may also accompany the reaction. The lungs at postmortem examination are found characteristically over inflated. In the rabbit, both cardiovascular and pulmonary functions are severely impaired with drop in systemic blood pressure, and constriction of airways. In the human, generalized anaphylaxis presents with itching, erythema, vomiting, abdominal cramps, diarrhea and respiratory distress. In severe cases, laryngeal edema and vascular collapse may result in death.

Wide ranges of antigens, which trigger anaphylactic reactions in susceptible humans, have been identified. For ex. Bee, wasp, hornet and ant stings, drugs-sulfonamides, penicillin, insulin, benzoates, salicylates, antitoxins, seafood, nuts, eggs and milk etc. If not treated quickly it can be fatal. To treat systemic anaphylaxis, epinephrine is administered. It acts as an antagonist of mediators like histamine and leukotrienes by relaxing the smooth muscles and reducing the vascular permeability. Epinephrine is also known to improve cardiac out put, which is essential to prevent vascular collapse during an anaphylactic reaction. Epinephrine also blocks degranulation of mast cells by increasing the cAMP levels.

PASSIVE TRANSFER ANAPHYLAXIS

Since the reaction is antibody mediated, anaphylactic sensitivity can be transferred to a normal recipient by means of serum. The source of antibody may be the same species, ex., the human, in which case the predominant immunoglobulin involved is of the IgE class, or a different species, as described below. For ex., a guinea pig sensitized by an intravenous injection of rabbit antibody to ovalbumin and challenged with ovalbumin 48 hours later will suffer a fatal anaphylactic shock. A similar reaction can occur following the use of homologous (i.e., guinea pig) antiserum.

CUTANEOUS ANAPHYLAXIS

It is classified into active and passive cutaneous anaphylaxis.

Active cutaneous anaphylaxis

Upon injection of antigen into the skin of a sensitized animal, a local anaphylactic reaction will occur within a few minutes. It consists of localized swelling and redness, a wheel and flare reaction. Skin tests in man for allergy to a wide variety of antigens (allergens) are characteristic of this phenomenon. The local increase in vascular permeability that is characteristic of this reaction may be demonstrated by the use of tracer dyes such as Evan's blue. This dye binds to albumin in the blood and when the blood vessels exhibit increased permeability, the albumin that leaks out is dyed blue and stains the tissues.

Passive cutaneous anaphylaxis

Specific types of antibody can also passively transfer localized anaphylaxis, most importantly, in the human, of the IgE class. In animals, this type of transferred reaction in the skin was described by Ovary and called passive cutaneous anaphylaxis (PCA). Sensitizing antibody is injected intradermally, and after an obligatory latent period (usually 24 to 72 hours), antigen is given intravenously with Evan's blue dye. The local permeability reaction as evidenced by bluing of the skin appears within minutes.

LOCALIZED ANAPHYLAXIS
Allergy and allergens

Allergy is naturally occurring anaphylaxis in man, which includes many of the disease conditions. It affects principally the skin, the respiratory tract and the gastrointestinal tract. Although sensitive state may arise spontaneously, in most cases it is possible to decide the manner in which hypersensitivity was incited. Coca subdivided the allergy into Atopic and nonatopic type. The atopic allergy is hereditary and can be seen in only the hereditarily predisposed individuals for hypersensitivity. The nonatopic allergy can occur in any individual.

The allergens are the agents that incite allergic reactions, which do not necessarily possess antigenicity. The body areas affected known as shock organs or shock tissues. Different allergens encounter different organs or tissues so a variety of clinical forms of allergy occur, namely, hay fever, asthma, urticaria, and angioedema, probably infantile eczema. Serum allergy may occur in individuals naturally sensitive to foreign animal proteins, such as horse danders and also frequently develops as a result of active sensitization by injection of foreign serum.

Atopic allergy

1. HAY FEVER (ALLERGIC RHINITIS)

It is characterized by the watery exudation from the mucous membrane of the upper respiratory tract and conjunctiva. The natural consequence of which includes violent and often protracted sneezing, nasal discharge and lacrimation. The allergen is some agent in the surrounding atmosphere that is either inhaled or comes in contact with the exposed mucous membrane. Plant pollens, house dust, mold spores and various substances may also produce the symptoms of hay fever. Seasonal hay fever is caused by pollens of grasses, such as, timothy rye, jute grass, ragweed, parthenium and various other weeds. So-called perennial hay fever occurs through out the year and bears a clinical resemblance to seasonal hay fever. It is caused by various inhaled or ingested materials, such as, animal dander's, vegetable powder, house dust, foods (milk, eggs, shell fish), drugs (quinine, aspirin, iodine etc.)

2. ASTHMA

It is a conditional and paroxysmal difficulty in breathing with wheezing or whistling sound produced during respiration due to obstructions of smaller bronchioles. It is either allergic or non-allergic. **Allergic asthma** may be caused by some inhaled substances as in hay fever together with certain drugs and chemical inhaled by the laboratory workers. Various ingested food substances may also incite asthmatic attack, among them eggs, wheat, and milk.

The non-allergic type is some times called **intrinsic asthma** and it is produced by unknown intrinsic factors of an individual, which include exercise or cold, apparently independent of allergen stimulation. Like hay fever, asthma is also triggered by degranulation of mast cells, which release the mediators in the lower respiratory tract. This results in contraction of bronchial smooth muscles, edema of airways, enhanced mucous secretion and inflammation of the bronchial passage. All this leads to bronchial congestion and difficulty in breathing.

Asthma is primarily considered to be inflammatory disease. The asthmatic response can be divided into two types, **early** and **late response** (Fig. 18.5). The early response is initiated by histamine, leukotriene (LTC$_4$) and prostaglandin D$_2$. It occurs within minutes after the allergen exposure. The late response

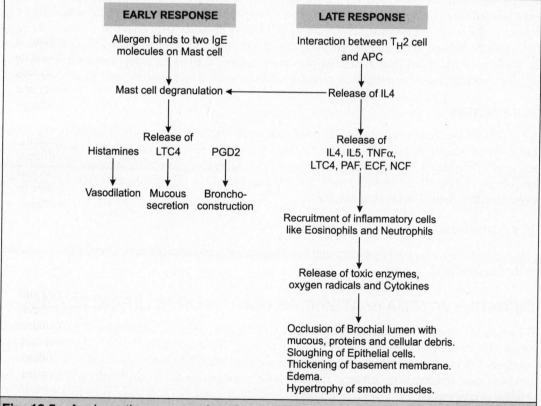

Fig. 18.5   A schematic representation of early and late inflammatory response during asthma. Key: LTC 4 = leukotriene; PGD2 = prostaglandin D2; PAF = platlet activation factor; ECF = Eosinophil chemotactic factor; NCF = Neutrophil chemotactic factor; TNF a = Tumor necrosis factor a; IL 4, IL 5 = Interleukin 4 and 5.

occurs, hours after allergen exposure. The mediators involved here are IL-4, IL-5, IL-6 and TNF-α, eosinophil chemotactic factor (ECF) and platelet activating factor (PAF). These mediators recruit inflammatory cells, including eosinophil and neutrophils into bronchial tissue.

The neutrophils and eosinophils are capable of inflicting severe tissue injury by releasing toxic enzymes, free radicals and cytokines. These events lead to flooding of bronchial lumen with mucus, proteins, cell debris and sloughed off epithelium. Fluid-build up (edema), thickening of basement membrane, hypertrophy of bronchial smooth muscle. More often mucus adheres to bronchial wall, which contains cellular debris, eosinophils and neutrophils and spirals of bronchial tissue known as Curshmann's spirals.

Treatment of asthma is similar to that of hay fever. Avoidance of the allergic substances is always the most desirable method when feasible. Some materials such as food and drugs can be avoided with out too much difficulty. House dust and pollens are practically inescapable. In these cases specific desensitization procedures may be attempted. For temporary relief or during severe symptoms, physician often employs adrenaline or epinephrine, ephedrine etc.

3. FOOD ALLERGIES

In allergic individuals, various foods also induce localized anaphylaxis. Cross-linking of allergens with IgE on mast cells along the upper and lower part of the alimentary canal can induce localized smooth muscle contractions. If the upper part of GI tract involves in anaphylactic reaction it would induce vomiting, whereas contraction of the lower part of GI tract will lead to diarrhea. Degranulation of mast cells along the GI tract increases, so that the allergens enter the blood stream. Depending on the region of deposition of allergen, an individual may show difference in symptoms of allergy. For ex. Some individuals may develop asthmatic attack after ingesting certain food. Others may develop atopic urticaria or angioedema.

A. URTICARIA

It is a skin disorder, characterized by the appearance of the intensely itching wheels or welts with raised often-white centers surrounded by an area of erethema. They are distributed widely over the body surface and tend to disappear in one or two days. Allergic urticaria is generally caused by ingestion of the allergens or more by inhalation or contact. Common food allergens include strawberries, citrus fruits, fish, shellfish, eggs, tomatoes, brinjal and chocolates, etc.

B. ANGIOEDEMA

It is similar to urticaria, but lesions are larger and more restricted in distribution. They often occur about in the head and neck region.

INFANTILE ECZEMA or ATOPIC DERMATITIS OR ALLERGIC ECZEMA

It consists of reddened vesicular blisters like lesions of the face, neck, and skin region of the inside of the elbow and knee joints. The lesions ooze and crust over. The usual allergens are thought to be eggs, coconuts, fish etc. It is an inflammatory disease associated with a family history of atopy. The disease is observed most frequently in children. The skin lesions are known to have T_H2 cells and an increased number of eosinophils.

LATE PHASE REACTION

Once the type I hypersensitive reaction subsides, the mediators released during the reaction often induce a localized inflammation, which is called late phase reaction (LPR). The LPR begins to develop4-6 hrs after the initial type I reaction and it persists for 1-2 days. LPR is characterized by localized infiltration of neutrophils, eosinophils, macrophages, lymphocytes and basophils. This infiltration is mediated by cytokines released by mast cells, namely GM-CSF (granulocyte-monocyte colony stimulating factor), TNF-α, IL-1, IL-3, IL-5, ECF and NCF.

During the LPR, eosinophil plays a principal role accounting for 30% of the cells that accumulate. ECF released by mast cells during the initial reaction attracts large number of eosinophils to the affected site. Eosinophils also possess Fc receptor for IgG and IgE isotypes. Allergens bound to antibody- coated eosinophil will activate much like mast cells and cause degranulation of eosinophil.
Degranulation of eosinophil leads to release of leukotrienes, basic proteins, and platelet activating factor, cationic proteins and eosinophil derived neurotoxins. These mediators play a protective role in parasitic infection, but in LPR they contribute to extensive tissue damage.

Similar to eosinophils, neutrophils are another major participants in LPR, also accounting for 30% of the inflammatory cells. They are also attracted to the site of type I reaction by neutrophil chemotactic factor, released by degranulating mast cells. In addition to this, IL-8 released at the site is also known to activate neutrophils, resulting in release of their granular contents, which include lytic enzymes, platelet activating factor and leukotrienes.

DETECTION OF TYPE I HYPERSENSITIVITY

In humans, type I hypersensitivity can be identified by *skin testing*. Small amounts of allergens are introduced at the inner region of skin (subcutaneous) of the forearm region or back of an individual either by intra-dermal injection or by scratching the skin. Several allergens can be tested simultaneously by serially injecting one after the other and marking the area with a pen, the code of the allergen. If a person is allergic to a substance, it will stimulate mast cells to undergo degranulation and release the mediators. This results in wheal and flare reaction within 30 min. The advantage of skin test is that, in a single sitting many allergens can be tested and the disadvantage is, it may sensitize the individual to a new allergen. In rare instances it may lead to systemic anaphylaxis. Sometimes it may show late manifestation, which appears 4-6 hrs after the injection and may last up to 24 hrs. As indicated earlier, late phase reaction may lead to tissue damage at the reaction site.

The other method of assessing type I hypersensitivity is to determine the serum level of IgE by *radioimmunosorbent test (*RIST*) or radioallergosorbent test (*RAST*).* These two techniques have been explained in Chapter 8.

TREATMENT OF TYPE I HYPERSENSITIVITY

First step is to identify the allergen and avoid contact if possible. Avoid contact with pollen grains and house dust by wearing mask. Often removal of house pets, avoidance of offending foods and dust control measures can eliminate type I response.

Hypersensitization is another approach involving repeated injection of increasing doses of allergens has been known to reduce the severity of type I reaction or even eliminate it completely. Such repeated administration of allergens appears to shift immune response by producing IgG or by inducing T cell mediated suppression. In this case, IgG antibody is referred to as blocking antibody, because it competes for allergen and depletes it by phagocytosis. As a result, the allergen is not available for cross-linking fixed IgE on the mast cells. Hence allergic symptoms decrease.

Another approach for treating allergies has emerged from the findings, that the soluble antigen tends to stimulate a state of anergy by activating T cells. Antihistaminic drugs are most useful in treating allergic symptoms. These drugs act by binding to the histamine receptors on target cells and blocking the receptor. There are two types of receptors, H_1, is blocked by classical antihistamines and H_2 is blocked by newer classes of antihistamines. The mechanism of action of different drugs involves interference at various biochemical steps in mast cell activation and degranulation (Table 18.3).

Table 18.3 Mechanism of action of some drugs used in treatment of type I hypersensitivity.

Drugs	Action
ANTIHISTAMINES	Block H_1 and H_2 receptors on target cells
CROMOLYN SODIUM	Blocks Ca^{2+} into mast cells
THEOPHYLLINE	Prolongs high cAMP levels in mast cells by inhibiting phosphodiesterase which cleaves cAMP to 5'-AMP
EPINEPHRINE (adrenalin)	Stimulates cAMP production by binding to β- adregernic receptors on mast cells
CORTISONE	Reduces histamine by blocking conversion of histidine to histamine that stimulates mast cell production of cAMP

TYPE II HYPERSENSITIVITY OR ANTIBODY MEDIATED CYTOTOXIC HYPERSENSITIVITY

This type of reaction is observed in blood transfusion reactions in which host antibodies react with foreign antigens present on the incompatible transfused blood cells. This reaction mediates destruction of transfused blood cells. Antibodies like; IgG and IgM can mediate cell destruction by activating complement system, which destroys the foreign cells (See Fig.15.4 and 15.6 in chapter 15). Cell destruction can be brought about by antibody dependent cell-mediated cytotoxicity (ADCC). In this process, cytotoxic cells with Fc receptors will bind antibodies and promote killing of the cells (see Fig. 13.4). Antibody bound to a foreign cell also can serve as an opsonin, enabling phagocytosis, because the phagocytic cells possess Fc or C3b receptors to bind. Certain autoimmune diseases also involve autoantibody-mediated cellular destruction via type II mechanism.

Blood transfusion reaction

ABO blood group antigens are a type of glycoproteins found on the membrane of RBCs and are encoded by different genes belonging to multiple allelic groups. An individual possessing an allelic form of blood group antigen can recognize other allelic forms on transfused blood and mount an immune response against the foreign blood group antigen. Antibodies against ABO blood group antigens are called *Isohaemagglutinins* and they belong to IgM category. Details are given in Chapter 2.

Isohaemagglutinins after binding to opposite blood group antigens on RBCs induces destruction of these foreign RBCs by complement mediated lysis. This is called *transfusion reaction*. The clinical manifestation of this may have immediate or delayed effect. Mainly massive intravascular hemolysis may often occur due to complement-mediated lysis of RBCs bound by antibodies. As a result, within hours free hemoglobin can be detected in the plasma and it escapes through the kidney into urine, resulting in hemoglobinuria. Accumulation of hemoglobin in the kidney due to over load may cause acute tubular necrosis. Some of the hemoglobin may get converted to bilirubin, which is toxic. Some other symptoms of transfusion reaction include fever, nausea and chill. Treatment involves prompt termination of transfusion and maintenance of urine flow by administering diuretics.

Delayed hemolytic transfusion reaction may occur in individuals who undergo repeated transfusion with compatible blood that is incompatible for some minor blood groups. The reaction sets in between 2 to 6 days after transfusion. The incompatible minor antigens such as Kidd, Kell and Duffy induce production of IgG rather than IgM. Therefore, complement mediated lysis of RBCs is incomplete hence many of the transfused cells are destroyed at extravascular sites. The destruction of cells is brought about by phagocytosis by macrophages. Symptoms of delayed hemolytic transfusion reaction include fever, anemia, mild jaundice and increased bilirubin. Since RBC destruction takes place in extravascular space, free hemoglobin does not make its presence in plasma and urine. Proper cross matching of the antigens between the donors and recipients blood will avoid the transfusion reaction.

Erythroblastosis fetalis or hemolytic disease of the newborn

This commonly occurs when the Rh factor incompatibility takes place between the mother and the fetus. When the mother is Rh- and the fetus is Rh+, during the first pregnancy the usually mother is not exposed to enough of fetal red blood cells to activate her Rh- specific B cells. However, at the time of delivery, separation of placenta from the uterine wall causes some amount of fetal umbilical cord blood to come in contact with mother's blood. These fetal RBCs activate Rh specific B cells, resulting in the production of IgM and IgG and memory B cells. IgM clears the Rh+ fetal red blood cells from mother's circulation, but memory cells remain. Activation of memory cells occurs in subsequent pregnancy, which results in the formation of IgG anti-Rh antibodies. IgG is capable of crossing the placental barrier and damage fetal RBCs. This results in mild to severe anemia, sometimes leading to fatality. Hemolysis of fetal RBCs may result in accumulation of hemoglobin and production of bilirubin. Bilirubin being lipid soluble may cross blood brain barrier and deposit in fetal brain leading brain damage.

It is possible to prevent erythroblastosis fetalis by administering antibodies to the mother against Rh antigen within 24 to 48 hrs after delivery. These antibodies are called **Rhogam**, which binds to fetal red blood cells that enter the mothers blood circulation and destroy them before the B cells recognize them and get activated as well as produce memory cells. In such cases, in the subsequent pregnancies, mother is unlikely to produce IgG anti-Rh antibodies, so that the damage to fetus is prevented.

Drug induced hemolytic anemia

Certain drugs such as penicillin, cephalosporin and streptomycin may bind to proteins on RBC membranes, forming a hapten-protein complex. In some cases, such complexes induce the formation of antibodies, which then react with drug bound to RBC membrane. This will initiate complement mediated lysis of such antibody bound RBCs resulting in anemia. When the drug is withdrawn, the anemia disappears.

TYPE III-IMMUNE COMPLEX MEDIATED OR ANTIBODY-ANTIGEN COMPLEX MEDIATED HYPERSENSITIVITY

Generally when antigen and antibody react, they generate immune complexes, which cleared from the body by phagocytic cells. In some case, large amount of immune complexes are formed, which cannot be easily cleared by phagocytic cells results in tissue damage. This type of immune complex mediated tissue damage reaction is called type III hypersensitive reaction. Depending on the region where these immune complexes are formed in the body, different types of tissue damaging reactions are observed.

Immune complexes are capable of activating complement system (Figs.15.2 and 15.3). As discussed in Chapter 15, the C3a, C4a and C5a complements split products are known to be anaphylactic, that cause localized mast cell degranulation and consequently increase the vascular permeability at the site of the reaction. Larger molecular weight immune complexes get deposited in the basement membrane of glomeruli of kidney and the walls of the blood vessels. Smaller complexes may pass through basement membrane and get deposited in the sub-epithelium. Therefore, the type of lesion caused depends on the site of deposition of immune complexes.

C3a, C5a and C5b, 6, 7 complement factors are also chemotactic actors for neutrophils. Immune complexes are capable of stimulating these complement chemotactic factors; hence neutrophils infiltrate at the site of reaction. Neutrophils produce lytic enzymes to dissolve the phagocytized immune complexes. The immune complexes attached to the basement membrane interfere with phagocytosis, allowing neutrophils to release the lytic enzymes due to unsuccessful attempt of phagocytosis. Release of lytic enzymes and the activation of membrane attack component of complement results in tissue damage at the vicinity. Formation of microthrombi may also take place due to release of clotting factors by the aggregation of platelets, which were activated by complement at the site of immune complex reaction.

Arthus reaction or localized type III hypersensitivity

It may be elicited in the rabbit by series of subcutaneous injections of foreign proteins at intervals of few days. There is no untoward response to early injections, but later injection produces local infiltration, which develops in to necrosis and abscess formation (Fig.18.7). A more striking picture is obtained by immunization through intravenous route. The intensity of the Arthus reaction in the rabbit, which is sensitized, varies with the concentration of the antibody in the serum. The phenomenon is not limited to skin reaction; inflammation and necrosis have been induced in the lung, heart, kidney, peritoneum, testes, brain and joints. Arthus reaction can be demonstrated in two ways, namely, 1) reverse Arthus reaction, 2) passive Arthus reaction.

Reverse Arthus reaction

This is produced in rabbits by injecting protein intravenously and homologous antiserum by the intracutaneous route either immediately or at any time within the next three or four days. The intensity of the local reaction at the site of the antiserum injection diminishes as the interval between injection increases. Reverse Arthus reactions may not be so severe as direct reactions, often producing severe local edema.

Passive Arthus reaction

Which can be induced in normal rabbits by injection of serum from other rabbits sensitized or immunized against foreign proteins. When the antiserum is injected intracutaneously, the reaction occurs at the site of antiserum injection.

Naturally after an insect bite or after coming in contact with the bristles of caterpillar or epidermal hairs of certain plants, a sensitive individual may develop localized type I reaction at the site in the form of wheal and flare reaction. Sometimes, 4-8 hrs later, atypical Arthus reaction may develop at the site with pronounced erythema and edema. Intrapulmonary contamination due to bacterial and mold spores and dried fecal proteins of bird droppings, cockroaches may also lead to pulmonary Arthus type reaction.

Serum sickness or generalized type III reaction or Non-atopic allergy

Serum sickness develops 8 to 12 days after injection of an amount of a foreign protein such as antitoxin containing foreign serum, such as horse anti-tetanus or anti-diphtheria serum. In such cases, the recipient of a foreign anti-serum develops antibodies specific for the foreign serum proteins; these antibodies then form circulating immune complexes with the foreign serum antigen. Serum sickness is characterized by

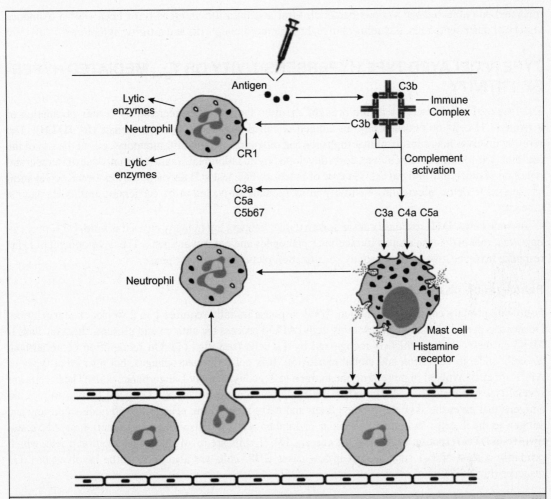

Fig. 18.7   Schematic representation of components involved in Arthus reaction (Type III hypersensitive reaction)

general swelling of lymph nodes and is accompanied by itching, urticarial erythematoses, eruption and often edema of eyelids, face and ankles. In severe cases fever and pain in the joints are also noted. The average duration of the symptoms is two days, but they may persist as long as two weeks. The antigen-antibody complexes, which are formed, get deposited in blood vessels, polymorphonuclear leukocytes also accumulate, and severe artiritis follows. When this affects the kidney, glomerulonephritis is produced with proteinuria.

Other than serum sickness, immune complexes mediated type III reactions also contribute to other type of pathogenic conditions. These include infectious disease such as, meningitis, malaria, trypanosomiasis and hepatitis, drug reactions such as allergy to sulfonamides and penicillin. It may also contribute to the autoimmune diseases such as rheumatoid arthritis and systemic lupus erythematosus. Immune complex mediated reactions against various bacterial, viral and parasitic antigens have been shown to induce variety of other symptoms, including skin rashes, glomerulonephritis and arthritic symptoms.

TYPE IV DELAYED TYPE HYPERSENSITIVITY OR T$_{DTH}$ MEDIATED HYPER-SENSITIVITY

The localized inflammatory reaction brought about by the cytokines secreted by certain population of activated TH cells on encountering an antigen is called **delayed type hypersensitivity (DTH).** The reaction involves major influx of macrophages and other nonspecific inflammatory cells at the site of the reaction. The localized tuberculin reaction developed by an individual, against a small dose of intradermal injection of tuberculin antigen is DTH type of reaction. This test was developed by Robert Koch in 1890 as a means to detect tuberculin sensitivity in individuals suspected to be carriers of antibodies against tuberculi.

In some cases, DTH response causes severe tissue damage, but in many cases it is mild. DTH plays an important role in defense against intracellular pathogens and contact antigens. The development of DTH response involves, two phases, namely sensitization phase and effector phase.

Sensitization phase of DTH

Following primary contact with antigen, DTH response initially requires 1 to 2 weeks of sensitization. During this period, the antigen presenting cells (APCs) process the antigen and presents them on class II MHC on their surface, which is recognized by T$_H$ cells (see Fig. 11). On recognition of an antigen T$_H$ cells undergo activation and clonal expansion. It is not only macrophages, but also other types of APCs are also involved in presenting the antigen to T$_H$ cells, namely Langerhance cells. These cells are special types of dendritic cells found in the epidermis (cutaneous layer). They are known to pick up antigens that enter the skin and process them and carry them to the nearest lymph node to present the antigen to the T cells. In humans, vascular endothelial cells are also known to function as APCs and involve in DTH response. In most of the cases, CD4$^+$ T cells are involved in sensitization phase, which primarily consist of T$_H$1 subtype, but in few cases CD8$^+$ cells are also know to be involved in DTH response (Fig. 18.8).

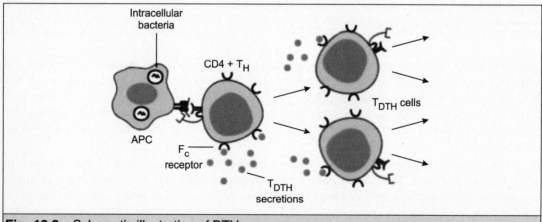

Fig. 18.8   Schematic illustration of DTH response.

Effector phase

This involves secondary contact with antigen and usually occurs, 24 hrs after the secondary contact. In this phase, the activated T cells (T_{DTH}) secrete variety of cytokines, which will be responsible for recruiting the cells of inflammatory reaction at the site of the reaction. Generally, the secondary response peaks at 48-72 hrs after the secondary contact with antigen. Since there is delay in onset of the response it is called delayed type hypersensitivity. This delay involves secretion of cytokines, which are responsible for recruitment of inflammatory cells. When the DTH response is fully developed only 5 % of the total population of cells involved in the reaction will belong to sensitized antigen specific T_{DTH} and the remainder are other nonspecific cells and macrophage. The cytokines produced by the T_{DTH} induce the monocytes found in the blood stream to adhere to the endothelial lining of blood vessels, which then migrate from blood to the surrounding tissue. In the tissue, the monocytes differentiate in to **activated macrophages.** As mentioned earlier (Chapter 3), activated macrophages show increased ability of phagocytosis and to kill microorganisms through various cytotoxic mechanisms. In addition to this, activated macrophages show enhanced expression class II MHC, therefore more efficient antigen presenting ability. Infiltration of macrophage during the DTH response provides an effective means of host defense against intracellular parasites. In most of the cases macrophage helps in clearing the antigen rapidly, but rarely certain antigens take long time to get cleared from the body. In such instances the DTH response is prolonged and the inflammatory reaction associated with DTH results in tissue damage, which is depicted by granulomatous development. This is due to continuous activation of macrophages, which in turn express excess of tissue adhesion molecules leading to aggregation of macrophages leading to **granuloma**, epitheloid structure. These granulomatous structures produce high concentration of lytic enzymes, which destroy the surrounding tissue.

Major cytokines involved in DTH reaction

1. IL-2 functions as an autocrine factor for T_{DTH} cells and helps in proliferation of these cells.
2. IL-3 and GM-CSF induce localized hematopoiesis of the granulocyte-monocyte lineage.
3. IFN-γ and TNF-β together with macrophage derived IL-1 and TNF-α act on nearby endothelial cells, inducing extravasation of monocytes and other inflammatory cells.
4. Activated T_{DTH} cells also produce, monocyte chemotactic and activating factor (MCAF) and migration inhibition factor (MIF). Both these factors are responsible for drawing the macrophages to the site of the DTH reaction and retaining them at the same place.

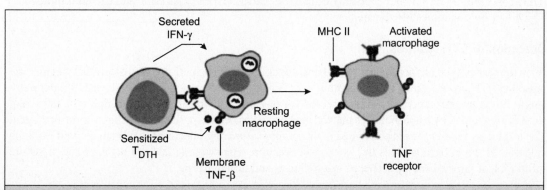

Fig. 18.9   Development of DTH reaction. Cytokines like IFN-γ, TNF-β released from sensitized T_{DTH} cells mediate in the reaction

The macrophages that accumulate at the site of DTH reaction secretes lytic enzymes, which destroy the cells harboring intracellular pathogens. Generally, the initial response will be more severe and results in damage to healthy tissue. This ultimately succeeds in getting rid of intracellular pathogen. For ex. *Mycobacterium tuberculosis* is an intracellular bacterium. The DTH response against this bacterium involves complete surrounding of the infected cells by macrophages and formation of granulomatous lesion called **tubercle.** This occurs in the lung tissue and the release of lytic enzymes by the activated macrophages causes tissue damage.

Protective role-played by DTH response

There are different types of contact antigens and intracellular pathogens, which stimulate DTH response (Table 18.4).

Table 18.4   Types of contact antigens and intracellular pathogens that initiate DTH reaction

Intracellular viruses	Intracellular bacteria
Herpes variola and Measels	Mycobacterium Tuberculosis Mycobacterium leprae Brucella abortus Listeria monocytogenes
Intracellular Fungi	**Intracellular parasites**
Pneumocystis carini Candida albicans Histoplasma capsulatum	Leishmania donovani
Contact antigens	
Poison ivy and oak Hair dye chemicals Picrotoxins Nickel derivatives	

The response to AIDS virus results in depletion of CD4$^+$ cells. Therefore, DTH response in full blown AIDS cases will be very poor, hence they suffer from various types of parasitic and bacterial infections, which may be sometimes life threatening.

Detection of DTH reaction

As in the case of type I hypersensitive test, here also skin test can be performed to determine whether the person is DTH prone against a particular antigen. For this test, the test antigen is injected intradermally and 48 to 72 hr later, injected site is observed for any lesion. A positive skin reaction will show red, slightly swollen; itchy patch indicates that the individual has been exposed to the antigen or the pathogen. The test for *M. tuberculosis* is performed in the similar manner by injecting the protein derived from the cell wall of the bacterium. This test is Montax reaction. The swelling and red patch is due to severe infiltration of injected site by activated macrophages and inflammation.

Type V-STIMULATORY HYPERSENSITIVITY

It is a kind of autoimmune response where autoantibodies bind to certain cell receptors and bring about stimulation of the receptor similar to that of natural receptor-ligand binding and bring about the same action in the target cell. In this case thyroid stimulating hormone receptor of the thyroid gland cells meant for binding of thyroid stimulating hormone (TSH) secreted by the adenohypophysis is bound by an autoantibody against the TSH receptor, which happens in Graves disease. The autoantibody after binding to the TSH receptor brings about the same changes in thyroid cell similar to TSH stimulation and excess of thyroid hormone is secreted resulting in Graves disease.

Recently, another receptor responding in the same manner has been found in patients suffering from gastric ulcers who are resistant to cimetidine drug therapy are found to have autoantibodies to histamine receptor-H_2, which causes excess release of histamine in the gastric epithelium.

Exercise

1. What is hypersensitivity? Write an account on IgE mediated hypersensitivity or What is anaphylaxis? Describe various types of anaphylaxis (20 marks).
2. Write notes on: (10 marks each)
   (a) Type II Hypersensitivity
   (b) Type III Hypersensitivity
3. Give an account of delayed type hypersensitive reaction (20 marks)
4. Write notes on: (5 marks each)
   (a) Atopic allergy
   (b) Cutaneous anaphylaxis
   (c) Arthus reaction
   (d) Serum sickness

Chapter 19

Transplantation Immunology

- Immunology of Graft Rejection
- Precautions against Graft Rejection
- Graft Versus Host Disease or (Reaction) (GVHD)
- Tissue and Organ Transplantation
- Strategies to Induce Graft Acceptance or Tolerance by Manipulating CD40
- Immunology of Tolerance
- Non-Autoreactive Nature of Positively Selected T Cells
- The Adaptation Concept: Nature of The Immature T Cells

- Methods of Graft Rejection
- Methods for Tissue Typing
- Mechanism of Graft Rejection
- CD40 in Allograft Rejection
- Immunosuppressive Agents
- Specific Immunosuppressive Therapy During Transplantation
- Tolerance in Tetraparental (Allophenic) Mice
- APL (Altered Peptide-Ligand) Concept: Nature of Selecting Antigens
- Anergy Concept: Nature of APC
- Active Termination of T Cell Immune Response

❏ ❏

The replacement of a diseased organ by a transplant of healthy tissue (organ) is called transplantation. In the early 1940s Medawar provided insight into nature of graft (transplant) rejection while working with burn patients of World War II. He observed that, graft of skin from one region of the body to another in the same patient was easily accepted, whereas grafts obtained from close relatives like brother or sister were rejected. He also observed that when a second graft was performed, by obtaining the tissue from the same donor, the rejection reaction occurred with greater intensity and much faster. Medawar performed certain animal experiments and discovered that prior sensitization with donor cells led to increased rejection of a subsequent graft. The transplant leads to various complications in the host, which is mediated through host body immune response, and very often the transplant gets rejected or may lead to graft verses host reaction or disease. Before discussing the nature and implications of this rejection phenomenon let us look into the terms involved in various types of grafts between individuals and species.

Classification of grafts

The graft can be classified into four major types: 1). Autograft, 2). Isograft, 3). Allograft, and 4). Xenograft.

1. *Autograft*: The tissue of the original donor is grafted back into the same donor. For example, skin graft from thigh to face in severely deformed cases of burnt individuals (plastic surgery).
2. *Isograft*: Graft between syngeneic individuals (i.e., identical genetic constitution). For example, clones or identical twins.

3. *Allograft:* (Homograft). Graft between allogenic individuals (i.e., members of the same species but of different genetic constitution or parent hood). For example, one human to another.

4. *Xenograft:* (Heterograft). Graft between xenogenic individuals (i.e., different species or individuals of different genetic lineage). For example, pig to human, baboon to human.

Immunology of Graft Rejection

First and second set rejection reactions

In the allograft, that the second contact with antigen would represent a more explosive response than the first and indeed, the rejection of the second graft is accelerated. The initial stage shows very poor vascularization or some times no vascularization at all. The graft area shows remarkably increased population of polymorphonuclear lymphocytes, which invade the area and lymphoid cells including plasma cells. Thrombosis and acute cell destruction can be seen by three to four days. All allograft need not show second set rejection reaction of graft, but only those derived from the original donor or a related strain would show rejection. Graft from unrelated donors are rejected in the first set of reactions.

Role of lymphocytes, in the graft rejection reaction is demonstrated in neonatally thymectomized animals, which have difficulty in rejecting skin grafts but their capacity is restored by injection of lymphocytes from a syngeneic normal donor, suggesting that T cells are implicated. The T cell recipients from a donor which has already rejected a graft will show accelerated rejection response to a further graft of the same type, showing that the, lymphoid cells are stimulated and retained in the memory cells of the first contact with graft antigens.

After rejection the host generally produces antibodies against the tissue antigens of the donor graft and it recognizes the same donor immediately on second transplant and cause accelerated rejection reaction.

Methods of Graft Rejection

(a) Lymphocyte mediated rejection

In an experiment where passive transfer of serum from an animal which has rejected skin graft (allograft) did not accelerate the rejection of the similar graft on the recipient animal, injection of lymphoid cells (particularly circulating lymphocytes) were effective in bringing about graft rejection immediately.

It has been well documented from the histological study of graft rejection area showing infiltration by mononuclear cells (phagocytes) with a very few polymorphs or plasma cells indicating that the lymphoid cells play a primary role in first set of rejection. More direct evidence has come from *in vitro* studies showing that T cells taken from mice rejecting an allograft could kill target cells bearing the graft antigens *in vitro*. The long survival of the graft in children suffering from thymic deficiency implicates the T-lymphocytes involvement in graft rejection reaction.

On close scrutiny of T cell sub-population $CD4^+$ and $CD8^+$ both are involved in graft rejection. The role of $CD4^+$ and $CD8^+$ T cell sub-populations in rejection of skin allograft was demonstrated in mice by injecting monoclonal antibodies to deplete one or both types of T cells and then measuring the rate of graft rejection. It was observed that blocking $CD8^+$ population alone had no effect on graft survival and the graft was rejected within 15 days, similarly, in the control mice. On the other hand blocking of $CD4^+$ T cell population resulted in prolonged graft survival from 15 to 30 days. However, blocking of $CD4^+$ and $CD8^+$ cells with monoclonal antibodies resulted in graft survival of allograft for a longer time, i.e. up to 60 days. This study indicates that collaboration of both $CD4^+$ and $CD8^+$ cells resulted in more pronounced graft rejection.

(b) The role of humoral antibody

Involvement of humoral antibody in the destruction of lymphocytes through cytotoxic (type II) reaction in allogenic graft has been well documented. However, there are certain exceptional cases such as skin and solid tumor grafts where humoral antibodies responsible for cytotoxic reaction are not involved. It is now clear that different organ transplants involve different rejection reactions. For the kidney allograft rejection reaction following methods of rejections may take place.

(1) Hyperacute rejection

This would occur within minutes of transplantation, characterized by microthrombi in glomeruli and sludging of red cells. This occurs in individuals with pre-existing humoral antibodies-either due to blood group incompatibility or pre-sensitization to class I MHC through blood transfusion. In this type of rejection the transplant is rejected so quickly that the graft never becomes vascularized. The complement system is activated due to antigen-antibody complex formation at the grafted site, resulting in an intense infiltration of the area by neutrophils. This further leads to inflammatory reaction, where blood clots appear within the capillaries, preventing vascularization of the grafted tissue.

Repeated blood transfusion, sometimes develop significant antibody titer against MHC antigens found on WBCs present in the transfused blood. By chance if the MHC antigens are the same as those on subsequent graft, it will lead to hyperacute rejection reaction due to the action of antibodies on the graft. In women, who had repeated pregnancies may develop antibodies to paternal alloantigens of the fetus and if they receive the graft carrying the same antigen, it is subjected to hyperacute rejection. Sometimes, hyperacute rejection of graft may occur due to the presence of antibodies against blood group antigens in the graft. Therefore, ABO blood group matching and tissue typing are carefully performed prior to transplantation to avoid hyperacute rejection reaction. Finally individuals who had received a graft previously will have developed high titer antibodies against some of alloantigens. These antibodies will mediate hyperacute rejection of subsequent graft that expresses some of the alloantigens.

(2) Acute early rejection

Graft rejections occurring up to 10 days or so after transplantation, which is characterized by severe infiltration of the graft by mononuclear cells and rupture of peritubular capillaries and appears to be a cell mediated hypersensitivity reaction involving T-lymphocytes.

(3) Acute late rejection

This occurs from 11 days onward in-patient's administered with immunosuppressive drugs such as prednisone and azathioprine. This is probably caused by deposition of immunoglobulins in the blood vessel walls, which induces platelet aggregation in the glomerular capillaries leading to acute renal shut down. This will further lead to destruction of antibody-coated cells through antibody dependent cell mediated cytotoxicity.

(4) Insidious and late rejection

This is associated with subendothelial deposits of immunoglobulin and C3 on the glomerular basement membranes, which may sometimes be on expression of an underlying immune complex disorder of possibly of complex formation with soluble antigens derived from the grafted kidney.

Precautions against Graft Rejection

Since major histocompatibility complex (MHC) is the major cause of most of the graft rejections, lot of work has been done into defining these antigen specificities. This has been done to minimize rejection by matching graft and recipient MHC in much the same way, as the individual's blood is cross-matched with the blood of other individuals before transfusion. Various antigens that determine histocompatibility are encoded by 40 different loci of HLA complex in human beings (Chapter 5). Because the MHC loci are closely linked, they are inherited as complete set known as haplotype from each parent. MHC inheritance in out bred population is very complex because the high polymorphism exhibited by each MHC locus, give a high probability of heterozygosity at most loci. Therefore, there is only 25% chance of inheriting identical phenotype between the parent and the child. Even if the MHC identity of donor and recipient may be almost the same there is a possibility of rejection due to differences at various minor histocompatibility loci (Chapter 5). MHC antigens are generally recognized by, T_H and T_C-cells, which is called as alloreactivity, whereas minor histocompatibility antigens are recognized in conjuncture with self MHC molecules. In addition, the tissue rejection reaction induced by minor histocompatibility antigens is less vigorous. Still graft rejection does occur. Therefore, immune suppression is necessary even if transplantation is carried out between HLA identical individuals. The cell surface antigens are always found associated with class I and class II MHC molecules in order that they may be recognized by T lymphocytes.

Tissue distribution of MHC molecule

Almost all nucleated cells, essentially carry Class I MHC molecules. These are abundantly expressed on lymphoid cells, less so on liver, lung and kidney and very sparsely on brain and skeletal muscle. Class II MHC molecules are more restricted being especially associated with B cells, antigen presenting cells and macrophages.

Methods for Tissue Typing

Tissue types (alleles) at the 3 class I loci, HLA-A, -B and -C are identified by complement dependent cytotoxic reactions by using operationally monospecific sera. These are selected from patients transfused with whole blood and who often become immunized by foetal antigens with specificities defined by paternally derived genes absent from the mother's genome. An individual's tissue is typed, by setting up his lymphocytes against a panel of such sera, in the presence of complement. Cell death normally being judged by the inability to exclude trypan blue or eosin. Different antigens are arbitrarily assigned numerical specificities; (Fig.19.1a) an individual heterozygous at each locus must express four major class I HLA specificities and two minor ones (HLA-C) derived from both the paternal and maternal chromosomes (Fig. 19.1b).

It is absolutely necessary to bear in mind the important distinction between typing based on T cell discrimination and all other types of analysis because the important initial event for transplantation is the recognition of the graft antigens by T cells, and antibodies do not necessarily define the same epitopes. Therefore, T lymphocyte typing into five different subgroups can subdivide individuals bearing the serologically defined DR4 specificities.

The latest data on well-established specificities at the three class I MHC and three class II MHC loci are presented in the Fig. 19.2a. Most transplanters favor a reasonable degree of matching especially at the DR locus. The consensus is that matching at the DR loci is of greater benefit than the B loci which in turn are of more relevance to graft survival than the A loci.

Because of the many thousands of different HLA phenotypes possible, it is usual to work with a large pool of potential recipients on a community or racial or country basis so that when graft material becomes available the best possible match can be made. Except for the bone marrow cells, which can be kept

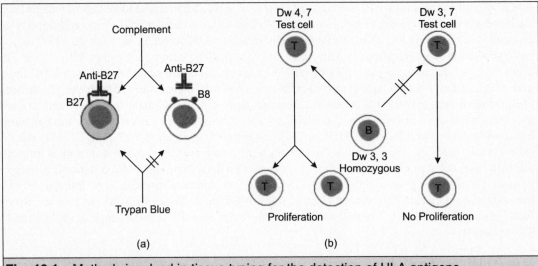

Fig. 19.1 Methods involved in tissue typing for the detection of HLA antigens.

viable even after freezing and thawing, other tissue storage facilities for long term are not good enough. With a paired organ such as kidney, living donors may be used; siblings provide the best chance of a good match. (Fig. 19.2b).

Graft versus Host Disease or (Reaction) (GVHD)

In the young rodents it is characterized by inhibition of growth, splenomegaly and hemolytic anemia (due to production of antibodies against red blood cells). In the humans, fever, anemia, weight loss, rash, diarrhea, and splenomegaly are observed. The stronger the difference in transplantation antigens, the more severe is the reaction. Where donor and recipient differ at HLA or H-2 loci, the consequences can be fatal. It should be also noted that reactions to minor and major antigens or combination of them might be equally dangerous and difficult to control.

Two possible situations leading to GVH reactions may occur in human beings. Immunologically anergic subjects receiving bone marrow transplants, for example, combined immunodeficiency, for red cell aplasia due to radiation accidents or as a possible form of cancer therapy. Competent T cells present in the GVH reactions; so could maternal cells, which passively cross the placenta.

It involves both activation phase and effector phase. In the activation phase, donor T_H cells from the bone marrow recognize the recipient antigen-MHC complexes displayed on APCs. Donor T_H cell gets activated due to antigen presentation and co-stimulatory signal by APC and starts producing IL-2 and undergoes proliferation. The cytokines produced by activated donor T_H cells will induce activation of variety of effector cells including NK-cells, CTLs and macrophages, which bring about effector phase of GVH disease. CTLs act directly to cause tissue damage. Cytokines such as TNF released by T_H cells, CTLs, NK-cells and macrophages has been shown to mediate direct cytolytic damage to cells.

At present various treatment methods have been employed to prevent GVH disease in bone marrow transplantation. Usually, the transplant recipient is placed on a course of immunosuppressive drugs, such as cyclosporin A and methotrexate. Another approach has been to treat donor bone marrow with monoclonal antibodies specific for T cells or anti-T cell anti-sera, before transplantation, thereby depleting the offending

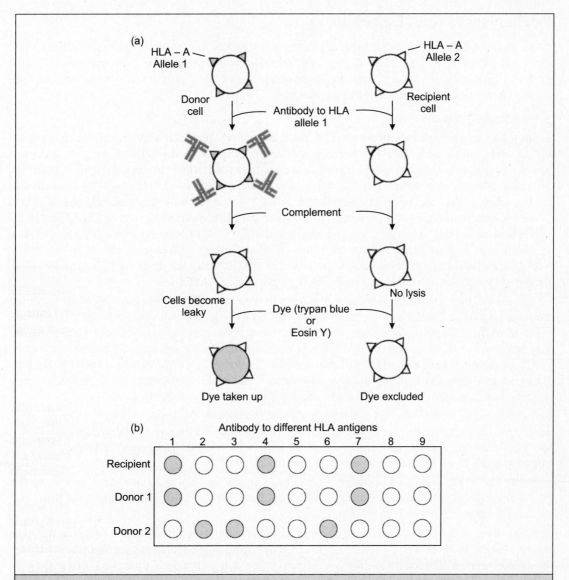

Fig. 19.2 A diagrammatic representation of microtoxicity method in tissue typing. (a) Potential donors white blood cells and the recipient are added to separate wells of microtitre plate. (b) Cells express numerous HLA antigens, they are separately tested with a battery of monoclonal antibodies to specific HLA antigens

T cells. Complete depletion of T cells from donor bone marrow may result in rejection. Therefore, partial depletion of T cells in donor bone marrow is done. Low level of donor T cell activity apparently results in a low level GVH disease. It is actually beneficial because it prevents any residual host T cells from becoming sensitized to the graft. It has been observed that, in leukemic patients with low level GVH disease seems to result in destruction of leukemic cells, thus there is less chance of recurrence of leukemia.

Mechanism of Graft Rejection

As mentioned earlier, graft rejection is principally by cell-mediated immune response against alloantigens expressed on the cells of the graft. During graft rejection, both delayed type hypersensitive and cell-mediated cytotoxic reactions are observed. Therefore, process of graft rejection can be divided into two stages: (1). Sensitization phase and (2) Effector phase.

1. Sensitization phase

In this phase, antigen reactive lymphocytes of the recipient undergo proliferation in response to alloantigens on the graft. CD4$^+$ and CD8$^+$ T cells recognize the alloantigens on the cells of the graft and start proliferating. Both minor and major histocompatibility antigens of graft will be responsible for stimulation of lymphocytes of the recipient. Even though, minor histocompatibility antigens are weak, sometimes, large number of them in unison can stimulate a strong immune response. Immune response to major histocompatibility antigens involve recognition of both the MHC molecules, namely Class I and II. In addition to these MHC molecules, the peptide present in the cleft of both the MHC molecules is also known to play an important role in sensitization reaction. Proteins of allogenic cells may be present within the cleft of class I MHC molecule, whereas class II MHC holds within its cleft, the proteins taken up and processed through the endocytic pathway of the allogenic APCs.

The TH cell through its TCR recognizes the antigens presented through the class II MHC molecule on the surface of APC. This interaction brings about activation of T_H cells, where co-stimulatory signals of APCs also play an important role. Depending on the tissue, different populations of cells within the graft may function as APCs. Dendritic cells are present in almost all tissues and in majority of cases they act as APCs, because they have highest level of class II MHC expression. Host APCs are also known to migrate into graft and endocytose the alloantigens (both minor and major histocompatibility molecules) and process them into peptides to be presented on self-MHC molecule to the host T_H cells.

In some organ transplants, APCs from donor tissue migrate into the regional lymph nodes and such leukocytes are called *passenger leukocytes*. Mostly these passenger leukocytes are dendritic cells, which express the allogenic MHC antigens of the donor graft cells, they are recognized as foreign and thus stimulating the T cells in the lymph nodes (Fig. 19.3).

In the skin grafts instead of passenger leukocytes, Langerhans cells and endothelial cells lining the blood vessels are implicated in presentation of alloantigens. MHC Class I and II antigens of the donor graft cells, are expressed on both these cells.

Depending on the type of transplant, involvement of immunologic response also differs in different tissues. For ex. In the skin graft, blood vessels are not present in the beginning. Lymphocytes carried by host blood capillaries encounter the foreign antigens of the skin graft, which are carried back to the host lymph nodes. This stimulates effector lymphocytes, which undergo proliferation and are carried by the lymphatics back to the grafted site, where they mount immune attack. During the transplant of kidney, liver or heart, the blood vasculature is immediately restored, by suturing the blood vessels of the host and the graft tissue. Due to this host lymphocytes circulating in the blood, immediately come in contact with alloantigens and undergo activation. Activated lymphocytes are carried back to host lymph nodes, spleen and bone marrow. In these lymphatic tissues the effector lymphocytes are generated and transported back to the graft by blood or lymphatics.

Graft induced T cells proliferation is brought about by dendritic cells and vascular endothelial cells, which express allogenic antigens. The major proliferating cell is the CD4$^+$-T cell, which recognize alloantigens directly or alloantigens presented by APCs. The amplification of T_H cells plays an important role in inducing other immunologic effector mechanisms.

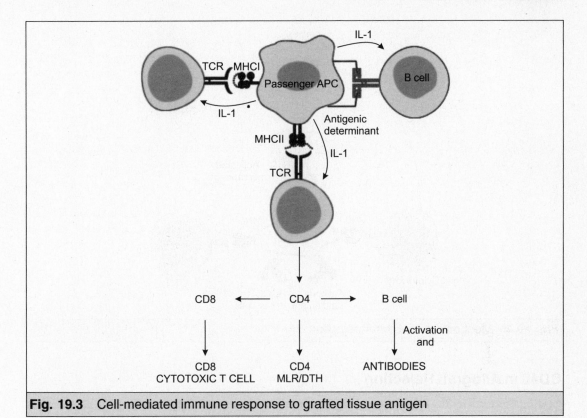

Fig. 19.3 Cell-mediated immune response to grafted tissue antigen

2. Effector stage

Various effector mechanisms involved in allograft rejection are illustrated in Fig. 19.4. In most of the cases, cell-mediated reactions involving delayed type hypersensitivity and CTL-mediated cytotoxicity are more common. Antibody-dependent cell-mediated cytotoxicity (ADCC) and antibody-plus-complement lysis are less common mechanisms. During cell-mediated graft rejection reaction, an influx of T cells and macrophages into graft occurs. Foreign class I MHC antigen recognition on the graft brought about by host CD8$^+$ T cells, which leads to CTL-mediated cytotoxicity or killing. In some transplants, CD4$^+$ T cells that function as class II MHC restricted cytotoxic cells will be responsible for graft rejection.

In both the effector mechanisms of graft rejection, cytokines secreted by T$_H$ cells play a crucial role in further magnification of immune graft rejection reaction (Fig. 19.4). For ex. IL-2, IFN-γ and TNF-β are important cytokine mediators of graft rejection. IL-2 is responsible for promotion of T cell proliferation and is generally necessary for the production of CTLs (Fig. 19.4). IFN-γ is known to play key role in DTH response and promotion of influx of macrophages into graft and their subsequent activation into destructive cells. TNF-β has direct cytotoxic activity on cells of the graft. Various cytokines like IFN-α, β and, γ, TNF-α and β are known to increase the expression of class I MHC and IFN-γ increases class II MHC expression as well.

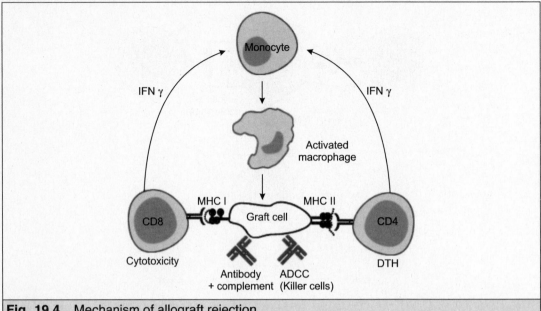

Fig. 19.4   Mechanism of allograft rejection.

CD40 in Allograft Rejection

CD40, the receptor for CD40L is expressed on a wide variety of cells, including dendritic cells (DCs), B cells, macrophages, and endothelial cells. This wide distribution of CD40 and several recent discoveries suggests that the CD40 pathway may play a critical role at many levels of the sensitization and effector phase of allograft rejection, as inhibition of this pathway with an anti-CD40L mAb dramatically prolongs murine islet and cardiac allograft survival. Other investigators have demonstrated the importance of the CD40 pathway in alloimmunity in rodent graft versus host disease (GVHD) models in which the disease is inhibited by either an anti-CD40L mAb or by CD40L gene disruption. In a Rhesus renal allograft model CD40 blockade with anti-CD40L antibody for 14-28 days resulted in an allograft survival time of greater than 90 days. However, an episode of renal allograft dysfunction, occurring 30 days after transplantation and after initial treatment with an anti-CD40L mAb, resolved with a second course of treatment. The predominant effect of a CD40 blockade in these models might be on the effector phase (Fig. 19.5).

Two recent reports suggest that the CD40 pathway, in addition to its role in the effector phase, may also play an important role in the sensitization phase of T cell dependent immune response *in vivo*. Studies in mouse autoimmunity and antiviral models suggest that the regulation of B7 expression on APCs is the major mechanism by which CD40 modulates the development of T cell dependent responses. This would involve B7-CD28 pathway for allograft rejection. Other studies have also shown that principal mechanism by which CD40L blockade inhibits rejection is not mediated through the B7-CD28 pathway.

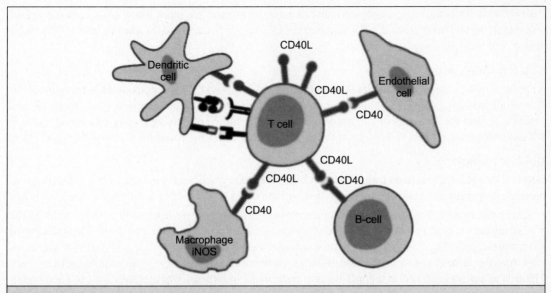

Fig. 19.5 CD40-CD40L interaction in the development of T cell dependent immune responses.

Tissue and Organ Transplantation

A. Corneal transplant

Cornea is considered to be immunologically privileged location, because of absence of blood vessels and lymphatic vessels as well. Therefore, corneal grafts survive without the need for immunosuppression. Because they are avascular, the alloantigens of the graft are not generally able to sensitize the recipient lymphocytes and the graft shows increased likely hood of acceptance, even when the HLA antigens are not matched. The corneal graft becomes cloudy if the individual has been pre-sensitized.

B. Kidney transplants

At present survival rate of kidney transplant individuals has remarkably improved due to proper patient management and tissue matching. Matching at the HLA-D locus has a strong effect on the graft survival but in long term cases (5 years or more) reasonable HLA-B and to a lesser extent HLA-A matching also becomes apparent. It has now been well established that multiple blood transfusions prior to grafting have a significant beneficial effect on survival but the explanation is still not forthcoming.

DR_{w6}-positive individuals are relatively poor at accepting DR_{w6} -negative grafts while their kidneys survive relatively well as grafts when DR_{w6} negative individuals are recipients. The conjuncture is that in the recipient, DR_{w6} is a good immune response gene for class II antigens and that when DR_{w6} is present on a graft is a good inducer of T suppression.

Patients are partially immunosuppressed at the time of transplantation because uremia causes a degree of immunological anergy. The combination of azathioprine and prednisone is commonly employed in the long-term management of kidney grafts but replacement of azathioprine with cyclosporin A has yielded good results. When transplantation is performed because of immune complex induced glomerulonephritis, immunosuppressive treatment does help to prevent a similar problem occurring in the transplanted kidney.

Patients with antibodies against glomerular basement membrane are more likely to destroy their renal transplants unless first treated with plasmapheresis (plasma deprived of antibodies) followed by immunosuppressive drugs.

C. Heart transplants

At present figures for heart transplants have reached 80% survival, helped considerably by cyclosporin A, therapy, which of course is nephrotoxic, however, with the combined treatment of azathioprine and prednisone after the 3 months of cyclosporin therapy have shown promising results. Matching of single DR class antigens has given 90% survival at 3 year compared with a figure of 65% for two-DR mismatches.

D. Liver transplants

Survival rate of liver and heart transplants is almost the same; particularly using combined cyclosporin/ prednisone therapy. Rejection crisis is avoided by high doses of steroids or anti-lymphocyte globulins.

Experiments with liver grafts between pigs revealed unexpected results. Many animals retained the grafted organs in a healthy state for many months without any form of immunosuppression. The transplanted liver represented a large antigen pool, which induced a state of unresponsiveness to grafts of kidney or skin from the same donor. The mechanism is not clear but may involve true tolerance or enhancement. There is as yet no evidence as regards hepatic transplants in humans whether they lead to such highly desirable state.

E. Bone marrow transplants

Individuals suffering from aplastic anemia and immunodeficiency disorders are given bone marrow transplants. In addition to this, acute leukemic patients who under go whole body irradiation and chemotherapy to kill the neoplastic cells are also the candidates for bone marrow transplants. For a successful result with bone marrow transplants, to avoid severe GVH reactions, siblings offer the best chances of finding a matched donor. For matching the antigens other than major HLA loci may prove to be essential. If the T cells from the grafted marrow are removed the incidence of GVH reaction is reduced, this could be achieved by treating the marrow with cytotoxic cocktail of anti-T cell monoclonals and significant improvements in concurring GVH reaction is achieved through treating the patients with cyclosporin A. It is interesting to note that leukemia patients with GVH disease have a lower incidence of relapse.

Immunosuppressive agents

Non-specific interference with the induction or expression of the immune response is called immunosuppression. Because of the non-specific nature of immunosuppressive effects of drugs the patient undergoing this therapy will be susceptible to infection; they are also more prone to develop lymphoreticular cancers. Immunosuppressive therapy is used for patients receiving grafts and those suffering from autoimmune diseases.

Immunosuppression can be brought about by 3 different ways.

(1) Surgical ablation; (2) Irradiation; (3) Drugs.

1. Surgical ablation

Thymectomy, spleenectomy and lymphadenectomy in adult recipients of grafts seem to help, but extracorporeal irradiation of blood and thoracic ducts have proved beneficial. Injection of anti lymphocyte immunoglobulin or monoclonal anti-T_3 antibodies seems to have successfully reversed the kidney graft rejection reaction in adult mice.

2. Total lymphoid irradiation (TLI)

For the past 20 years, people suffering from Hodgkins disease (an auto-immune disorder of the lymphoid tissue) have been treated with TLI, where bone marrow is shielded and the individuals lymphoid tissue, lungs and other vital non lymphoid tissues are subjected to fractionated irradiation. When mice treated in similar manner were injected with allogenic bone marrow they fully accepted the graft and show signs of graft-Vs-host reaction symptoms, which would normally occur. The irradiation induces the formation of large granular lymphocytes lacking T, B and macrophage markers which non specifically suppress the cytolytic reaction involved in allogenic graft, while at the same time facilitating the development of antigen specific suppressor which maintains tolerance. At present the application of this technique to humans is still awaiting for the want of FDA permission.

3. Immunosuppressive drugs

Many of the drugs employed at present for immunosuppression were earlier used for cancer chemotherapy, because these drugs are highly toxic to dividing cells. These anti-mitotic drugs are toxic even to bone marrow cells and highly proliferative intestinal cells and must therefore be used with great care. The drugs commonly used for immunosuppression during tissue transplants are a) azathioprine, b) methotrexate, and c) N-mustard derivative of cyclophosphamide, d) cyclosporin A, e) steroids like prednisone.

(a) Azathioprine or Imuran

This drug has preferential effect on T cell mediated reaction. It is broken down in the body first to *6-mercaptopurine* and then further converted to *ribotide*. The ribotide has similar structure like that of *inosinic acid* except that it has a SH group on the 6th position (Fig. 19.6). It is a competitive inhibitor of the enzyme concerned in the synthesis of *guanilic acid* and *adenylic acid*; it also inhibits the synthesis of *5-phosphoribosylamine*, a precursor of inosinic acid by a feed back mechanism. The net result is inhibition of nucleic acid synthesis.

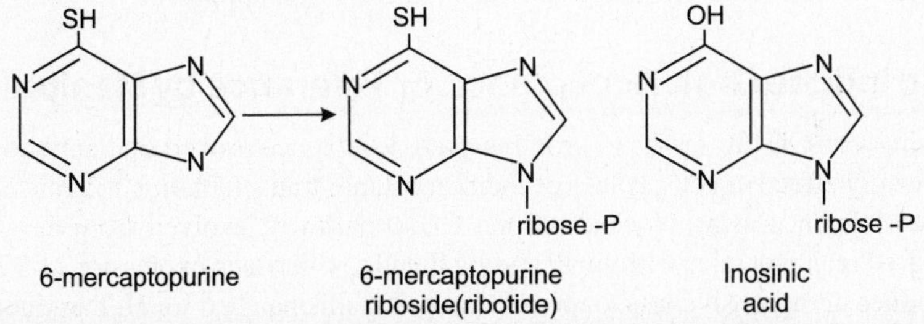

Fig. 19.6   Structural differences in 6-mercaptopurine and inosinic acid.

(b) Methotrexate

It is an inhibitor of folic acid, which in turn inhibits nucleic acid synthesis. Folic acid is responsible for production of dihydrofolate, which is one of the precursors of nucleic acid synthesis.

(c) N-mustard derivative of cyclophosphamide

This compound probably attacks the DNA directly by alkylating its nitrogenous bases and cross-linking, therefore, preventing correct duplication during cell division.

All these drugs discussed above appear to exert their toxic effect on cells during mitosis and this reason are most effective when administered after the presentation of antigen (after the graft) when the antigen sensitive cells are dividing.

(d) Cyclosporin A, FK506 and Rapamycin

It is a neutral hydrophobic cyclical peptide containing 11 amino acids, obtained from fungi as one of the metabolite. Cyclosporin A is capable of penetrating antigen sensitive T cells in the G_0-G_1 phase and selectively block the transcription of lymphokine mRNA. It is not toxic to memory cells of immune response and to the cells of bone marrow and intestinal epithelia. In some cases of immune reactions it has been shown that cyclosporin treatment has led to the development of specific T-suppressor cells which could actively maintain tolerance.

Cyclosporin has its own side effects such as nephrotoxicity. It has to be continuously monitored in the blood of a patient to keep the dose below toxic levels.

(e) Prednisone

It is a steroid, which intervenes at various points in the immune response affecting lymphocyte reticulation and generation of cytotoxic effector cells. In addition to this, it is also anti-inflammatory where it inhibits neutrophil adherence to vascular endothelium in an inflammatory area and suppression of macrophage/monocyte functions such as microbicidal activity and response to lymphokines.

Croticosteroids act in four areas of the immune system. They have effects on leukocyte circulation; they influence the immune effector mechanism in lymphocytes; they modulate the activities of inflammatory mediators; they directly influence gene expression. When steroids are administered to humans, it leads to depletion in circulating eosinophils, basophils and lymphocytes. As a result of steroid induced decreased adherence in neutrophils, their population increases. Corticosteroids suppress the chemotaxis in monocytes, neutrophils and eosinophils and also cytotoxic and phagocytic abilities of neutrophils. Corticosteroids also suppress production of IL-1 by macrophages and IL-2 by T_H cells. At high doses, corticosteroids cause thymic atrophy and trigger T cell apoptosis.

Strategies to Induce Graft Acceptance or Tolerance by Manipulating CD40

Initial studies using anti-CD40L mAbs to promote graft acceptance proved that antibody therapy alone was neither uniformly effective nor capable of inducing stable transplantation tolerance. An alternative strategy to induce tolerance-using blockade of the CD40 pathway, evolved from the observation that treatment of allograft recipient mice with small resting B cells, which lack expression of B7 co-stimulatory molecules can induce unresponsiveness to mouse skin grafts mismatched for H-Y antigen. The rationale of this approach is that CD40 blockade will prevent CD40-mediated B cell activation and B7 expression in vivo, thereby enhancing the tolerogenicity of the B cell inoculum. This treatment regimen has been shown to diminish the ability of mice to mount an alloimmune response and to prolong the survival of fully allogenic pancreatic islets. Other studies have confirmed the fact that transfusion of donor specific splenocytes in combination with anti-CD40L mAb treatment may prolong allograft survival independently of any effect on the B7-CD28 pathway.

As an alternative strategy to promote allograft acceptance, Larsen and his team have reported that simultaneous blockade of the CD40L-CD40 and B7-CD28 pathways would effectively inhibit allograft rejection by preventing T cell clonal expansion. This promotes long-term survival of fully allogenic skin grafts and inhibits the development of chronic vascular rejection of primarily vascularized cardiac allografts.

More recently they have found that by using this strategy, it is possible to prolong the survival of rat and porcine xenogenic skin transplanted in murine recipients. The extremely potent inhibition of alloimmunity achieved by simultaneous blockade of the CD40L-CD40 and B7-CD28 pathways has exciting prospects for clinical application and also further illustrates that while interrelated, these two pathways serve as critical independent regulators of T cell dependent immune response.

Specific Immunosuppressive Therapy during Transplantation

Immunosuppressive therapies discussed so far are non-specific hence they produce generalized immunosuppression. Generalized immunosuppression has its own effects, such as, increasing the risk for other infections in graft recipients. At this juncture, ideally antigen-specific immunosuppressive therapy against alloantigens of graft is required, while preserving the normal response to unrelated antigens. Some partially successful attempts made for developing specific immunosuppression include monoclonal antibodies to T cells, agents that block co-stimulatory signals, microchimerism of donor cells.

In some cases, it has been shown that, monoclonal antibodies to CD3 of T cell receptor complex, is known to block T cell activation. Rapid depletion of T cells in circulation is brought about by CD3 monoclonal antibodies. The mechanism involved in T cells depletion is that, the antibody coated T cells bind to Fc receptor on phagocytic cells, which then phagocytose and clear the T cells from circulation. U. S. F. D. A has approved the use of monoclonal antibodies to CD3 receptors in humans to reverse acute rejection reaction.

Activated T lymphocytes are known to express high affinity IL-2 receptors on their membrane. Monoclonal antibodies to high affinity IL-2 (anti-TAC) receptor have been used successfully to increase graft survival. Exposure to anti-TAC prior to grafting is known to block proliferation of T cells activated in response to the alloantigens of the graft.

Anti-CD4$^+$ monoclonal antibodies are known to prolong graft survival. Interestingly, anti-CD4$^+$ does not decrease the population of T cells, instead it induces the T cells to enter into immunosuppressive state.

Simultaneous treatment with monoclonal antibodies to the adhesion molecules ICAM-1 and LFA-1 for 6 days following transplant have been known to increase the survival of cardiac transplant in allogenic mice. However, when monoclonal antibodies to one of the adhesion molecule are administered, it could not prevent the rejection of cardiac transplants. Only when both pairs of adhesion molecules were blocked at the same time, the signal transduction is blocked. Therefore, activation of T cells is also blocked.

Monoclonal antibody therapy to treat bone marrow before it is transplanted is practiced to deplete the immunocompetent T cells in the bone marrow transplant, so as to prevent GVH disease. The efficiency of monoclonal antibodies against T cells can be increased, by selecting those isotypes capable of stimulating complement system.

So far, monoclonal antibody therapy used for transplants in humans is of mouse origin. The recipient develops antibodies against mouse monoclonal antibodies and clears them from the body quickly. To avoid this, chimeric antibodies have been attempted, where mouse and human hybrid monoclonal antibodies (Fig. 19.7) are being tried in experimental trials.

At present, attempts have been made to inject animal monoclonal antibodies against different

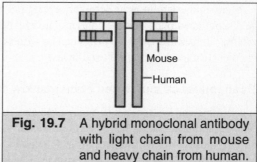

Fig. 19.7 A hybrid monoclonal antibody with light chain from mouse and heavy chain from human.

cytokines, which play an important role in graft rejection. For ex. TNF-α, IFN-γ and IL-2 are being investigated. Monoclonal antibodies against TNF-α are known to prolong bone marrow transplant in mice and prevent GVH disease. Monoclonal antibodies against IFN-γ and IL-2 have each been shown to prolong cardiac transplant in rats. So far monoclonal antibodies against cytokines have not been tried in human transplantation.

Agents that block the co-stimulatory signals

As mentioned earlier (Chapter 10) T_H cell activation occurs through co-stimulatory signals in addition to the signals mediated through TCR. One such co-stimulatory molecule is B7 found on the APCs, which interacts with CD28 or CTLA-4 molecule on T cells (see Fig. 11.5). In the absence of co-stimulatory signal, T cells become anergic. CD28 has moderate affinity to B7 molecule and it is expressed both on resting and activated T cells. On the other hand, CTLA-4 is expressed only on activated T cells and has 20 folds higher affinity to B7 molecule. Therefore, blocking the Co-stimulatory signal following transplantation would cause the host T cells to become anergic, thus enabling the grafted tissue to survive. Lenschow and Bluestone tested this approach by transplanting human pancreatic islet cells into mice that were injected with CTLA-4 antibody (CTLA-4 Ig). Xenogenic graft survived in the mice for long time, but was quickly rejected in untreated control animals. The effect may be brought about by the binding of B7 molecule on APC by CTLA-4 Ig, so that co-stimulatory signal is not generated when the host T cells try to recognize the graft antigens.

Microchimerism of donor cells

After the transplantation of solid organs, passenger leukocytes can be detected in the peripheral circulation of the recipient during the first few days after the transplant, and can persist for many years.

Survival of the donor leukocytes or dendritic cells, which, migrate from grafted tissue into host lymphatics and induce a kind of tolerance to allogenic cells is called *microchimerism*. This suggests that graft acceptance depends upon establishment of a microchimeric state.

Studies from the biopsies of still functioning kidney graft, which were examined 32 years after the transplant revealed that the interstitial cells of the allograft were from the recipient, whereas nephrons were from the donor. In this study it was also revealed that the presence of dendritic cells from the donor in the skin and lymph nodes of the recipient. In another study, 25 individuals who had received liver transplants 22 years ago, who were immunosuppressed with azathioprine or cyclosporin-A revealed donor cell microchimerism in the skin, lymph nodes, heart, lung, spleen, intestine, kidneys, bone marrow and thymus. Widespread distribution of donor cells suggests that substantial numbers of them survive within the recipient.

Microchimerism in graft acceptance suggests that administration of immunosuppressive drugs may be discontinued once a stable chimera is achieved. At present, clinical trials are underway to determine whether immunosuppressive drugs can be withdrawn without inducing graft rejection in liver transplant recipients, after chimerism is established.

T cell tolerance and mixed bone marrow chimerism

When allogenic or xenogenic haematopoietic cells are transplanted to animals in which pre-existing peripheral immune cells have been intentionally eliminated, donor haematopoietic cells migrate to the host thymus where they induce clonal deletion of developing thymocytes expressing T cell receptors that recognize them. If both donor and host cells contribute to hematopoiesis (state of mixed chimerism), the new T cell repertoire generated in the recipient thymus is rendered tolerant of antigens of the both the donor and the host. Such mixed chimeras do not require host myeloablation unlike in the case of fully allogenic chimeras.

NK cell tolerance in mixed bone marrow chimeras

NK cells in mixed chimeras originate from both the donor and the host bone marrow, a failure of NK cells to undergo an adaptive or selective process that makes them mutually tolerant could result in the gradual loss of haematopoietic reconstitution of the donor, the host or both. It is found that NK cells possess a receptor known as Ly-49, which is responsible for recognition of self-MHC class I molecules. The Ly-49 expression in both donor and host NK cells was markedly altered in the chimeric situation.

B cell tolerance and mixed bone marrow chimerism

Like T cells, developing B cells can be tolerized by a clonal deletion mechanism. Production of some antibodies, particularly those directed against repetitive carbohydrates is T cell independent. Tolerization of this group of B cells becomes highly essential with respect to xenotransplantation, because human serum contains natural antibodies that recognize endothelial cells of highly disparate species, such as pig.

IMMUNOLOGY OF TOLERANCE

Immune tolerance or unresponsiveness as defined by Sir. Macfarlane Burnet means the natural process by which, an animal or individual tolerates or fails to react to its own genetically proper substances. For those experiments carried out in adult animals in which, by certain manipulation, the animal fails to respond to some standard antigenic stimulus, in such cases the word unresponsiveness suits well. It can be conveniently separated from Immune tolerance, which is strictly a natural phenomenon.

Natural immunologic tolerance

Natural immune tolerance is not a genetically laid down process, but a physiologically learnt process. Here almost all body components, during early stage of development are exposed to immune system and induce the immune system to realize it as **"self"** component. Therefore, preventing the immune system from mounting an immune response in the later part of life.

Cattle breeders observed that, when a male and female twin calf develops in the same womb with single placenta and bifurcated umbilical cord are born, the female will be sterile and dies. It is called Freemartin cattle. In 1945 Ray Owen found that non-identical bovine twins (male and female) each had the same complex of blood groups, which corresponds to mixture of blood types that would be expected if each calf had born separately. In most instances, the mixture of circulating red blood cells remained almost same in composition in each individual for years. Yet if calves of identical genetic character had been born individual births, blood of **A** injected into **B** or vice versa, would have provoked an immune response and would have been eliminated during the pregnancy (termination of pregnancy).

An analogous situation in humans occurs, where non-identical twins share a common placental circulation in the uterus, which is a rare phenomenon. Since they are non-identical, they need not possess same blood group, and on testing they show two genetically different blood groups and tolerated. In addition to this, they accept mutual skin graft, which otherwise would never be possible between non-identical twins from separate placentae, therefore, have independent circulation.

These findings are in themselves sufficient to prove that, provided there is mingling of stem cells and lymphocytes from an early stage of development, genetically indifferent cells can be implanted and remain tolerated indefinitely. Tolerance is of genetic origin, because genetically controlled cellular mechanisms are installed and ready to react appropriately to whatever potentially antigenic patterns may be encountered. In 1957, Burnet suggested that the simplest mechanism to account for tolerance was to assume that the newly differentiated immunocytes-T and B cells if destroyed or rendered incapable of multiplication when it recognized and reacted with a corresponding antigenic determinant. Only when it reached certain maturity would the T and B cells react positively, upon encountering the antigenic determinant. The recognition of antigen by the T and B cells and cooperation between them is very essential for the production of circulating antibody and memory T and B cells. When there is no cooperation between the T and B cells, an animal would develop tolerance to the antigen and does not produce antibodies.

Tolerance in Tetraparental (Allophenic) Mice

Beatrice Mintz deliberately constructed mouse whose cells are of two genetically distinct types. Two immunologically distinct breeds of mice, **A** and **B** females are mated each to male of their own type and 24 hrs later the fertilized ova are collected in the early stage of cell division. The ovum **A**, was fused with **B** ovum consisting of blastocyst stage comprising of an equal number of diploid **A** and **B** cells. If the blastocyst is transferred to the uterus of a foster mother, it will develop into physiologically normal mouse, whose every organ is a mosaic of **A** and **B** derived cells. Under ordinary circumstances, **A** and **B** mouse are incompatible and actively reject skin transplants within each other. However, transparental mice accept each type of cell (**A** or **B** strain) as self. It should be emphasized that, this synthetic mouse is quite different from an F1 **A** X **B** hybrid; it is a chimera of two different cell types, in contrast to the hybrids, in which all cells will contain **A** and **B** chromosomes. If a, piece of skin from **AB** hybrid is transplanted to **A** mouse, each cell is recognized for the foreign **B** antigen it contains and the whole graft is rejected. If a similar experiment is done with the **A+B** chimera, the graft is partially rejected and it appears like worm eaten patch, which allows an approximate visualization of the mosaic of **A** and **B** cell patches in the skin. There are two interpretations of tetraparental tolerance. Mintz and Silvers thought it likely that there was complete tolerance in the chimeric mice and an absence of active lymphocytes. Another group, I. Hellstrom, K. E. Hellstrom and J. J. Trentin found evidence that there were T cytotoxic cells, whose activity was suppressed by a serum factor. Whatever may be the mechanism of tolerance in chimeric mouse, the tolerance shown by them is just as complete as it is in any normal mouse.

Burnet proposed the **clonal selection** for the production of clones of T and B cells during the normal course of development of immune response against a particular antigen. These cells are stimulated by the antigen on interacting with it and undergo proliferation into many clones, from which, one of them is selected for the immune response. Burnet also proposed that immune tolerance may occur, when foetal immunocytes recognize an antigen, which is in abundance, it leads to **clonal deletion** of those immunocytes. More accurately, few years later Joshua Lederberg in the context of B cell tolerance put forward a concept that lymphocytes at an immature stage are eliminated or functionally suppressed if they recognize self. Early experiments conducted by Bellingham and Medawar supports this theory of clonal deletion. They infused lymphoid cells from inbred strain **A** mice into another neonatal inbred strain **B** mice. After some time they performed skin graft in strain **B** mice from strain **A.** Under normal circumstances the strain **B** mice would reject the skin graft, but in this experiment strain **B** mice accepted the graft. Thereafter, many skin grafts performed on strain **B** mice from strain **A** did not sensitize the strain **B** mice and it continued to accept the graft without showing any signs of graft rejection. This tolerance in strain **B** mice against the graft from strain **A** mice was due to neonatal transfusion of **B** cells from strain **A** mice into strain **B**. Possible explanation for this can be given on the basis of Burnet's theory of clonal selection and tolerance. Since the strain **B** mice in the neonatal stage were exposed to the antigens of strain **A** mice in excess, strain **B** mouse immune system learnt to recognize the antigens of strain **A** as its own because they were abundant in number. Hence the tolerance was developed in strain **B** mice for the antigens of strain **A** mice.

Deletion of T cells was first demonstrated some 30 years later for noncognate interaction of TCR belonging to certain family with Vβ6. The interaction between Vβs and MHCs behave as high affinity contacts that result in deletion. Finally, deletion of potentially autoreactive T cells when the αβ TCR on maturing CD4$^+$ and CD8$^+$ thymocytes is engaged by a peptide ligand of high affinity for the TCR presented by MHC encoded molecules on thymic medullary epithelium, dendritic cells, or macrophages. The proportion of T cells that are deleted by high affinity interactions with these thymic antigen-presenting cells (APC) range from 5% to over 50% of T cells that had undergone positive selection in the thymic cortex. In 1988 Philippa Marrack and other workers demonstrated that certain self-reactive clones of maturing T cells were deleted from the thymus and never reached circulation. It is apparent now that the immature T cells that enter the thymus are subjected to two selection processes. In the first process also called **positive selection**, T cells are taught to recognize the MHC peptides, which is highly essential for self-recognition. The second step, **negative selection**, is critical for self-tolerance. The developing T cells are exposed to different combinations of self-antigens. Young T cells that bind to self-antigens die by apoptosis in the thymus, hence they do not reach circulation. Only when this mechanism fails, it results in autoimmune disease. Rubin and Rommel, recently proposed another concept for development of tolerance. According to them positive selection and self-tolerance must always be coupled. For clonal deletion to be principal mechanism for avoiding autoimmunity, this independent machinery evolved separately from the positive selection machinery and would need to be in place before the positive selection developed. At the same time, without the positively selected cells to act on, the clonal deletion machinery would have no survival advantage. Therefore, positive selection is the key for development of self-tolerance. The various concepts that explain the principal role played by positive selection are dealt as follows.

Non-autoreactive Nature of Positively Selected T Cells

For positive selection, specialized stromal cells in the cortex of thymus that express class I and II MHC complexes and antigen presentation by thymic epithelial cells (TEC) are required. For the MHC molecules to be stable on the cell surface, they need to bind to peptides and assume proper three-dimensional structure. In the thymus the environment if sterile and only peptides available for occupancy of the MHC would be derived from self-material. It is important to note that, the peptide defined as **cognate** or **index** antigen of mature peripheral T cells in circulation (because it shows agonistic properties) would not be a part of intrathymic population of peptides. In the thymus, T cells that encounter such peptides are the cognate T cells, which would be eliminated. Positive selection appears to be mediated by peptide analog, which consists of complex mixture of self-peptides. These peptides may have similar conformation and charge to the cognate antigen and that can have much lower affinity for the TCR (Fig. 19.8).

The selecting antigens cannot activate positively selected T cells, even though the complex between the self-peptides and MHC is required for further maturation. Therefore, thymocytes that develop to the CD4$^+$ or CD8$^+$ phenotype can be presumed to have encountered endogenous antigens(s) on TEC of low affinity for their TCR. These naive T cells have an extended life span after emigration to the periphery.

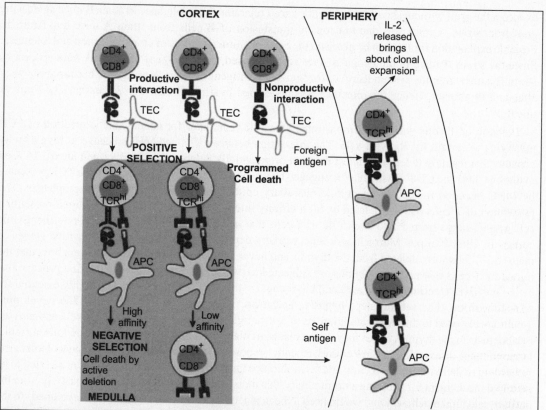

Fig 19.8   T cell selection and acquisition of self-tolerence in the thymus. Shown are the possible developmental fates of pre-T cells in the thymus cortex bearing T-cell receptors (TCRs) differing in affinity for self antigens. Those T- cells with no affinity for self-peptides and MHC die by neglect. Any TCR engaged by self antigens presented by Thymic Epithelial Cells (TEC) induces signal transduction pathways. This initiates a programme of cellular differentiation that induces enhanced expression of TCR and CD69 and production of factors responsible for tolerence to the selecting antigens. Positively selected T-cells migrate from cortex into the thymic medulla and are exposed to similar set of antigens presented on dendritic cells, which bear co-stimulatory molecule B7 of professional APC. T-cells with high affinity for self antigens presented on dendritic cells will be subjected to death by apoptosis. T-cells with low affinity for self-antigens are ignored due to their recently acquired ability for increased threshold for activation. These cells go on to differentiate into CD4⁺ or CD8⁺ mature T-cells. These cells migrate to the periphery (circulation), where, if a T-cell encounters self-antigen with same degree of affinity to that of the antigens involved in positive selection, it fails to respond. Only antigens of higher affinity for the TCR, typically derived from foreign sources, would be able to surpass the activation threshold established during positive selection.This results in interleukin-2 (IL-2) production and clonal expansion. The term negative selection depicts clonal deletion.

These cells retain the capacity to respond to a non-self antigen of high affinity for their TCR. There is ample evidence to indicate that, T memory cells require persistence of cognate antigen to provide low-level signaling through the TCR. In the mean time, MHC and self-peptides involved in the positive selection of naive T cells may also maintain a very low threshold of signal. It should be noted that, random rearrangements of the genetic elements encoding TCR could create infinite number of specificities in the T cell repertoire. These T cells may go waste because a pathogen could never be encountered that engages their TCR. It is by linking positive selection with recognition of self-antigens, the T cell repertoire is restricted to respond to molecular subunits found in all biological structures. In this way, mature T cells will have higher probability to respond to pathogens than those T cells that respond to purely random TCR repertoire. Some evidence suggests that organ-specific- antigens may reach the thymus through the circulation, either directly or after the uptake and processing by APC. Furthermore, failure to protect nonthymic antigens from exposure to the peripheral immune system may be the basis for common occurrence of certain organ-specific autoimmune diseases such as autoimmune thyroiditis and insulin dependent diabetes.

At present there are three major concepts, namely, APL (altered peptide-ligand) concept, adaptation concept and anergy concept.

APL (Altered Peptide-ligand) Concept: Nature of Selecting Antigens

The first example of differential ligand signaling was reported by Evavold and Allen, who found that single amino acid difference from the cognate antigen, while stimulating the IL-4 production and B cell helper activity of T_H2 clone, failed to cause its proliferation. Later studies showed that alteration of one or two conservative amino acids at the TCR contact residue of the index ligand failed to induce proliferation, instead caused altered cytokine response or blocking the response to non-mutant antigen when simultaneously present (antagonism) or in a subsequent challenge (anergy). These APLs tend to be low affinity ligands for the TCR since they dissociate rapidly, but at the same time retain the similar capacity to bind to MHC as that of non-mutant ligand. When the APLs engage the TCR, they induce very low protein tyrosine phosphorylation of CD3ε, presumably because their interaction lasts only for short duration. This may also result in failure in signaling other multimeric signal transduction molecules involved in intracellular signaling events.

In the thymus, endogenous self-peptides may act as APLs, serving as antagonists or as partial or weak agonists. These agonists and antagonists, may induce differential gene expression during pre-T cell differentiation. For instance, weak agonists induce activation of additional transcription factors and at high ligand concentrations sufficient signaling to induce apoptosis or death.

On the other hand, strong agonists cause full signaling, resulting in cell death associated with clonal deletion. Taking into account the capacity of weak agonists to support positive selection, APLs might play an important role in promoting or inhibiting thymocyte development. In addition, potentially autoreactive T cells in the periphery, that escaped central tolerance, may be anergized or antagonized by the APLs in the periphery (Fig. 19.9).

Support for the APL concept in positive selection is obtained from studies with analog peptides, without involving CD4, CD8 or other adhesion molecules and where the positive selection ligands have less than 50 fold higher affinity for TCR than the nonselecting ligands. The endogenous peptides can be remarkably different from the agonist ligands, sometimes bearing minimum structural similarity with the cognate peptide. Such analogs would be inactive as APLs of mature T cells.

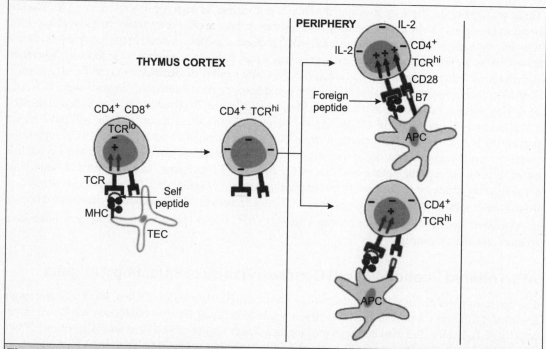

Fig. 19.9 A schematic diagram to explain the altered peptide ligand (APL) concept for acquisition of self-tolerance. Note the self-peptides in the thymus may behave as APLs, which interact with TCR and may cause partial signaling through the TCR as shown by gray arrows. This low activation signal is sufficient for further differentiation of pre-T cell. Failure to fully involve the multiple signaling pathways required for mature T cell activation results in the accumulation of negative regulators that increase the activation threshold in the developing thymocytes. In the periphery antagonistic peptides may continually establish self-tolerance by subthreshold stimulation and the non-self (foreign) peptides have sufficient ability for full T cell activation through strong signaling pathway.

Source: RUBIN, R. L. AND ROMMEL, A. K. *crit. Rev. Immunol.* **19**: 199-218, 1999.

Recent reports indicate that, antagonists APLs affecting T cell differentiation in the thymus required 3 to 4 orders of magnitude higher concentration than that required for agonist peptides to induce deletion. Therefore, it will be necessary for TCRs of immature T cells to discriminate among low affinity thymic peptides in order for the APL concept to be applicable for positive selection. With a diverse population of MHC-bound peptides being available in the thymus for positive selection, there exist considerable specificity in their interaction with the TCRs on pre-T cells. In this manner, APLs that behave as low affinity peptides could produce differential signaling through the TCR, so that continually signals are transduced to sustain development of T cells without activating it.

The Adaptation Concept: Nature of the Immature T Cells

Mature CD4$^+$CD8$^+$ thymocytes and peripheral T cells express the TCR-CD3 complex at approximately 20 fold higher density than the immature CD4$^+$ or CD8$^+$ cells, which express negligible or low-density

TCR-CD3 complex. Transition from immature CD4$^+$CD8$^+$ TCR$^{-/lo}$ thymocytes to cells expressing medium or intermediate levels of TCR-CD3 complex (TCR^{med} or TCR^{int}) takes about 1 day. It is presumed that, in this initial contact, TCR would have initiated downstream signal transduction events, but because the T cells have relatively few TCRs the excitation level of the cell is below the threshold required to activate or delete it. Grossman and Singer proposed that, in addition to maintaining the cells viability, the stimulus received by the immature T cells is sufficient to induce developmental responses, which includes an increase in number of surface TCRs as well as *de novo* production or modification of molecules that can inhibit the excitation state of the cell. As a result of encountering sufficient number of high affinity ligands, if the stimulus reaches the maximum threshold, immature T cells die because the adaptive response cannot be produced fast enough. It is presumed that, T cells may be programmed to adapt to sub-threshold intracellular disturbances induced by transient TCR engagement by reestablishing the threshold required to subsequent antigen mediated stimulation or activation. In response to TCR engagement increased TCR α chain synthesis occurs, which gradually leads to increased TCR α/β expression in developing T cells.

More detailed studies have shown that, further differentiation and maturation of CD4$^+$CD8$^+$TCR$^{med/hi}$ into mature CD4 and CD8 single positive thymocytes is dependent on continual engagement of TCR by the positively selecting ligand and not just the engagement of CD4 and CD8 coreceptors. Because the T cells are continuously exposed to self-peptides, an increasing number of TCRs are engaged by self-antigens, but the response of the developing T cells would be limited by the coordinate production of inhibitory molecules. Further development of CD4 and CD8 single positive cells can take up to 2 more days of continuous contact with TEC. Therefore, for the maturation of developing T cells, sustained interaction between the TCRs and their ligands in low affinity aggregate is essential and not just the contact with antigen on TEC.

Positive selection is complete as the developing T cells finally move out of the cortical compartment of the thymus and the full endowment of TCRs has been reached. At this stage of differentiation T cell is tuned to be unable to respond to self-peptides at the concentration and affinity it encountered during the positive selection. In other words, the T cell that emerges from the thymus is desensitized to its selecting antigen and only foreign ligands with sufficient binding ability to exceed the acquired activation threshold will cause full activation. In the periphery, naive T cells that encounter the self-peptides to those participating in its selection may provide weak signaling through the TCR, resulting in continual tuning of the activation threshold to prevent self-reactivity. This also leads to long-term survival of T cells (Fig. 19.10).

Anergy Concept: Nature of APC

Normally, epithelial cells do not present antigens to T cells in the periphery, but TEC have special ability to present the self-antigens on their MHC to immature T cells. TECs do not have the ability to function as full APCs, because they lack B7-1 (CD80) and B7-2 (CD86) co-stimulatory molecules on their surface. TCRs produced after the productive rearrangement of theirs α and β chain, TCRs on CD4$^+$CD8$^+$ pre-T cells will start engaging self-peptides presented by MHC on TEC. This will be signal 1 as the first occupancy requirement of TCRs, where antigen ensures the specificity of the response. Second signals-are elicited by microbes, either directly or by the initial innate immune response, which identifies the antigen as a potential pathogen. The second signal for T cells include costimulators and cytokines that promote clonal expansion of the specific T cells and their differentiation into effector and memory cells. The best defined costimulators for T cells are the two members of the B7 family, B7.1 (CD80) and B7.2 (CD86), which are induced on antigen presenting cells (APCs) by microbes and by cytokines produced during innate immune response. The CD28 receptor on T cells recognizes B7 molecules and delivers activating signals; a second receptor for B7, called CTLA-4, functions to terminate T cell

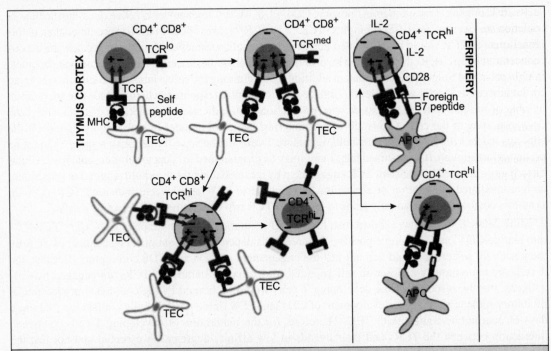

Fig. 19.10   A schematic representation of adaptation concept for acquisition of self-tolerance. Because of the low level of TCR expression on pre-T cells, the excitation induced after initial engagement of TCR will be modest. In response T cells increase the production of TCRs and inhibitors of excitation and activation threshold. Accumulation of inhibitory factor increases due to continual excitation of TCR together with greater expression of TCR and the TEC + peptide interaction. Because of this continuous activation threshold, the mature T cells are tolerant to similar self-peptides encountered in the periphery. Weak signaling through the TCR may maintain the acquired activation threshold and only foreign ligands with sufficient binding ability and those, which exceed the threshold of activation, will succeed in full activation.

Source: RUBIN, R. L. AND ROMMEL, A. K. *crit. Rev. Immunol.* **19**: 199-218, 1999.

responses and is discussed later in this section. It is suggested that mature T cells that enter in to anergic state or unresponsive state not because of the absence of B7-mediated costimulatory signals but because T cells use the CTLA-4 receptor to recognize B7 molecule.

T cell anergy may also be induced under conditions at which adequate costimulation is available but at which antigen receptor signal is suboptimal. For ex., when a T cell encounters an altered peptide ligand, which does not bind to the T cell receptor optimally. These cells also enter into a refractory state to subsequent activation by same antigen even when presented by better-equipped APC. This state is called anergic and such anergic T cells will not produce cytokines that elaborate entire cell-mediated immune response. Hence such T cells will fail to recognize self-antigens. Rubin and Rommel (1999) proposed this new concept of anergic response of T cells for self-antigens during positive selection. Anergy to high-affinity peptides may be overwhelmed by the costimulatory power of the deletional machinery and these cells are killed after encountering the bone marrow-derived or medullary epithelial cells. In this case clonal deletion may be advantageous for removing T cells with high affinity TCR for self. Even if these cells are functionally tolerized for self, they are at greater risk of autoactivation if cognate antigen at localized high concentration becomes accessible in the periphery to its TCR as a consequence of infection. Surviving single positive CD4 or CD8 T cells will leave thymus as resting naive T cells, imprinted with the message of inability to respond to selecting peptides or a stimulus of equivalent strength (Fig. 19.11).

Ohashi proposed that mature T cells have the capacity to respond only to agonists of higher affinity than that of selecting ligands. Therefore, the capacity of peripheral T cells to distinguish between self and the non-self ligands lies only in the exclusion of foreign antigens during the T cell development. The association of an anergy-like process with positive selection is based on the well-accepted two-Vs-one signal paradigm that underlies peripheral T cell activation Vs anergy. Many molecular events associated

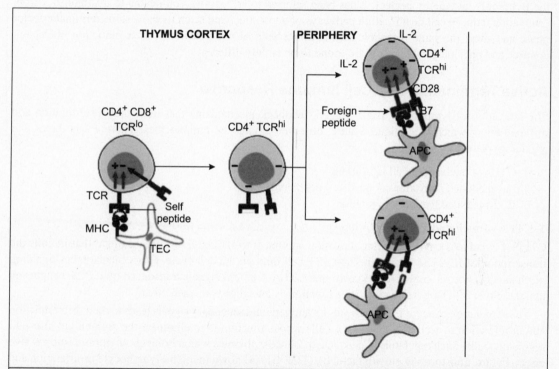

Fig. 19.11   A schematic representation of anergy concept of acquisition of tolerance. Pre-T cells on exposure to TEC + self-antigen will undergo further differentiation in the thymus cortex. In the absence of costimulatory signals as shown by black arrow, more inhibitory factors are produced, including negative regulators of cytokine genes. In the periphery, occasional encountering of selecting antigens may refresh the partial anergic state. At the same time negative regulators of cytokine genes allow the mature T cells to be activated by antigens of higher binding ability than that of the selecting peptides.

Source: RUBIN, R. L. AND ROMMEL, A. K. *Crit. Rev. Immunol.* **19**: 199-218, 1999.

with signal 1 in the absence of signal 2 have been identified in peripheral T cells, which is thought to be useful for anergy induction during positive selection.

Nature some how has designed a redundant mechanism for regulating T cell function after engaging the TCR in the absence of co-stimulation, which is the key for T cell tolerance through positive selection.

Loss of activated lymphocytes due to death by neglect

This is another concept put forward by Parijs and Abbas (1999) that the frequency of mature T lymphocytes for any one antigen is in the order of 1 in 10^6. It has been observed that on exposure to appropriate antigen that is capable of eliciting specific immune response, this frequency can increase to 1 in 1000 or more within a day or two and return to normal levels within 4 to 12 weeks. This rapid decline in lymphocyte populations is designated to elimination of lymphocytes by apoptosis. The lymphocytes that are deprived of costimulatory and cytokine stimuli are known to lose expression of antiapoptotic proteins, mainly of the Bcl family and die by neglect. It has been referred to as "passive cell death" to distinguish it from "activation induced cell death". Both pathways of apoptotic death seem to show same terminal effector phase and show the same morphological and biochemical manifestations, their induction, molecular controls and physiological controls are found to be largely different

Active Termination of T Cell Immune Response

The activation of lymphocyte itself triggers feedback mechanisms that limit their proliferation and differentiation, which is a unique feature, observed among the lymphocytes. There exists three such regulatory pathways in T cells.

(1) CTLA-4 mediated T cell inhibition,
(2) Fas-mediated activation-induced cell death and
(3) IL-2-mediated feedback regulation.

1. CTLA-4-mediated T cell inhibition

CTLA-4 is induced on T cells after activation and binds to B7 and transduces a signal that inhibits the transcription of IL-2 and the progression of T cell through the cell cycle. Exact biochemical signaling mechanism is not yet known. It is known that CTLA-4 blocks signals transduced by CD28, suggesting that these two B7 recognizing molecules function as antagonists of each other.

The stimulation of naive T lymphocytes by antigens and secondary signals leads to their differentiation and proliferation as well as into effector cells whose function is to eliminate the antigen but also into regulatory cells. Such regulatory T cells may produce cytokines, which bring about immunosuppressive effect. For ex. transforming growth factor β1 (TGF-β1) is known to inhibit lymphocyte proliferation and IL-10 is known to inhibit macrophage activation and expression of costimulators. These inhibitory cytokines are said to limit the expansion of specific lymphocytes and return the activated macrophages and other inflammatory cells to their resting state. An important point to note is that the existence of multiple mechanisms for feedback inhibition of immune response, where a molecule or pathways may function to amplify and terminate immune responses. For ex. IL-2 and B7 molecule, both of which are capable of delivering activation and inhibitory signals as and when needed.

2. Mechanism of homeostasis: Returning the immune system to basal state

The immune response against an antigen is characterized by increased population of lymphocytes and antibodies at the initial state, which falls to basal state after some time. The decline in immune response is characterized by remarkable decrease in population of lymphocytes accompanied by decrease in effector functions leaving long-lived memory cells as surviving indicators of previous antigen exposure. It is presumed that the passive cell death is the cause of loss of antigen-stimulated lymphocytes. As the innate immune response to antigen (microbe) and the antigenic stimulus is eliminated by the immune response, the stimuli that are needed for lymphocyte survival i.e., costimulators and cytokines gradually decrease, resulting in reduced expression of antiapoptotic Bcl family proteins. The control of potentially harmful T cell (T cytotoxic cells) and macrophage reaction by immunosuppressive cytokines such as IL-10, TGF-β1 is important for limiting the inflammatory reaction. Much less is known about the function of T cell anergy or CTLA-4 or Fas mediated regulation in normal homeostasis. It is observed that T cells lacking CTLA-4 or Fas show normal kinetics of expansion and decline after exposure to an antigen in vivo. It shows that there is a possibility that CTLA-4 and Fas mediated regulation is more important for the maintenance of self-tolerance that for the regulation of responses to foreign antigens.

3. Prevention of autoimmune reactions: Mechanism of tolerance

The mechanism of self-tolerance falls into three categories as proposed by Parijs and Abbas. A) Central tolerance; (B) Peripheral tolerance; (C) Clonal ignorance.

A. Central tolerance: It is due to the death of developing lymphocytes when they encounter self-antigens in the generative centers of the lymphoid organs and it is important for tolerance to self-antigens that are present at high concentrations in the bone marrow and thymus.

B. Peripheral tolerance: It is brought about by mechanisms that act on mature lymphocytes that have left the generative organs and encounter self-antigens in peripheral tissues.

C. Clonal ignorance: It happens when certain self-antigens may induce neither central nor peripheral tolerance but are simply ignored by the immune system. It may be because the self-antigen is anatomically sequestered from the immunocompetent lymphocytes or because the antigen is presented to lymphocytes in the absence of second signals that are needed to trigger the effective immune response. Another important feature is, self-antigens do not normally elicit innate immune reactions, therefore they may be ignored by the immune system. It is still not known which or how many self-antigens induce central or peripheral tolerance or are ignored and which characteristics of the self-antigens determine which of these mechanisms self-tolerance.

If the compartment of mature B and T cells encounter the self-antigens in the absence of second signals or if the self-antigens trigger mechanisms that actively block lymphocyte activation or induce apoptosis may induce self- tolerance in these cells. It is widely believed that self-antigen recognition without costimulation induced functional anergy. The frequently noted association between infections and autoimmunity has been attributed to the activation of anergic self-reactive lymphocytes by adjacent cells reacting to microbial antigens. It may also result from the activation of autoreactive lymphocytes that have remained ignorant of the antigen until second signals are up-regulated as a consequence of second infection. Since the response of lymphocytes to self-antigens is tightly regulated by specific molecular interactions maintenance of self-tolerance is possible. This can be exemplified from a knock out mice model for autoimmune disease, where it lacks the ability to produce proteins that are crucial for terminating immune response. It is observed that, mutations in Fas or FasL results in lupus like autoimmune disease, which is due to abnormally prolonged survival of autoreactive helper T cells and inability to remove autoreactive B lymphocytes by apoptosis. In human beings also mutation in fas gene is associated with an autoimmune syndrome with lymphoproliferation. The regulatory function of CTLA-4 is illustrated by targeted disruption of the CTLA-4 gene in mice, which results in massive accumulation of activated lymphocytes in the spleen and lymph nodes and infiltration of multiple tissues by activated lymphocytes leading to tissue injury that sets in within 3 to 4 weeks of age. These lesions are suggestive of autoimmune disease but to date there are no evidences that indicate that the infiltrating lymphocytes actually recognize and respond to self-antigens. Mice lacking IL-2 and the α and β chain of the IL-2 receptor develop lymphadenopathy and various manifestation of autoimmunity including autoimmune hemolytic anemia. The role of regulatory T cells in preventing autoimmunity is best exemplified in animal's models, in which selective depletion of T cells with an activated phenotype allows the development of multiorgan autoimmune lesions. Such results indicate that, a subsets of T cells respond to self antigens and keep in check other, potentially pathogenic autoreactive lymphocytes. The immunosuppressive cytokines may be performing the regulatory functions, but the critical molecules have not yet been identified.

The single gene models of animals have provided valuable information regarding the mechanism of T cell-mediated autoimmune disease. In these models, central tolerance or negative selection of developing T cells, is not found to be affected but mainly peripheral tolerance is under attack. All the genes involved play an important role in T cell regulation. Any defects in lymphocyte regulation may result in autoimmune disease without any change in the way the self-antigens are presented to the immune system. This also implies that specific recognition of self-antigens is a normal phenomenon and that key to the maintenance of self-tolerance is the control imposed on specific lymphocytes after they have encountered the self-antigens. It is observed that, the regulatory mechanisms depending on Fas-FasL interactions, CTLA-4 and IL-2 are actually triggered by antigen recognition, suggesting that the self-tolerance develops, if the responses to self-antigens are initiated and then aborted. Most intriguing finding is that the existence of multiple mechanisms of self-tolerance disruption of any one pathway leads to autoimmunity. In other words these mechanism can not compensate for one another. The available evidences indicate that Fas-FasL interactions are responsible for activation-induced apoptotic death of mature T cells in vivo, CTLA-4 plays a role inducing functional inactivation apoptototic process and induction of anergy, and IL-2 potentiates Fas-mediated cell death and possibly other regulatory mechanisms. Possibly because different self-antigens may induce peripheral tolerance by different mechanisms, the roles of the regulatory proteins may be nonredundant. For instance, tissue restricted self-antigens present at low concentrations may induce anergy, and widely spread and abundant self-antigens may trigger activation induced cell death. It is still not known, because target antigens have not been clearly identified, which have been a major problem in human autoimmune diseases.

Exercise

1. Write notes on (5 marks each):
    (a) Classification of grafts and first and second set rejection
    (b) Role of lymphocytes and humoral antibody in graft rejection
    (c) Methods of tissue typing
    (d) Graft verses host disease
    (e) Manipulation of CD40 for graft acceptance
    (f) Natural immunological tolerance
    (g) Tolerance in tetraparental allophenic mice
    (h) Mechanism of tolerance
2. Write briefly on: (10 marks each)
    (a) Role of CD40 in graft rejection
    (b) Tissue and organ transplants

    (c) Conventional immunosuppressive agents
    (d) Altered peptide-legand concept of tolerance (illustrate)
    (e) Adaptation concept of tolerance (illustrate)
    (f) Anergy concept of tolerance (illustrate)
    (g) Active termination of T cell immune response in immune tolerance
3. Give an account of mechanism of graft rejection (20 marks)
4. Explain the specific immunosuppressive therapies during transplantation (20 marks)
5. Write an account on Non-autoreactive self tolerant nature of T cells (20 marks)

Chapter 20

Immunology of Tumors

- Clinical Evidence of Immune Response in Malignancy
- Tumor Antigens
- Tumor Antigens Recognized by T-Lymphocytes
- Tumor Antigens Defined by Xenogenic Antibodies
- Immune Response to Tumor Antigens
- Immunological Surveillance
- Immune Therapy of Cancer

A tumor is said to be an abnormal growth of cells to form a lump or mass of transformed cells. This abnormal growth occurs due to loss of regulatory control on cell division and the genes responsible for certain characteristics of the cell have undergone mutation. There are two types of tumors, **benign tumor** and **malignant tumor.** Benign tumor is usually encapsulated and confined to a single site, whereas the malignant tumor, the cells break off from the main tumor mass and travel through the blood system and lodge themselves elsewhere and initiate new tumor formation at the site where they have lodged. The malignant cells are provided with such abilities due to change in surface adhesive molecules. In addition, malignant cells also express certain special receptors on the membrane for their autocrine factors, which endows cancer cells with special antigenic property. The immune system recognizes these changed surface molecules and attacks the tumor cells as though they are foreign invaders. In spite of the immune response being developed against cancer cells, they still survive and thrive in the body by evading the immune response. Evasion of immune response by cancerous cells is achieved by changing the antigenic molecules repeatedly thereby confusing the immune system. This chapter deals with the properties and types of tumor antigens, how tumor cells evade immune response and the new strategies of immune-mediated gene therapy for the treatment of cancer is discussed.

I. CLINICAL EVIDENCE OF IMMUNE RESPONSE IN MALIGNANCY

Cancers or malignant tumors grow in an uncontrolled manner, which invade the normal tissues due to metastasis and often grow at sites distant from the tissue of origin. In general, cancers are derived from only one or a few normal cells that have undergone a poorly defined process called malignant transformation. Cancers are known to arise from any tissue in the body. Those derived from epithelial cells are called *carcinomas,* are the most common kind of cancers. *Sarcomas* are malignant tumors of mesenchymal tissues arising from cells such as fibroblasts, muscle cells, and fat cells. Solid malignant tumors of lymphoid tissues are called *lymphomas*, bone marrow and blood borne malignant tumors of lymphocytes or other hematopoietic cells are called *leukemias*.

Although tumors are derived from tissues of ones own body, the malignant transformation process leads to the expression of molecules on the tumor cells that are recognized by ones own immune system as foreign bodies. Such molecules are called tumor antigens, which may induce immune responses directed at the tumor cells that express them. In fact, several clinical and experimental evidences suggest that tumors can stimulate immune responses in their hosts.

Histological observations of the tumors suggests that the tumors are immunogenic by the presence of mononuclear infiltrates, composed of T cells, natural killer cells (NK

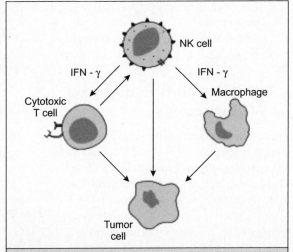

Fig. 20.1 The three key cells that may be involved in killing tumor cells and the central role played by interferon in regulating the process.

cells) and macrophages (Fig 20.1). Such cells are found around any tissue during inflammatory reaction or during tissue injury, but they are also most frequently seen around certain types of tumors, medullary breast carcinomas, malignant melanomas of the skin, thymomas, testicular seminomas. Another histopathological evidence is that the hyperplasia of lymphocytes in the lymphnodes draining the tumor growth site. Furthermore, there is over expression of class II major histocompatibility complex (MHC) molecules and intracellular adhesion molecule-1 (ICAM-1), suggesting an active immune response at the site of the tumor.

Clinicopathologic correlations show that the presence of lymphocytic infiltrates in some tumors (e.g., medullary breast carcinomas and malignant melanomas) is associated with a better prognosis compared with histologically similar tumors without infiltrates. Experimental evidences strongly indicate that tumor cells can initiate specific T cell mediated immune response. Recently several tumor antigens that are recognized by class I MHC restricted cytotoxic T lymphocytes (CTL's) *in vivo* have been identified as mutant forms of normal cellular proteins

II. TUMOR ANTIGENS

Malignant tumors behave abnormally due to expression of mutated or viral genes and /or deregulated expression of normal genes of a cell. Therefore, cancerous cells express proteins that either are not expressed at all or are present in much lower quantities in normal cells (Fig. 20.2). These proteins may appear foreign to the host body because they were never there on the tissue (cell) surfaces prior to tumor development or were expressed in such low quantity that they did not induce immune tolerance. Such proteins can stimulate immune responses to tumor cells. In addition, surface proteins characteristic of tumors may serve as targets for natural killer cell (NK cells) attack.

The fact that the tumor cells express antigens that can stimulate immune response in the host has been clearly demonstrated in both experimental animal models and in human cancer patients. Tumor antigens can be classified into two main groups based on the types of immunological probes used to detect them.

1. Tumor antigens recognized by T-lymphocytes.
2. Tumor antigens defined by xenogenic antibodies.

I. Tumor Antigens Recognized by T- lymphocytes

These tumor antigens may stimulate T cell mediated rejection of tumor transplants in animals previously immunized with the tumor. These tumor antigens are cell-proteins that MHC complexes to either CD4 or CD8 T lymphocytes. Some tumor antigens recognized by T lymphocytes are unique and specific to certain tumors and some are present on many cancers of different types involving different tissues.

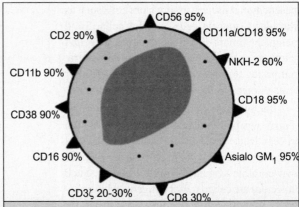

CD56 95%
CD11a/CD18 95%
CD2 90%
NKH-2 60%
CD11b 90%
CD18 95%
CD38 90%
CD16 90%
Asialo GM$_1$ 95%
CD3ζ 20-30%
CD8 30%

Fig. 20.2 Some antigen markers that develop on the surface of the cancerous cells and provoke an immune response.

Tumor antigens recognized by T-lymphocytes include a wide variety of cellular and viral proteins. The major categories of these antigens are:

A. Tumor specific transplantation antigens (TSTA's) on carcinogen or radiation induced rodent tumors.
B. Tumor antigens expressed on in vitro mutagenized tumor cells.
C. Tumor antigens encoded by normally silent cellular genes in spontaneous tumors.
D. Tumor antigens encoded by oncogenes or tumor suppressor genes.
E. Tumor antigens encoded by genomes of oncogenic viruses.
F. Tumor antigens resulting from mutations.

A. Tumor specific transplantation antigens

In 1950's studies carried out on rodent tumors induced by chemical carcinogens or by radiation provided the first evidence regarding the expression of tumor antigens on the tumor cells that induce specific and protective immune responses. In an experiment, a sarcoma was induced by smearing *methylcholanthrene* (MCA) on the skin of inbred variety of mice. These tumors could be easily removed and transplanted onto other mice or re-transplanted back on the same original host. Transplantation into new syngeneic mice leads to successful growth of tumors and eventual death of new host. In contrast re-transplantation on the original host results in specific immunological rejection of the tumor. This is found to be caused by tumor specific cytotoxic T-lymphocytes (CTL's). In another experiment, the cells of the tumors from one mouse were irradiated and killed and used to immunize the second syngeneic mice. Subsequent introduction of live cells from the original tumors into the immunized mouse with irradiated cells will result in immunologic rejection of the tumor transplant.

These experiments demonstrate an important feature of the transplanted tumors is that they show specific immune response and memory. Since the tumor antigens in this experimental system are detected by rejection of transplanted tumor cells, they are called *tumor rejection antigens or tumor transplantation antigens*. One remarkable feature of these tumor rejection antigens is their enormous diversity. For example, one MCA induced sarcoma will not induce protective immunity against another MCA induced sarcoma, even if both the tumors are obtained from the same mouse. Therefore, they are called *tumor specific transplantation antigens (TSTA's)*.

B. Tumor antigens expressed on in vitro mutagenized tumor cells

It has been identified that some tumor antigens expressed on experimental tumors are mutant cellular proteins with single amino acid substitutions. This has been shown by tumor specific CTL clones, which were used to isolate genes encoding tumor antigens. The strategy adopted in this study was to artificially mutagenize a tumorigenic mouse cell line *in vitro* and isolate non-tumorigenic variant cell lines that were immunologically rejected when transplanted into syngeneic mice. Note that tumorigenic cell line does not express tumor rejection antigens, but the mutagenized cell line does. That is why mutagenized tumor is rejected (Fig. 20.3). Mixed lymphocyte tumor cultures were prepared by mixing spleen cells from mice that had rejected tumors with cells from the same non-tumorigenic variant line. Active CTL's that specifically recognized and lysed the variant tumor grew out of the culture and cloned lines of these CTL's, each derived from a single lymphocyte were propagated. These clones are powerful tools for the identification of tumor antigens.

Tumor specific CTL clones have been used for isolating the genes that code for tumor antigens (Fig. 20.3). In one such study, a cosmid library of tumor antigen genes was derived from the non-tumorigenic line (as described earlier) and these genes were transfected into the parental tumorigenic line. The transfectants were screened for their sensitivity to lysis by the tumor specific CTL clones. The genes identified in this manner are the cellular genes that have undergone point mutations. These genes are

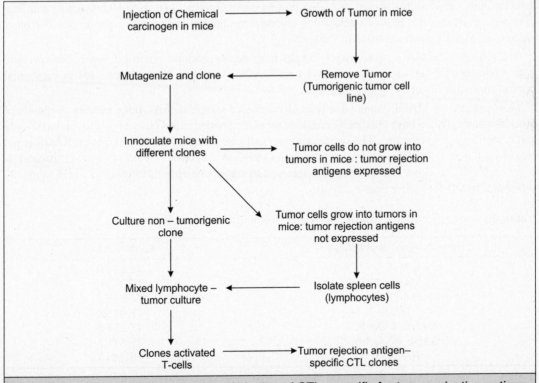

Fig 20.3   Schematic representation of cloning of CTLs specific for tumor rejection antigen

unrelated to one another and their function is also unknown; they do not involve in malignant transformations of the tumor cell. The proteins produced by these mutated genes are endogenously synthesized, processed and presented to the host immune system, usually in association with class I MHC molecules. If these proteins are normal self-proteins, they do not induce immune responses because of the absence of self-reactive T cells. However, if these proteins are altered forms of normal proteins, they will be recognized by specific CTL's and will be lysed and rejected. Proteins coded by the mutated part of the tumor antigen gene can bind to self-MHC or are not recognized by self-tolerant T cell population. Initially the number of cells expressing the mutated gene product might be too low to stimulate an immune response; proliferating clone of malignant cells may produce enough of the mutant protein to stimulate T cell population.

C. Tumor antigen encoded by normally silent cellular genes in Spontaneous tumors (Tumor Specific Shared Antigens) (TSSA)

Some genes are usually silent and do not express in normal cells or they are expressed in the early stage of development, during differentiation and embryogenesis, before the onset of self-tolerance mechanism. When these genes are switched on as a result of malignant transformation of a cell and are expressed inappropriately in the wrong tissue at a wrong time in the life of an individual, they may behave as tumor antigens and evoke immune responses. These tumor antigens may be shared by many different tumors. The strategy for isolating these genes employed is the same as explained earlier where tumor antigen specific CTL clones are used. A human gene called MAGE-1 (for melanoma antigen I) was isolated from malignant melanoma cell line and codes an antigen recognized by a melanoma-specific CTL clone derived from the melanoma-bearing patient. MAGE-1 protein is expressed on up to 50% of melanomas and 25% of breast carcinomas and has been detected in placental trophoblast and testicular germ cells. The other antigens of MAGE group are listed in Table. 20.1.

The activation of MAGE gene usually results from demethylation of their promoters that correlate with a non-specific genome-wide demethylation. MAGE expression has been detected in substantial number of human tumors.

Most antigens of MAGE group have been characterized on melanomas, but a number of tumors of other histological types have also been found to express such antigens. RAGE was recently found to code for an antigen recognized by CTLs on human renal cell carcinomas. Like MAGE genes, RAGE is not expressed in most normal tissues, except retina, but is activated in number of tumors of various histological types (Table 20.1). These human antigens expressed by tumors bearing the appropriate MHC type are promising targets for cancer immunotherapy.

Table 20.1 Human Tumor Specific Antigens Shared by different tumors

Gene/Antigen expression	Normal tissue
MAGE-1	TESTES
MAGE-3	TESTES
MAGE-6	TESTES
BAGE	TESTES
GAGE-1 OR 2	TESTES
GAGE –3 OR 6	TESTES
RAGE-1	RETINA

Source: B. J. Van den Eynde and P. Van der Bruggen: T cell defined tumor antigens. *Curr. Opinion in Immunol.* **9**: 684-693 (1997).

D. Tumor antigens coded by oncogenes or tumor suppressor genes (Oncogenic proteins)

This class of tumor antigens includes non-mutated oncogenic molecules whose expression is at least partially responsible for the tumor's malignant phenotype. These proteins are frequently growth factors or growth factor receptors and they can be expressed at low levels by normal cells. Sometimes, only during certain stages of differentiation, they are constitutively expressed, usually at high levels, particularly by malignant cells.

Most of the tumors express genes whose products are required for malignant transformation as well as maintenance of the malignant phenotype. In most of the cases, these genes have been found to be altered or mutated form of normal cellular genes that regulate cell division and differentiation process. Carcinogen induced point mutations, deletions or chromosomal translocations may alter the status of proto-oncogenes to oncogenes whose products have transforming activity. Moreover, integration of viral oncogenes into normal cellular genes (proto-oncogenes) can result in production of structurally abnormal products that have oncogenic activity. There are other genes called as tumor suppressor genes, which also code for proteins for normal cellular growth and differentiation. Point mutation at any site on these genes will result in production of non-functional products or may render the gene inactive, with the result malignant transformation may occur. The altered products of mutated proto-oncogenes or tumor suppressor gene expressed in tumors may stimulate immune response in the host. These altered protein products are usually intracellular molecules that are likely to be processed and presented as peptides in association with class I MHC molecules, but phagocytosis or internalization of tumor cells may also result in class II MHC associated presentation (Table 20.2).

As target antigen for immunotherapy, non-mutated oncogene products have a major advantage: immunotherapy frequently selects for tumor antigen loss variants that are resistant to the host immune response. If an over expressed oncogenic protein is the target antigen, its loss would produce a less malignant or non-malignant tumor cell. Immunity to these self-proteins is therefore, inducible and because of their relationship to malignant phenotype, such molecules may be desirable target antigens for immunotherapy.

E. Tumor antigens encoded by genomes of oncogenic viruses

Both RNA and DNA viruses are known to induce tumor formation in both experimental animals and humans. Virally induced tumors usually contain integrated proviral genomes in their cellular genomes and these tumors often express viral genome coded proteins. These endogenously synthesized proteins undergo processing and produce complexes of processed proteins with MHC molecule (class I) and expressed on the tumor cell surface. Such tumor cells expressing viral proteins become the targets of T cell immune response. There are various types of protein products produced by DNA and RNA viruses.

DNA viruses such as papova viruses (including polyoma virus and semian virus SV-40) and adenoviruses induce malignant tumors in neonatal and immunodeficient adult rodents. There are many genes in these viruses which interact to bring about malignant transformation. In humans, DNA viruses such as Epstein-Barr virus (EBV) is associated with B cell lymphomas, Hodgkins lymphoma and nasopharyngeal carcinoma. Human papilloma virus (HPV) is associated with most human cervical carcinomas.

Specific immunity to DNA virus coded nuclear antigens protects against tumor development in animals. For example, SV-40 induced tumors in mice express certain antigens that induce specific immunity against subsequent SV-40 induction of tumors, but not against other virally induced tumors. Therefore, these virally expressed antigens are called as tumor rejection antigens. One such virally coded tumor rejection antigen is the T antigen; a nuclear protein in SV-40 transformed cells. Human adenovirus induced rodent tumors express a virally coded protein called E1A, which is found largely in the nucleus, when class I restricted CTL's specific for a processed peptide of the E1A protein are adaptively transferred in to mice with adenovirus induced tumors, these CTL's kill the tumors (Fig. 20.4).

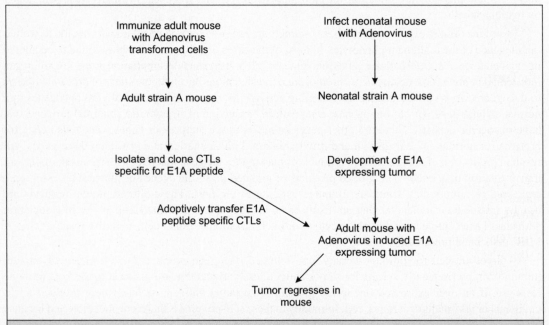

Fig. 20.4   Schematic representation of mechanism involved in viral antigen-specific cytolytic T-lymphocytes that kill virally infected tumors in vivo

RNA tumor virus's retroviruses induce tumors in days to weeks after infection and are called *acute transforming retroviruses*. Examples are Rous sarcoma virus (carrying Src oncogene), avian myelocytomatosis virus (carrying myc oncogene) and Kirsten murine sarcoma virus (carrying K-ras oncogene). Other retroviruses such as murine leukemia viruses, cause tumors months after infection and do not carry any well-defined oncogenes.

This shows transforming retroviruses bring about misregulation of cellular genes by inserting their genome in the cellular genome and bring about loss of cell growth control and differentiation.

In humans well-established RNA tumor virus is T cell lymphotropic virus-1 (HTLV-1), which is the etiologic agent for adult T cell leukemia/lymphoma (ATL) an aggressive malignant tumor of CD4 T cells.

F. Tumor antigens resulting from mutations

Antigens of this category correspond to peptides derived from regions of ubiquitous proteins that are mutated in tumor cells. Two of these mutations affecting the human genes *cyclin dependent kinase* (CDK)4 and β-catenin respectively may be involved in oncogenesis, as they were found in several independent tumors. The CDK4 mutation prevents the protein from binding to its inhibitor, *p16*. This appears to alter the regulation of the cell cycle, favoring uncontrolled growth of the tumor cells. The β-catenin mutation results in the stabilization of the mutated proteins, which favors the constitutive formation of complexes with transcription factors such as Lef-1. Constitutive β-catenin-Lef-1 complexes may result in persistent tansactivation of as yet unidentified target genes, thereby stimulating cell proliferation or inhibiting apoptosis. Another mutation, which may antagonize apoptosis, was identified recently with CTLs specific for a human squamous cell carcinoma. A mutated form of the CASP-8 gene, which codes for protease caspase-8, encodes the antigen. Myeloid leukemia often expresses the chimeric protein bcr-abl, which results from a chromosomal translocation t(9:22). Identical translocations occur frequently in certain type of leukemias, these antigens should be shared by many leukemias.

II. Tumor Antigens Defined by Xenogenic Antibodies

Many cell surface molecules on tumors, which are identified by antibodies raised in other animals after immunizing the animals with tumors, are called tumor antigens. These antigens that are found in different types of tumors arising from the same type of cells and most if not all may also be found on some normal cells or benign tumor cells. These antigens do not stimulate immunologic response in the host, hence are called *tumor-associated antigens* (TAA's). Several classes of these antigens may be expressed on the same tumor. Despite the fact that they may not play a role in protective immune reactions in the host, these TAA's are important for diagnosis and possible treatment of cancers. There are three classes of TAA's, namely:

(a) Oncofoetal antigens,
(b) Altered glycoproteins and glycolipid antigens,
(c) Tissue specific (differentiation) antigens on tumor cells.

(a) Oncofoetal antigens

These are proteins normally expressed on developing (foetal) tissues but not on adult tissues. Oncofoetal antigens are expressed on tumor cells due to derepression of genes by unknown mechanisms. The importance of oncofoetal antigens is that they provide markers that aid in tumor diagnosis other than this, their importance in tumors is not well known. Furthermore, the oncofoetal antigens are not antigenic in the host, because they are expressed as self-proteins during development. The study of oncofoetal antigens has proved useful for diagnostic purpose and has provided some insight into tumor biology. The two most well studied oncofoetal antigens are alpha-foetoprotein (AFP) and carcinoembryonic antigens (CEA).

1. Alpha-foetoprotein (AFP)

It is a 70 kD alpha globulin glycoprotein normally synthesized and secreted in foetal life by the yolk sac and liver. In adults it is replaced by albumin, and only low levels are present in the serum. Serum levels of AFP can be significantly elevated in patients with hepatocellular carcinomas, germ cell tumors and occasionally gastric and pancreatic cancers. AFP is also found to show increased levels in the serum of patients suffering from liver cirrhosis.

2. Carcinoembryonic antigen (CEA)

This is a member of immunoglobulin super family and is highly glycosylated. It is 180kD integral membrane protein. CEA expression is greatly enhanced in colonic cancer and it is also released into extracellular fluid. Serum CEA levels is used to monitor the occurrence or recurrence of metastatic colon carcinoma after primary treatment. Recent studies have demonstrated those CEA functions as an intercellular adhesion molecule, promoting the binding of tumor cells to one another.

(b) Altered glycoprotein and glycolipid antigens

Abnormal surface glycoproteins or glycolipids are expressed on most humans and experimental tumors as a result of defects in the sequential addition of carbohydrate moieties to core proteins or lipid molecules. For example, abnormal glycosides such as GD3 on human melanomas and aberrantly high expression of blood group antigens such as group A and Lewis Y on many human carcinomas. Abnormal glycolipid and glycoprotein synthesis is associated with tissues invasion and metastatic behavior of many tumors.

Some CTLs detected against breast, ovarian and pancreatic carcinomas recognize an epitope of mucin, a surface protein composed of multiple tandem units of 20 amino acids. Whereas in normal cells mucin is heavily glycosylated, in these tumors the peptide repeats are unmasked by under glycosylation, resulting in CTL recognition. These mucin antigens therefore, appear to be very specific for tumor cells and the lack of HLA restriction should facilitate therapeutic vaccination trials. On the other hand, the mucin molecule has recently been shown to be very potent inhibitor of T cells, a mechanism that could account for an inefficient anti-tumor response and a best candidate for evaluation in tissue transplants.

This class of TAA's continues to be a preferred target for antibody-based approaches to cancer therapy.

(c) Tissue specific (differentiation) antigens on tumors

These antigens are a part of normal cell surface and are characteristic of particular tissue type at a particular stage of normal tissue differentiation. Tumors arising from a particular tissue often express the differentiation antigens of that tissue. Since these antigens are part of normal cells, they do not stimulate immune response against the tumors on which they express. The clinical significance of differentiation antigens on tumors relates to their use as targets for immune therapy. For example, malignant lymphomas arising from the malignant transformation of a developing B cell may often be diagnosed as B cell lineage tumors by the detection of surface marker characteristic of normal pre-B cells, called CD10.

A large number of CTLs isolated from melanoma patients were found to recognize not only a majority of melanomas but also normal melanocyte. A good example is *tyrosinase,* a melanocyte protein that gives rise to different peptides that are presented by either MHC class I or class II molecules to CD8$^+$ or CD4$^+$ T cells respectively. The tyrosinase peptide amino acids at 369-377 presents an interesting post-translational modification that was observed when the naturally occurring peptide was analyzed. The **asparagine** residue at 371 was found to have transformed into an aspartic acid, presumably due to glycosylation of asparagine and subsequent deglycosylation by an enzyme, which removed the amino groups with the glycan.

IMMUNE RESPONSE TO TUMOR ANTIGENS

Both humoral and cell mediated immune response to tumor antigens have been shown *in vivo*. The main effector mechanisms in anti-tumor immunity can be classified as follows:

(1) T-lymphocytes, (2) Natural killer cells, (3) Macrophages, (4) Antibodies.

1. T-lymphocytes

As has been discussed earlier in tumor transplantation studies that cytotoxic T-lymophocytes (CTLs) provide effective anti-tumor immunity *in vivo*. CTLs mediated rejection of transplanted tumor is the only well established example of specific anti-tumor immunity *in vivo*. It has been well established that the anti-tumor activity is predominantly shown by CD8 CTLs, that are similar to those CTLs, that show anti-viral activity in viral infection, and development of cell mediated immune response. As discussed earlier,

CTLs may perform immunesurveillance function by recognizing and killing potentially malignant cells that express peptides coded by mutant cellular genes and are present in association with class I MHC molecules. CTLs can be isolated from animals and humans who already possess well-established tumors. For example, patients with advanced carcinomas and melanomas contain CTLs in their peripheral blood system, which can lyse explanted tumors from the same patients. Mononuclear cells found in human solid tumors as infiltrates are called tumor- infiltrating lymphocytes (TILs), also include CTLs with the capacity to lyse the tumors from which they were derived.

CD4 helper T cells even though do not show direct anti-tumor cytotoxic activity they are known to play a important role in anti-tumor response by enhancing the secretion of cytokines for effective development of CTLs. In addition, CD4 cells are also known to secrete tumor necrosis factor (TNF) and interferon gamma (IFNγ) on activation by tumor antigens, which can increase tumor cell class I MHC expression and render the cells sensitive to lysis by CTLs.

2. Natural killer cells (NK cells)

These are produced as a natural acquired immune response to tumors. The mechanism of lysis of tumor cells by NK cells is the same as that of CTLs, but they do not express T cell antigen receptors, and they kill targets in an MHC unrestricted manner. The tumoricidal activity of NK cells is enhanced by cytokines, including interferons, TNFα, interleukin-2 (IL-2) and interleukin-12 (IL-12). Hence, NK cell activity depends on the concurrent stimulation of T cells and macrophages, which in turn produce these cytokines. Lymphokine activated killer (LAK) cells are derived from peripheral blood cells or TILs from tumor patients with high doses of IL-2. LAK cells show remarkable nonspecific activity to lyse other cells, including tumor cells. T cell deficient nude mice have normal or elevated number of NK cells and they do not have high incidence of spontaneous tumors.

3. Macrophages

Like NK cells, macrophages are known to preferentially lyse the tumor cells and they are known to possess Fcr receptors, which can be targeted to tumor cells coated with antibodies. Macrophages involve various mechanisms to kill the tumor cells, which include the release of lysosomal enzymes, relative oxygen metabolites and in mice nitric oxide. Activated macrophage is known to secrete the cytokine tumor necrosis factor (TNFα), which is capable of selectively killing tumor cells and not normal cells. TNFα kills tumors by two different mechanisms. First, the binding of TNFα to cell surface receptors is directly toxic to tumor cells. TNFα induces the production of free radicals there by causing cell death. On the contrary, normal cells produce superoxide dismutase in response to TNFα and this enzyme inactivates free radicals. The tumor cells fail to produce superoxide dismutase hence they are susceptible to free radical toxicity caused by TNFα. TNFα may also involve in disruption of cytoskeletal proteins and gap junction proteins. Second, TNFα can cause tumor necrosis by mobilizing various host responses. TNFα selectively attacks vascularized tumors and is much less effective in killing avascular implants. Histologically it resembles hemorrhagic necrosis in response to TNFα; this has led to the suggestion that TNFα acts selectively on tumor vessels to produce a Schwartzman-like reaction causing thrombosis of the vessels and ischemic necrosis of tumors.

4. Antibodies

Tumor bearing hosts do produce antibodies against tumor antigens even though T cells mediate effective anti-tumor immune responses. In some cases, the antibody production is specific for viral antigens. For example, patients with Epstein-Barr virus (EBV) associated lymphomas show antibodies against EBV coded antigens expressed on the surface of their tumor cells. Human cancer patients produce antibodies against their own tumors, and these antigens are also present on certain normal tissues as well. There is no evidence for a protective role of such humoral antibody responses against tumor development and growth. The potential for antibody-mediated destruction of tumor cells has largely been demonstrated *in vitro* through complement activation or antibody dependent cell mediated cytotoxicity in which, Fc receptor bearing macrophages or NK cells mediate the killing.

IMMUNOLOGICAL SURVEILLANCE

Early in 1950's Paul Ehrlich coined the term immune surveillance for the immune system, which is continuously looking for abnormal cells and their antigens in the host and destroy these abnormal cells before they grow into tumors or could kill tumors after they are formed. In 1960's Sir Macfarlane Burnet and Lewis Thomas further expanded this idea of immune surveillance, they proposed that the immune system played an important role in delaying the growth or causing regression of established tumors. A variety of evidence has accumulated to support these ideas:

1. Postmortem data suggest that there may be more tumors than become clinically apparent.
2. It has been observed that many tumors contain lymphoid cell infiltrates and in some tumors this is the indication of immune responses.
3. Once in a while spontaneous regression of tumors may occur.
4. Tumors are known to occur more frequently in the neonatal period and old age, when the immune system shows very low response.

Although at first glance this appears to be impressive evidence in favor of the theory on closer examination, the association between immunosuppression and increased tumor incidence is less conclusive. In all the cases of immunodeficiency or immune suppression in man, the spectrum of tumors, which arise, is limited and there is evidence that viruses are involved in causing many tumors (Table 20.2).

Table 20.2 Tumor viruses and immunodeficiency

Causes of immune deficiency	Common tumor types	Viruses involved
Inherited immunodeficiency	Lymphoma	EBV
Immunosuppression for organ transplants or AIDS	Lymphoma	EBV
	Cervical cancer	HPV
	Kaposis sarcoma	Maybe HIV itself
Malaria	Burkitt's lymphoma	EBV
Autoimmunity	Lymphoma	EBV

This suggests that the immune response may be important in preventing the spread of potentially oncogenic viruses, rather than surveillance against all tumors. Normal tumors, which become infected with EBV carry the virus for life and show a strong cytotoxic T cell response to the virus. Increased virus replication and shedding of viral particles in secretions has been demonstrated in immunodeficient individuals, so it is clear that the immune response limits virus replication under normal circumstance.

Animal experiments support the view that immune surveillance is largely directed toward viruses rather than tumors. A large study of athymic nude mice did not show a general increase in tumor frequency. However, a high proportion of the mice developed tumors caused by the small DNA polyoma virus, which rarely causes tumors in normal animals.

None of this evidence necessarily implies that there is no immune response to the majority tumors. It is therefore, likely that immune responses to tumors are often weak and relatively late.

IMMUNE THERAPY OF CANCER

The treatment of cancer patients by immunological approaches has held a great promise for the next decades to come. There are five ways in which immune therapy against cancer can be worked out. Which are as follows:

1. Nonspecific stimulation of the immune system.
2. Active immunization against tumors.
3. Adoptive cellular therapy.
4. Passive therapy with anti-tumor antibodies.
5. Cytokines.

1. Nonspecific immune stimulation of the immune system

In this case, stimulation of cancer patients with adjuvants, such as Bacille Calmette -Guerin (BCG) mycobacterium, injected at the site of tumor growth has been tried for many years. This treatment leads to the stimulation of macrophages.

2. Active immunization against tumors

The first attempt to immunize patients against defined tumor antigens were undertaken in B cell lymphoma patients, who were immunized with idiotypic epitope of the immunoglobulin expressed by their lymphoma cells. Tumor regressions were observed in several patients immunized with idiotypic protein mixed with adjuvant or pulsed with dendritic cells and injected into the patient. Such a treatment of B cell lymphoma required the preparation of a different vaccine for each patient.

The MAGE-like antigen can be also used to develop common vaccines. A few HLA-A1 melanoma patients whose tumor cells express MAGE-1 were injected with autologous blood monocytes pulsed with MAGE-1 encoded peptide. Some CTL response was observed but no tumor regression was observed. Twelve patients with most advanced melanoma have received subcutaneous injection of an antigenic peptide, encoded by MAGE-3 and presented by HLA-A1, in the absence of adjuvant. Tumor regression was observed in 3 patients, but no CTL response could be detected in the blood of these three patients.

In another trial, large number of patients have been injected with peptides corresponding to melanoma differentiation antigens mixed with either incomplete Freud's adjuvant or granulocyte-macrophage colony stimulating factor (GM-CSF). Objective tumor regressions were documented in few patients and enhanced delayed type hypersensitivity reactions were observed when GM-CSF was injected.

Injecting the killed or irradiated tumor cells together with nonspecific adjuvants will induce active immunization against the particular tumor. Memory T cells expanded by such immunization would hopefully limit the growth of already established tumors. Unfortunately methods adopted so far for active immunization are unsuccessful, probably because tumor cell vaccines do not effectively activate specific T cell responses. Two experimental areas that may help to make tumor vaccination more effective and specific are the introduction of genes into tumor cells, which renders the cells more immunogenic and the identification of tumor specific antigens recognized by T lymphocytes.

Recent experiments demonstrate that when exogenous genes that code for either cytokines or co-stimulators are introduced into animal tumor cells, and these cells are reintroduced into the host from which they were derived (*ex vivo approach*) significant reduction in tumors or complete disappearance of tumor occurred (Fig. 20.5).

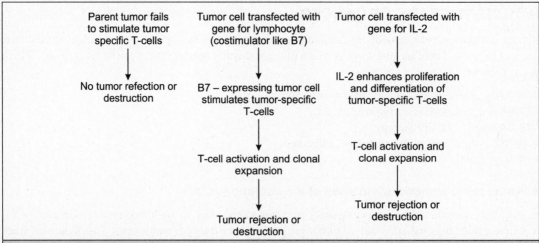

Fig. 20.5   Schematic representation of mechanism involved in tumor cell destruction by transfection of co-stimulation molecule B7 or by IL-2 gene into tumor cells makes them more prone to destruction by T-cells (cytotoxic).

For example, when rodent tumors transfected with IL-2, IL-4, IFN-γ, or granulocyte macrophage colony stimulating factor (GM-CSF) genes are injected into animals, the tumors are rejected or regress. Eosinophils and macrophage accumulate around IL-4 producing tumors, macrophages will be seen infiltrating in large numbers around IFN-γ secreting tumors, and IL-2 producing tumors are generally surrounded by massive lymphocytic infiltrates. The tumors surrounded by inflammatory cells recruited by different cytokines may provide different effector functions and the activation of T cells against the tumor antigens.

(a) Immunization with DNA or RNA encoding tumor antigen/peptide

As an alternative to immunization with protein, DNA encoding tumor antigen/peptide has been used for the immune therapy of cancer. The DNA can be introduced either via direct injection into the target tissue or following immunization with dendritic cells (DCs) that are stably transfected with tumor antigen encoding genes. Several types of viruses, including poxvirus, adenovirus and retrovirus have been used to insert tumor antigen genes into DCs. In another strategy, DCs have been pulsed with tumor cell RNA and used as immunogens. This approach has the advantage that it is not necessary to characterize a relevant tumor antigen(s) and that only a small number of autologous tumor cells are necessary to provide the required RNA.

(b) Enhancement of anti-tumor immunity by antibody treatment

Improved understanding of T cell activation has led to two novel antibody treatment approaches for enhancing anti-tumor immunity in the tumor-bearing host. One approach involves, blocking the inhibitory receptor, CTLA4 on T cells. T lymphocytes express two counter receptors for B7.1 and /or B7.2 with CTLA4. Interaction of B7.1/B7.2 with CTLA4 leads to T cell anergy or apoptosis, whereas interaction with CD28 results in T cell activation. Administration of antiCTLA4 monoclonal antibodies to tumor-bearing mice induces a potent anti-tumor immunity, presumably by blocking the inhibitory pathway and favoring the T cell activation pathway.

In a second approach, monoclonal antibodies have been used to directly activate tumor reactive T cells.

(c) Manipulation of co-stimulatory signal

Several experiments carried out in different laboratories have demonstrated that, co-stimulatory signals necessary for activation of CTL precursors (CTL-Ps) can enhance tumor immunity. When mouse CTL-Ps are incubated with melanoma cells *in vitro* in the presence of co-stimulatory signal, antigen recognition occurs, but in the absence of co-stimulatory signal, the CTL-Ps do not proliferate and differentiate into effector CTLs. However, when the gene encoding B7 ligand is transfected to melanoma cells, the CTL-Ps differentiate into effector CTLs. These findings offer a possibility of using B7-transfected tumor cells to induce a CTL response *in vivo*. For ex. In an experiment Linsley et al injected melanoma-bearing mice with B7$^+$ melanoma cells and observed that melanomas completely regressed in 40% of the mice. In a similar approach, Towsend and Allison vaccinated mice against melanoma. Normal mice were first injected with irradiated B7-transfected melanoma cells and then challenged with unaltered malignant melanoma cells. Large numbers of mice were protected against melanoma by this vaccine (Fig. 20.5). It is hoped that similar approach may help in treating melanoma in human patients.

(d) Tumor antigens as targets for adoptive therapy

Studies utilizing melanoma reactive CTLs have characterized many potential tumor rejection antigens, some considered essential tumor specific, such as MAGE-1, MAGE-3, NA17A, mutated cyclic dependent kinase (CDK)4, and mutated β-catenin. In addition to melanomas, a significant percentage of glioma cell lines, breast tumors, non-small cell lung carcinomas and head or neck carcinomas express MAGE-1, 2 or 3. These shared antigens could be exploited for clinical treatment.

3. Adoptive cellular therapy

In this immunotherapy cultured immune cells that have anti-tumor reactivity are introduced into a tumor-bearing host. There are two approaches, which have been tested, in clinical trials. a). Lymphokine activated killer (LAK) cell therapy. b). Tumor infiltrating lymphocyte (TIL) therapy.

(a) Lymphokine activated killer cell (LAK) therapy

Peripheral blood leukocytes removed from tumor patients are cultured *in vitro* for the generation of LAK cells under the influence of IL-2. The LAK cells are injected back into the cancer patients. LAK cells are derived from NK cells, and adoptive therapy with autologous LAK cells in combination with *in vivo* administration of IL-2 or chemotherapeutic agent has yielded good results in mice, with repression of solid tumors. Human LAK cell therapy trials have so far been largely restricted to advance stages of metastatic tumors, and the success of this approach is highly variable from patient to patient.

(b) Tumor infiltrating lymphocyte (TIL) therapy

Inflammatory infiltrates present in and around the solid tumors, obtained from surgical resection specimens, usually contain mononuclear cells from which LAK cells are derived. This approach result in enrichment of TIL's for tumor specific killer cells. In fact, TIL's include activated NK cells and CTL's, but the specificity of these mixed population of cells is not really established (Rosenberg et al., 1987).

(c) Enhancement of APC activity for immune therapy of cancer

Dendritic cells derived from mouse cultured in GM-CSF and incubated with tumor cells have been shown to activate both T$_H$-cells and CTLs specific for the tumor antigens. These cells were injected back into mice and when challenged with liver tumor cells, they displayed tumor immunity.

A more effective approach on similar lines has been tried, where tumor cells are transfected with gene encoding GM-CSF. These transfected cells are injected back into the same patient from whom the tumor cells were obtained. Genetically engineered cells start secreting GM-CSF, which enhances the differentiation of APCs, namely dendritic cells. Dendritic cells start accumulating around the tumor cells, where tumor antigens are presented to T_H-cells and CTLs by dendritic cells.cliniical trials are underway in melanoma patients, whose melanoma cells are transfected with GM-CSF (Fig. 20.6).

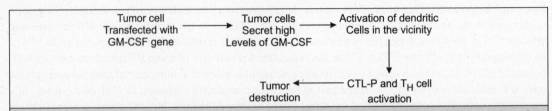

Fig. 20.6   Schematic representation of mechanism involved in tumor cells destruction after transfection of tumor cells with gene encoding GM-CSF. Active secretion of this cytokine by tumor cells activates dendritic cells, which present tumor antigens to both CTL-Ps and T_H cells.

Another approach is to expand peripheral blood dendritic cell population in culture in the presence of GM-CSF, TNF-α and IL-4. Highly proliferated dendritic cells are pulsed with tumor fragments and introduced back into the patients. These dendritic cells now activate T_H-cells and T-cytotoxic cells specific for tumor antigens.

4. Passive therapy with anti-tumor antibodies

In this approach antibodies that bind to antigens on tumor cells are coupled with toxic agents to be carried to the tumor surface and selectively kill tumor cells. Several types of these antibody treatments to tumor cells are described below.

(a) Anti-tumor antibodies coupled with radionucleides and drugs

Anti-tumor antibodies coupled with radioisotopes and drugs have all been tried for immunotherapy of cancer in humans and experimental animal models. Another approach is to covalently attach anti neoplastic drugs or cytocidal radioisotopes to anti-tumor antibodies. In all these cases the substance needs to be endocytosed by tumor cells and delivered to appropriate intracellular site of action.

Toxin and radionucleide-conjugated antibodies with specificities for TAA's on melanomas and carcinomas have been tried in humans. In addition, antibody conjugates specific for CD19, CD22 and CD30 receptors have been used for treating lymphomas. Adult T cell leukemias are treated with antibodies against IL-2Pα (interleukin-2, receptor α) because the T cell leukemias usually over express IL-2Pα. Anti IL-2R antibodies are conjugated with diphtheria toxin and the radionucleide **yttrium 90**, which are used to treat T cell lymphomas. In general, very small percentage of patient's show decreased burden of tumor; hence the efficacy of this procedure is limited.

(b) Anti-idiotypic antibodies and monoclonal antibodies

These have been used in the treatment of B cell lymphomas that express on their surface immunoglobulins with particular idiotypes. An idiotype is a highly specific tumor antigen since it is expressed only on the clones of B cells produced against neoplastic cells. Anti-idiotype antibodies are raised in rabbits by immunizing them with the patient's B cell tumor and depleting the serum of reactivity against all other human immunoglobulins. The strategy involved here is complement fixation or antibody dependent cell mediated toxicity (ADCC) to kill the lymphoma cells. Success of this approach is very limited, because surface immunoglobulin expression is not functionally related to the malignant tumor cells alone. Selective outgrowth of non-immunoglobulin expressing tumor cells can occur. Moreover, the high degree of mutations known to occur in immunoglobulin gene expression could result in the selective outgrowth of tumor cells with altered idiotypes no longer reactive with the anti-idiotypic antibody. Furthermore, since rabbit antibodies are foreign proteins, the tumor patients may develop antibodies against rabbit immunoglobulins, and these may interfere with the efficiency of the rabbit anti-tumor antibodies.

Levy et al produced mouse monoclonal antibody specific for B cell lymphoma idiotype and this anti-idiotype antibody was injected into the patient suffering from terminal B cell lymphoma. At the time of treatment, the lymphoma had metastasized into liver, spleen, bone marrow and peripheral blood. The monoclonal anti-idiotype antibody did specifically bind to B cell lymphoma, because these cells expressed that particular idiotype. Monoclonal antibodies activated complements and lysed the lymphoma cells without harming other cells. The patient underwent treatment with monoclonal anti-idiotypic antibody four times and at present has been in complete remission.

Another approach involving monoclonal antibodies in immunotherapy against cancer is to involve activated T cells directly to a tumor. In this approach two different monoclonal antibodies are produced: one specific for a tumor cell membrane antigen and one specific for CD3 membrane molecule of TCR complex. A hybrid monoclonal antibody or heteroconjugate was able to cross-link and activate T cells directly on the surface of the tumor cells (Fig. 20.7.)

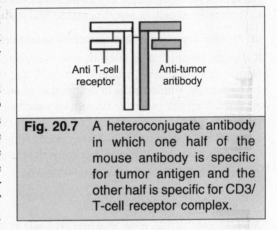

Anti T-cell receptor   Anti-tumor antibody

Fig. 20.7 A heteroconjugate antibody in which one half of the mouse antibody is specific for tumor antigen and the other half is specific for CD3/T-cell receptor complex.

Monoclonal antibodies can also be used to prepare tumor specific immunotoxins. In this case monoclonal antibodies against tumor specific or tumor-associated antigens are linked to a toxin of bacterial origin, ex. Diphtheria toxin. (Fig. 20.8). Immunotoxins prepared in this manner against variety of cancers, such as melanomas, colorectal cancers, metastatic breast cancers, various lymphomas and leukemias have

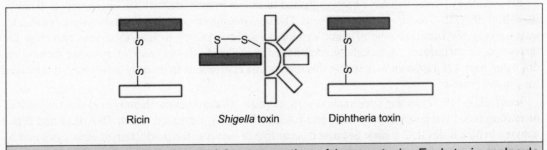

Ricin   *Shigella* toxin   Diphtheria toxin

Fig. 20.8 Toxins of bacteria used for preparation of immunotoxin. Each toxin molecule contains an inhibitory chain (dark gray shaded) and a binding component (unshaded). To make an immunotoxin, the unshaded part is replaced with a monoclonal antibody.

been evaluated in phase I and phase II trials. In eight separate trials 12-75% of leukemia and lymphoma patients exhibited complete remission. In contrast, the clinical response in patients with larger tumor was not favorable.

(c) Heteroconjugate antibodies

In this approach, an antibody specific for a tumor antigen is covalently coupled to an antibody directed against a surface protein on cytotoxic effector cells, such as NK cells or CTLs are targeted against tumor cells. Therefore, this approach is called heteroconjugate, which can promote binding of these effector cells to tumor cells. A heteroconjugate consisting of an anti CD3 antibody coupled to an antibody against a cell surface protein has been used to enhance CTL mediated lysis of the target cell. In this case, the anti-CD3 antibody not only serves to bring the CTL into contact with the target cells but also it activates the CTL. In order to treat melanomas, anti-CD3 antibodies coupled to melanocyte stimulating hormone enhance *in vitro* destruction of human melanoma cells by CTLs. These types of antibody therapies have so far been tried only in experimental animal studies (Fig. 20.7).

(d) *In vitro* depletion of bone marrow tumor cells by antibody plus complement-mediated lysis

It is useful for autologous bone marrow transplants in B cell lymphoma patients. In this procedure, bone marrow from the cancer patient is removed, and the patient is subjected to lethal dose of radiation and chemotherapy, which results in destruction of normal marrow cells and tumor cells. The bone marrow removed from the patient is treated with antibodies directed against B lymphocyte specific antigens, which are specifically expressed on B cell derived lymphomas. Complement is then added to promote lysis of the lymphoma cells that have bound antibodies. The treated marrow, having been purged of B cell lymphoma cells, is transplanted back into the patient who restores the hematopoietic system, which was destroyed by radiation and chemotherapy.

5. Cytokines in tumor therapy

At present high grade, pure cytokines are made available through recombinant DNA technology and they are in sufficient quantity, hence, treatment of various tumors through cytokine-mediated therapy has become feasible recently. The reason for using cytokines is based on their ability to enhance one or more components of cellular immune response and their effect is not specific for anti-tumor directed immune effector cells. The transfection of tumor cells with cytokine gene makes them more susceptible for immune response.

Among the cytokines that have been evaluated in cancer immunotherapy are interferons α, β and γ, IL-1, IL-2, IL-4, IL-5 and IL-12, GM-CSF and TNFα. Cytokine immunotherapy has its own drawbacks, such as systemic administration of some cytokines has been shown to lead to serious and even life threatening consequences. Although, several experimental and clinical trials of cytokine therapy are discussed here it is important to note that this therapeutic approach is in its early stage and not approved for general practice.

Interleukin-2 (IL-2) used in combination with adoptive cellular immune therapy or alone is capable of increasing blood lymphocytes, NK cells and LAK cell activity, increased serum TNF, IL-1 and IFN-γ activity. In high doses IL-2 is toxic because it is capable of inducing the production of other cytokines by T cells, which cause deleterious effects such as pulmonary edema, fever and often shock. This therapeutic approach has been approved by United States Food and Drug Administration for the treatment of advanced melanomas and renal cell carcinomas and has shown regression of tumors in 10 to 15% patients.

Tumor necrosis factor α (TNFα) and TNF β, both are known to exhibit anti-tumor activity. Both are capable of inducing hemorrhagic necrosis of tumors. TNF α is also known to inhibit tumor-induced angiogenesis by damaging vascular endothelial cells in the vicinity of tumors, there by starving the tumor of nutrition, blood-flow and oxygen leading to death of tumor cells. TNF α therapy has its own limitations because of its short half-life repeated injections are necessary, which leads to many side effects like fever, blood pressure and decreased WBC count. Only the drawback with this treatment is TNFα is highly toxic and causes many undesirable side effects. Recommended dose for human treatment is 0.04 mg/Kg body weight.

Alpha-interferon (IFN-α) is a type I interferon capable of increasing the lytic potential of NK cells and increases class I MHC expression on various cells types. It is largely produced by leukocytes. Clinical trials of humans showed that daily administration of IFN-α causes complete regression of tumor in some patients with myelomas, leukemias and lymphomas (hematopoietic malignancies) and solid tumors such as melanomas, kaposis sarcoma, renal tumor and breast cancer.

IFN-α, β and γ are known to increase the expression of Class I MHC on tumor cells. Increased expression of class II MHC on macrophages is known to occur due to the influence of IFN-γ. Tumor cells are known to express decreased levels of class I MHC and interferons restore MHC expression by tumor cells, hence make them prone to CTL action.

IFN-γ (Interferon-γ) is capable of activating macrophages and NK cells and it upregulates MHC molecule expression, which would enhance anti-tumor immunity. Intraperitoneal administration of IFN-γ for the treatment of ovarian cancer is currently being evaluated.

Growth factor of hematopoietic tissue, such as *granulocyte-macrophage colony stimulating factor* (GM-CSF) and *granulocyte colony stimulating factor* (G-CSF) are used in cancer treatment. Generally after chemotherapy or autologous bone marrow transplantation, the patient suffers from neutropenia (decreased neutrophil population). GM-CSF or G-CSF is known to stimulate maturation of granulocyte precursor thereby indirectly enhancing tumor immune response.

Evasion of Immune Response by Tumors

Although an individual has innate ability to build an immune response against cancer, the fact suggests that the death due to cancers is because of failed immune response. It is observed that tumor cells have the ability to evade immune system. Some of the evasion mechanisms adopted by tumors are discussed in this section.

(a) Immune mediated enhancement of tumor growth

Since the time of discovery that antibodies can be produced against tumor specific antigens, many attempts have been made to protect animals against tumor growth by immunizing the animals with tumor antigens or by passive immunization with anti-tumor antibodies. It was observed that instead of inhibiting tumor growth, in many cases, it actually enhanced the growth of tumors. Serum taken from these animals with progressive tumor growth was found to block cell-mediated lympholysis (CML) reaction, whereas serum taken from animals with regressing tumors had little or no blocking effect. Anti-tumor antibodies themselves act as blocking factors in some tumors. Most probably the antibody binds to tumor specific antigens and masks the antigens from cytotoxic cell action. Exact mechanisms involved in blocking reactions are not known. Immune complexes also may inhibit ADCC by binding to Fc receptor on NK cells or macrophages and blocking their activity.

(b) Antigenic modulation of tumors

In some tumors it has been observed that, certain tumor specific antigens disappear from the tumor cells in the presence of serum antibody and then reappear after the antibody is no longer present. This phenomenon is called **antigenic modulation.** It is observed that, when mice is immunized with leukemic T cell antigen

(TL-antigen), will develop high titer of anti-TL antibody, which binds to leukemic cells and induces blocking, endocytosis, and/or shedding of the antigen-antibody complex. As long as antibody is present, the leukemic T cells do not display the TL-antigen on the T cells, hence cannot be eliminated.

(c) Down regulation of class I MHC molecule production

Malignant transformation of cells is very often associated with down regulation of class I MHC molecule. In many cases the decreased expression of class I MHC molecules is accompanied by tumor growth. Since CD8$^+$CTLs recognize only antigens associated with class I MHC molecule, reduced class I MHC expression leads to failure in immune response by CD8$^+$CTLs.

(d) Absence of co-stimulatory signals

A co-stimulatory signal is triggered by the interaction of B7 molecule of APCs with CD28 on T cells together with interaction of TCR with antigen-MHC complex. Both these signals induce the T cell to produce IL-2 cytokine, which also helps in proliferation of T lymphocytes. In most of the individuals suffering from tumors show poor immunogenicity to tumors may be largely due to lack of co-stimulatory signals. T cell anergy may also occur in individuals suffering from cancer due to lack of sufficient number of APCs in the vicinity of tumor and improper T cell activation.

Exercise

1. Write an essay on tumor antigens (20 marks)
2. Give detailed account of immune therapy of cancer (20 marks)
3. Write notes on (5 marks each)
   - (a) Clinical evidence for immune response to malignant cells
   - (b) Immune response to tumor antigens
   - (c) Immune surveillance
   - (d) Cytokine therapy of cancer
   - (e) Evasion of immune response by tumors
   - (f) Antiidiotypic and monoclonal antibodies in cancer treatment
   - (g) Adoptive cellular immune therapy of cancer
4. Write briefly on (10 marks each)
   - (a) Tumor antigens defined by xenogenic antibodies
   - (b) Passive immune therapy of cancer
   - (c) Active immunization against tumors

Chapter 21

Autoimmune Diseases

- Organ-Specific Autoimmune Diseases
- Diseases Mediated by Direct Cellular Damage
- Diseases Mediated by Stimulating or Blocking Antibodies
- Systemic Autoimmune Diseases
- Insight Into Mechanism of Autoimmune Disease Based on Clinical Findings
- Autoantibodies to T Cell Receptors
- Cell and Nuclear Penetration by Autoantibodies
- Treatment of Autoimmune Diseases
- Experimental Therapeutic Approach

□ □

When the immune system goes against the self-components of the body it is called **Autoimmunity**. Normally the immune system has the mechanism to recognize the self-components form the non-self, for which the T and B-lymphocytes since their origin in the immune system of an individual are conditioned and taught to discriminate between the self and non-self. Due to various reasons this fine-tuning of the immune system cells to recognize the self and non-self component fails and leads to autoimmune disease. Generally, during the development and maturation process of T and B cells, they go through a process of selection. Those lymphocytes, which show reaction to self-components, are committed to clonal anergy or apoptosis and those committed to foreign antigens are selected and go through clonal expansion. Autoimmune disease in humans can be divided into two broad categories: **organ-specific** and **systemic autoimmune** disease. Table 21.1 gives an out line of different types of autoimmune diseases in humans.

ORGAN-SPECIFIC AUTOIMMUNE DISEASES

In this autoimmune disease, the immune response is directed against a specific antigen corresponding to a single organ. The target organ as a result of autoimmune attack by humoral or cell-mediated mechanism may suffer severe damage or alternatively, the function of the organ may be enhanced due to autoimmune attack resulting in hyperfunctioning, or the autoantibodies may block the function performed by the cell or organ and result in failure of the particular function.

Table 21.1 Classification of some autoimmune diseases in humans

Disease	Self-antigen
Organ-specific Autoimmune Disease	
Hashimoto's thyroiditis	Thyroid proteins and cells
Autoimmune hemolytic anemia	RBC membrane proteins
Goodpasture's syndrome	Renal and lung basement membrane
Graves disease	Thyroid-stimulating hormone receptor
Addison's disease	Adrenal cells
Idiopathic thrombocytopenia purpura	Platelet membrane proteins
Insulin-dependent diabetes mellitus	Pancreatic beta cells
Pernicious anemia	Gastric parietal cells
Myasthenia gravis	Acetylcholine receptors
Myocardial infarction	Heart
Post-streptococcal glomerulonephritis	Kidney
Spontaneous infertility	Sperm
Systemic Autoimmune Disease	
Multiple sclerosis	Brain or white matter
Rheumatoid arthritis	Connective tissue, IgG
Ankylosing spondylitis	Vertebrae
Scleroderma	Nuclei, heart, lung, kidney, gastrointestinal tract
Systemic lupus erythematosus (SLE)	DNA, nuclear proteins, RBC and platelet membrane
Sjogren's syndrome	Salivary gland, liver, kidney, Thyroid

Diseases Mediated by Direct Cellular Damage

Autoimmune cellular damage may occur when autoantibodies or lymphocytes bind to cell membrane antigens causing cellular lysis or initiate inflammatory response in the organ. As a result, the cellular structure of the organ is lost and is replaced by connective tissue leading to organ failure. Some of the human autoimmune diseases of such types are discussed in this section.

Hashimoto's thyroiditis

This disease frequently afflicts middle-aged women, due to production of autoantibodies and sensitized T_{DTH} cells specific for thyroid antigens. DTH response results in severe inflammatory reaction, where the thyroid gland is infiltrated by lymphocytes, macrophages and plasma cells leading to the formation of lymphocytic follicles and germinal centers. As a result of inflammation, thyroid develops **goiter** (visible enlargement). Autoantibodies are also produced against thyroglobulin and thyroid peroxidase, both of which are involved in uptake of iodine. Binding of autoantibodies to these protein products of thyroid severely impairs iodine uptake resulting in **hypothyroidism.**

Autoimmune anemias

It includes drug induced, pernicious and hemolytic anemia. **Drug induced anemia** is caused by sulfa drugs and antibiotics, where certain cell receptors are bound by drugs and stimulate cytolytic reaction leading to autolysis of the cells or some times some drugs form hapten complex with serum and cellular proteins and initiate autoimmune reaction against the hapten component. **Pernicious anemia** is caused by autoantibodies to intestinal **intrinsic protein factor**, which is responsible for uptake of vitamin B12. Binding of autoantibody to intrinsic factor protein leads to lack of absorption of vitamin B12 from the intestinal surface. Decreased vitamin B12 level in the body affects hematopoiesis, thus number of functional mature RBCs decrease.

Autoantibodies against RBC membrane-proteins causes complement mediated lysis or antibody-mediated opsonization and phagocytosis of RBCs by the phagocytes.

Goodpasture's syndrome

In this disease, autoantibodies attack the basement membrane of the kidney glomeruli and the lung alveoli. This initiates complement activation and cellular lysis accompanied by inflammatory response due to build up of complement split products. Continuous insult to the kidney and pulmonary basement membrane leads to kidney damage and lung hemorrhage ultimately leading to death.

Insulin-dependent diabetes mellitus

Pancreatic islet β cells are under attack by the autoantibodies, which destroys these cells completely by antibody-mediated complement lysis or by antibody-dependent cell-mediated cytotoxicity (ADCC) resulting in decreased insulin production. This disease is also characterized by infiltration of islets of Langerhans by large number of TDTH cells. DTH response leads to severe infiltration of islets by macrophages, which release certain cytokines like IFN-γ, TNF-α and IL-1 and these have been implicated in destruction of β cells.

Diseases Mediated by Stimulating or Blocking Antibodies

In certain autoimmune diseases, autoantibodies act as agonists, and bind to receptors of hormones and bring about similar effects like the hormone. This results in over production of a particular cellular product or increase in cell growth. Certain autoantibodies act as antagonists and block the receptor from actual hormonal or neurotransmitter action, thereby impairing the cellular function.

Graves' disease

Thyroid stimulating hormone (TSH) produced by the pituitary, binds to thyroid cells and initiates the synthesis of two thyroid hormones, thyroxin and triiodothyronine. In Graves' disease, autoantibodies are produced against TSH receptors. Binding of these receptors by autoantibodies mimics the action of TSH, resulting in the production of excess of thyroid hormones. Since there is no feed back regulation in such a condition, autoantibodies continuously stimulate the thyroid for the secretion of hormones. Therefore, these autoantibodies are called as Long-acting thyroid-stimulating antibodies (LATS).

Myasthenia gravis

This autoimmune disease is produced by antagonistic antibodies, which bring about negative action by blocking the receptor of a neurotransmitter that is acetylcholine. Acetylcholine receptors are abundant on skeletal muscles, and autoantibodies on binding to these receptors inhibit muscle action. Prolonged exposure of receptors to autoantibodies leads to complement mediated degradation of receptors, resulting progressive weakening of skeletal muscle response.

SYSTEMIC AUTOIMMUNE DISEASES

In this type of autoimmune disease the autoantibodies are directed against broad range of antigen and target organs. It is due to defective immune regulation of T and B-lymphocytes, which leads to widespread tissue damage from cell mediated and humoral antibodies as well immune complex mediated response.

Systemic Lupus Erythematosus (SLE)

It is prevalent in females between 20 and 40 years of age, characterized by butterfly rash on face, whole body rash, and arthritis and kidney dysfunction. SLE affected individuals may produce autoantibodies to wide variety of self-antigens such as DNA, thrombocytes, RBC, histone, leukocytes and clotting factors etc. Interaction of autoantibodies with these antigens can initiate complement reaction as well as immune complex mediated type III hypersensitive reaction. Complement activation leads to membrane attack complex formation, which ultimately results in cell damage. Complement split products (C3a and C5a) produced as a result of hyperactivation of complements, of which C5a increases the expression of CR3 receptor on neutrophils, facilitating neutrophil aggregation and attachment to vascular endothelium. As a result number of circulating neutrophils decrease and various occlusions of the small blood vessels develop leading to vasculitis. These occlusions cause wide spread tissue damage.

Multiple Sclerosis (MS)

It is an autoimmune disease that affects the central nervous system and causes neurological disability. Individuals afflicted with these disease produce autoreactive T cells that involve in causing inflammatory lesions along the myelin sheath of nerve fibers. Cerebrospinal fluid tapped from these patients will contain autoactivated T lymphocytes, which destroy the myelin sheath. Since myelin serves as insulatory sheath of nervous system, on breakdown leads to various types of neurological disorders.

Rheumatoid Arthritis (RA)

It is an organ specific but often-systemic autoimmune disease most common among women and afflicts them between 40 to 60 years of age. Most common symptom is inflammation of the joints and painful joints accompanied by other symptoms like cardiovascular, hematologic, and respiratory system. Afflicted individuals produce autoantibodies called **rheumatoid factors** that are reactive in the Fc region of IgG. A classic rheumatoid factor is IgM antibody, which reacts with IgG to form IgM-IgG complex and deposits in the joints. These complexes activate complement reaction leading to type III hypersensitive reaction and chronic inflammation of the joints. Early synovial histopathology resembles classic delayed type hypersensitivity (DTH) and includes prominent infiltration consisting of antigen presenting dendritic cells clustered with $CD4^+$ T cells in a perivascular location. Genetic susceptibility to RA is strikingly associated with certain MHC class II alleles, which may either control peptide presentation to T cells or influence T cell repertoires during thymic maturation.

Pathogenesis of RA

(a) Genetics

Genetic analysis in families with RA suggests that many genes are involved in the pathogenesis of the disease of which MHC is one locus. A striking association with HLA DRB1 alleles has been implicated. In a recent American study, up to 96% of patients with RA have one of these alleles and in a similar Scandinavian study, the incidence was 93%. However, in Greek patients only 43% has these alleles, and there was no association in these patients group with disease severity, as in other patient population. Thus RA susceptibility alleles may not be identical in different ethnic populations, as is often observed in studies of HLA association with autoimmune disorders. The susceptibility alleles share a motif in the third hypervariable region of DRβ chain: QKRAA.

(b) Environment

Only 30 to 50 % of identical twins are concordant for RA. This simple fact proves unequivocally that environmental factors, such as microbial infections, are one of the important causative factors of RA. Conditions like stress might predispose to subclinical microbial infections. Various candidate microbes have been considered over the years. These include mycobacteria, mycoplasma, Lyme disease-like bacteria, herpes viruses, Epstein Barr virus (EBV), parvoviruses, lentiviruses, and rubella virus, retroviruses, and enteric bacteria. The putative mechanisms can be divided in to two groups: either direct synovial infection or indirect immunopathogenic mechanisms. Some of the endemic viruses in association with RA are discussed below.

(i) *Parvovirus B-19*   Antibodies against this virus have been detected in the blood of patients with early RA. Viral DNA has also been detected by PCR in synovial tissue and bone marrow of RA patients.

(ii) *Human T cell leukemia virus type I (HTLV-I)*   HTLV-1 is an endemic virus in southern Japan and in the West Indies. An extensive study in Japan has documented serological, histological and PCR evidence indicating an association between the presence of the virus and a clinical disease indistinguishable from idiopathic RA. HTLV-1 transactivator or tax protein is implicated for the development of RA in endemic populations.

(iii) *Cytomegalovirus*   Among the most common endemic viruses worldwide are the herpes viruses. By analogy with HTLV-1, this family of viruses might participate in causing RA by transactivation of host cell genes without a requirement for the production of infectious virus in synovial tissues. Clinical investigations are still on to find out the association of cytomegalovirus association with development of RA.

(iv) *Epstein-Barr virus (EBV)*   High titers of antibodies against EBCV antigens have been found in patients with RA. In RA patients the frequency of B cell infected by EBV in the peripheral blood is high. Recently, a PCR study showed that EBV and human herpes virus 6 (HHV6) DNA is present at a higher frequency in saliva but not in blood of RA patients.

INSIGHT INTO MECHANISM OF AUTOIMMUNE DISEASE BASED ON CLINICAL FINDINGS

The first example of a human autoimmune disease, paroxysmal cold hemoglobinuria (PCH) described by Donath and Landsteiner in 1903, still serves as a prototype for our understanding of the mechanism of pathogenesis in autoimmune disease. In PCH, the patient produces antibody that binds his own RBCs. It is found that the PCH antibody is usually directed to a widely distributed alloantigen of the P blood group system. It is remarkable that the target antigen is actually an alloantigen to which autoantibodies are produced under the special circumstances of this disease. Thus, from this example one can say that autoimmunity is common, but autoimmune disease is unusual. It is attributable to the breakdown of a number of homeostatic safeguards designed to prevent harmful consequences of autoimmunity. The circumstances that favor the development of harmful or pathologic autoimmunity as well as the underlying mechanisms that contribute to autoimmunity are described in the section below.

Autoimmunity and autoimmune disease

Initiation of autoimmune disease of humans depends upon two types of risk factors, genetic and environmental. Genetic factors provide a disposition, whereas environmental agent is the immediate trigger of the disease.

In most human autoimmune diseases, there is a significant skewing of the MHC repertoire toward particular HLA haplotype: For ex. Graves disease is associated with the HLA B8/DR3 haplotype; insulin dependent diabetes is associated with HLA B8/DR3/DR4 with DR2 serving as protective allele. In all of the human autoimmune diseases studied, genetic traits account for about half of the risk of developing an autoimmune disease. This evidence is primarily based on a comparison of genetically identical monozygotic twins with nonidentical dizygotic twins.

Most human autoimmune diseases are complex, involving number of antigens of the target tissues. Part of the complexity is owed to epitope spread. Another common feature of human autoimmune disease is the presence of antibodies to a number of unrelated, organ specific antigens, which is also called as immunological escalation. For ex. In thyroidits, one commonly finds antibodies not only to thyroglobulin, the antigen responsible for initiation of the disease process, but also to thyroid peroxidase, and another antigenically unrelated constituent of the thyroid.

There is strong evidence that T cell-mediated immunity is of major importance in the pathogenesis of many autoimmune diseases, based on the experimental evidences from animals through adoptive transfer of T cells. Credence to this assumption comes from the autoimmune insulin dependent diabetes and multiple sclerosis. Human patients with myocarditis produce an autoimmune response to adenine nucleotide transporter or to cardiac myosin. Antibodies to these cardiac antigens may produce a functional defect in the cardiac myocyte and play an important role in the cardiac failure.

Chemicals as the cause of autoimmune disease

Several drugs, including hydralizines and procainamide, are known to induce lupus like disorders in genetically susceptible individuals. Penicillamine has been associated with myasthenia gravis as well as with a number of other autoimmune diseases. Exposure of miners to silica is described, as precipitating factor in the autoimmune disease, scleroderma, and mercury salts has been associated with autoimmune glomerulonephritis. One of the best-documented environmental factors related to autoimmune disease is dietary iodine, which is known to induce autoimmune thyroid disease. Preliminary evidence suggests that iodinated haptens in the thyroglobulin molecule, probably the active thyroid hormone tetraiodothyronine, increase the immunoreactivity of thyroglobulin.

Molecular mimicry

A number of viruses and bacteria have been shown to possess antigenic determinants that are identical or similar to normal host cell components. Molecular mimicry has been suggested as one of the mechanism leading to autoimmune disease. For ex. Post rabies encephalitis in individual who received rabies vaccine developed from rabbit brain cell culture. The vaccine prepared from this culture contained rabbit brain cell antigen along with it, to which human body developed antibodies and activated T cells leading to encephalitis. Mimicry between MBP peptides and viral peptides, such as that of measles, influenza, polyoma, Rous sarcoma, Abelson leukemia, poliomyelitis and adenovirus etc does occur and could be one of the causes. Molecular mimicry would also occur with heat-shock proteins, which are produced by mammalian cells during extreme stressful conditions.

B – Cell effector mechanisms

The critical role of autoantibodies initiating PCH can be viewed as a prototype of the pathological processes of autoimmune disease. In the more common forms of hemolytic anemia, autoantibody to erythrocytes is also a key factor in initiating disease. In the warm-type hemolytic anemia, autoantibodies to the red blood cells act at body temperature. Often this antibody is directed against one of alloantigens of Rh factor. This antibody does not initiate complement-mediated lysis; rather it shortens the life span of RBCs by enhancing their phagocytosis. In the cold antibody hemolytic anemia, the union of antibody with erythrocytes is demonstrable at laboratory temperature but difficult to demonstrate in the patient. Often in this case C3a is bound to erythrocytes, which facilitates opsonization and phagocytosis. The other major cells of blood, leukocytes and platelets may also be depleted by autoimmune mechanisms, leading to autoimmune leukopenia and thrombopenia. In autoimmune thrombopenia, presence of antibody to phospholipids or to β-2-glycoprotein-I is a valuable clinical indicator of thrombotic problems.

Another possible pathological consequences of autoantibody production are the development in vivo of immune complexes. Antigen-antibody complexes tend to localize in capillary beds in several locations, such as lung, brain and skin. The most damaging problems generally arise from immune complexes deposited in the glomeruli of kidneys. This damage can be easily distinguished from the autoimmune glomerulonephritis produced as a result of autoantibodies to the antigens of glomerular or tubular basement membranes.

A topic receiving great deal of attention and discussion recently is the ability of antibodies to produce damage to intracellular or even intranuclear antigens, which is contrary to the belief that antibodies cannot reach inside the cell. Much more details of this topic are dealt in another section of this chapter.

Another mechanism by which autoantibodies can inflict damage to the tissue is through cooperative action with lymphoid cells. This mechanism is called antibody-dependent cell-mediated cytotoxic reaction (ADCC), involves attachment of antibody to lymphocytes or macrophage through Fc receptor. Exactly till today, which autoimmune disease involves this mechanism is not known.

T – cell effector mechanisms

Among human autoimmune diseases, there is general consensus that cytotoxic T lymphocytes (CTLs) are the major effectors of damage to the organ-localized autoimmune disorders. They include insulin-dependent diabetes, chronic thyroiditis and multiple sclerosis. Most studies show evidence of T cell clonal expansions in the inflamed RA joint. CD4$^+$ CD57$^+$ CD28$^-$ T cells were five times more prevalent in RA than in age-matched normal controls.

Macrophage effector mechanism

The activated macrophage is an important effector mechanism in cell-mediated immunopathological reactions. Macrophages are a source of cytokines, such as IL-1, and IL-12 that enhances the production of TH1 subset of CD4 T cells. IL-12 is particularly important, because it enhances T cell-mediated immunity as well as the production of complement-fixing isotypes of antibody. Another important product of activated macrophage is interferon-γ. There is some evidence that indicates the involvement of IFN-γ in certain epithelial cell damage such as thyroid follicle cells. IFN-γ is also known to enhance the activity of nitric acid synthase, which synthesizes nitric acid. Nitric acid together with reactive oxygen intermediates can bring about remarkable tissue damage. Although there is no direct evidence of involvement of nitric acid and reactive oxygen intermediates in autoimmune response, but there is reason to suppose that they will turn out to be major effector agents.

Other effector mechanisms

Many of the mechanisms of innate immunity are involved in the damaging effects of autoimmune responses. For ex. NK cells are important in the early stages of viral infection. NK cells are found in autoimmune myocarditis. They are attracted by the interferon-γ by the infiltrating inflammatory cells. In turn, NK cells produce additional IFN-γ, with potential immunopathological consequences ascribed to this cytokine. In addition, cell injury and necrosis attract NK cells, polymorphonuclear nutrophils. Complement cascade activated through alternative as well as classical pathway may also contribute to the immunopathological consequences of autoimmune reactions.

AUTOANTIBODIES TO T CELL RECEPTORS

Autoantibodies against TCR have been previously found in two alloimmunization situations in humans: renal transplantation and pregnancy. In the pregnant women autoantibodies to TCR α and β chains especially to CDR3/J segment have been detected. These antibodies play an important role in suppressing T cell reactivity against fetal determinants where fetus acts as a natural allograft. Majority of RA patients studied so far displayed elevated levels of IgM autoantibodies directed against TCR determinants, with the major reactivity directed towards the CDR1 peptide segment of Vβ sequence. SLE patients contained IgG autoantibodies directed against numerous peptide sequences of the TCR β chain, TCR α chain and CDR1.

CELL AND NUCLEAR PENETRATION BY AUTOANTIBODIES

The idea that some antibodies possess the ability to penetrate both the cell and nuclear membranes of living cell is still considered to be a controversial concept. However, there is considerable body of literature to support the idea that penetration of cells by certain antibodies can and does occur. In vivo antinuclear antibodies (ANA) with a variety of autoimmune antibodies, including those to ribonucleoprotein RNP), smith antigen (Sm) Sjogren's syndrome A antigen (Ro/SSA), Sjogren's syndrome B antigen (La/SSB), and double stranded DNA (dsDNA) was elucidated. Anti dsDNA antibodies are found specifically in SLE and their levels correlate strongly with lupus nephritis. Extracellular matrix components such as heparan sulfate and laminin have been proposed to interact directly with anti-DNA antibodies primarily on the basis of anionic charge of heparan sulfate and cationic nature of anti-DNA antibodies. In most of the cases, anti-DNA antibodies and anti-RNP antibodies enter the cells through Fc receptor. Autoantibodies are thought to enter the nucleus through DNA/nucleosome receptor. In SLE, there is also evidence for direct binding to nucleosome receptors.

TREATMENT OF AUTOIMMUNE DISEASES

Some therapies available to date are only palliative but do not cure the patient completely. The relief experienced by the patient due to these therapies is far superior to the continuous sufferance. Immunosuppressive drugs like corticosteroid; azathioprine and cyclophosphamide are often given to slow down the proliferation of lymphocytes. They do decrease the severity of autoimmune symptoms but puts the patient at greater risk for infection or the development of cancer. Removal of thymus in autoimmune disease like myasthenia gravis yielded positive results because in this disease thymic hyperplasia or thymomas are common feature. Patients suffering from Graves' disease, myasthenia gravis, rheumatoid arthritis, and systemic lupus erythematosus from plasmapheresis have gained short-term benefits. In this procedure, plasma is removed from the patient's blood by continuous flow centrifugation and the red blood cells are given back by resuspending them in a suitable medium.

Experimental Therapeutic Approach

Many experiments conducted on autoimmune animal models have shed some light on possible therapies for autoimmune diseases in humans. Several of these approaches have been discussed in this section.

T cell vaccination

For this experiment, experimental autoimmune encephalomyelitis (EAE) rats were used. The animals were injected with very low dose ($<10^4$) of cloned T cells specific for myelin basic protein (MBP). The animals became resistant to development of EAE when later challenged with activated MBP-specific T cells or MBP in adjuvant. Later it was found that, such autoimmune T cell vaccine effect could be enhanced if the T cells membranes are cross-linked with glutaraldehyde or formaldehyde. When such cross-linked T cells were given to active EAE rats, permanent remission was observed. Cross-linked T cells acts as regulatory T cells to suppress the autoimmune T cells that mediate EAE.

This approach has been tried in few human patients, where a patient suffering from multiple sclerosis was injected subcutaneously with T cells that had been isolated from her own cerebrospinal fluid, grown in vitro and cross- linked with formaldehyde. At present her progress is being monitored.

In a different approach TCR-V region peptide was administered to rats going through severe EAE symptoms, disease progression was arrested and the animals recovered within 3 days.

Peptide blockade of MHC molecules

Given the central role of CD4$^+$ T cells in the perpetuation and pathology of many autoimmune diseases, and given the essential role of the TCR: peptide: MHC II interaction in the activation of these T cells, the blocking of this interaction is a logical target for therapeutic intervention. Polyclonal and monoclonal antibodies to MHC II molecules have ameliorated many animal models of autoimmunity, including systemic lupus erythematosus, EAE, myasthenia gravis; thyroiditis and collagen induced arthritis. In humans natural anti-MHC II antibodies are detected in the serum of many healthy individuals and autoimmune patients, and anti-DR/DQ antibody titers to paternal MHC II molecules correlate with pregnancy induced RA remissions during pregnancy. The development of MHC II vaccine to RA patients who showed similar MLR was undertaken recently. It was observed that these patients have common expression of a subset of HLA-DR1 or DR4 subtypes. Over 90% of RA patients, regardless of ethnic origin, express at least one HLA-DR allele encoding a shared sequence within amino acids 67-74 of the DRB1 gene. This region corresponds to the third hypervariable domain of the β chain, a TCR contact region adjacent to the peptide-binding region of MHC II molecules. Within this region, expression of the sequence LXXQKRAA is shared by susceptible alleles, but is not found in alleles that are not RA associated. These peptides have been found to be highly immunogenic in most of the cases. Therefore, a feasibility of generating an anti-MHC II allele specific antibody response by vaccination with peptide containing this LXXQKRAA motif has undergone phase I trial in humans and 25% of the patients mounted measurable DR4/1 peptide antibody response to this single immunization and now it is going through phase II trials.

In other studies, synthetic peptides differing by only one amino acid from their MBP counterpart have been shown to bind to the appropriate MHC molecule. When sufficient amount of such peptides were administered to EAE animals, the clinical development of EAE was blocked. In another study blocking peptide complexed to soluble class II MHC molecules reversed the clinical progression of EAE in mice.

Stimulation of T cells only by class II MHC without involving costimulatory signals would lead to clonal anergy in T cells.

Treatment with Monoclonal antibodies

Monoclonal antibody approach to treat several autoimmune diseases in animal models has been successful. Monoclonal antibodies directed to α subunit of the high affinity IL-2 receptor (anti-TAC) was found to block preferentially autoreactive T cells in the rats injected with activated MBP specific T cells. The control rats died of EAE, whereas animals treated with anti-TAC survived and did not develop any symptoms. Monoclonal antibodies against Vβ 8.2 T cell receptor are also known to reverse the EAE symptoms in mice. In nonhuman primates, monoclonal antibodies to HLA-DR and HLA-DQ have been shown to reverse EAE.

Tolerance induced by oral antigens

It is observed that mice fed on MBP do not develop EAE following subsequent injection with MBP due to development of tolerance. To develop tolerance HLA-DR and DQ complex of an individual plays an important role was observed from tolerance test in heterogeneous group study of human unrelated subjects.

Exercise

1. Give a detailed account of organ specific autoimmune diseases (10 marks)
2. Explain the mechanism of autoimmune diseases (10 marks)
3. Write notes on (5 marks each)
   (a) Systemic autoimmune diseases
   (b) Treatment of autoimmune diseases

Chapter 22

Immunodeficiency Diseases

- Phagocytic Deficiencies
- Defective Phagocytic Functions
- Humoral Deficiencies
- Cell-mediated Deficiencies
- Combined Immunodeficiencies

Immunodeficiency diseases arise from various abnormalities of the immune system, which result from congenital defects or due to acquired defects. Individuals suffering from immunodeficiency, permanently suffer from severe infections by pathogens, which are often caused by organisms of low pathogenicity. Congenital immunodeficiencies are due to abnormalities in certain genes that control hematopoiesis or development of leukocytes or immunoglobulin production (Fig. 22.1). Acquired immunodeficiencies are due to prolonged viral or bacterial infections, malnutrition or due to drug treatment. Acquired immuno-deficiency syndrome (AIDS) is one of the best example of significant immunodeficiency arising from retroviral infection, which infects the CD4$^+$ T$_H$ cells and causes depletion of cell mediated immune response ultimately leading to complete deficiency of cellular as well as humoral immune response. Table 22.1 lists the prevalent immunodeficiencies and the defects associated with each of them.

PHAGOCYTIC DEFICIENCIES

Phagocytes constitute an important arm of the immune system and they play a major role in natural or innate immunity. Any defects in the phagocytic defense mechanism will result in immunodeficiency. Defects in phagocytic defense could result from reduction in the number of phagocytes or from reduction in their function. Functions of the phagocytes would be, contacting the pathogen, phagocytosis, chemotaxis, extravasation, and killing of pathogen. Defects in any of these characters would lead to immunodeficiency. Individuals suffering from phagocytic defects constantly suffer from bacterial or fungal infections. The clinical manifestation may range from mild skin infection to life threatening systemic infections with various complications. Staphylococcus aureus, Streptococcus pneumoniae, Escherichia coli, and different species of Candida, Pseudomonas and Aspergillus cause most common infections in phagocytic deficiencies.

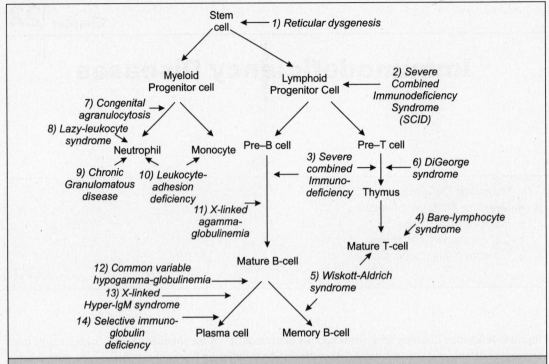

Fig. 22.1 Schematic representation of immunodeficiency diseases resulting from congenital defects that interrupt hematopoiesis or impair functioning of immune system.

Table 22. 1 Types of immunodeficiency diseases

Disease	Immune system deficiency	Possible mechanisms
Phagocytic Deficiency		
Congenital agranulocytosis	Decreased neutrophil count	Decreased production of (G-CSF)
Leukocyte adhesion deficiency	Failure of extravasation of Neutrophils and Monocytes Defective CTL killing Defective T cell help in B cell activation	Defective synthesis of β- chain of Integrin adhesion molecule
Lazy leukocyte syndrome	Decrease neutrophil chemotaxis	Not known
Chronic granulomatous disease	Defective killing of bacteria by neutrophils	Decrease H_2O_2 production due to NADPH oxidase
Humoral Deficiencies		
X-linked agammaglobulinemia (XLA)	Reduction in B cell count Absence of Ig	Block in B cell maturation due to defective V-D-J gene rearrangement

Contd.

Table 22. 1 Contd.

Disease	Immune system deficiency	Possible mechanisms
X-linked hyper IgM (XHM)	Low level of IgG and IgA	Defects in class switching
Common variable hypogammaglobulinemia	Decreased plasma cell	Defective differentiation of B cells to plasma cells
Selective immunoglobulin deficiency	Decreased levels of one or more Ig isotopes	Defects in maturation of plasma cells
Cell-Mediated Deficiencies		
DiGeorge Syndrome	Decreased T cell counts	Lack of T cell maturation due to absence of thymus
Nude mice	Decreased T cell count	Lack of T cell maturation due to absence of thymus
Combined Immuno Deficiencies		
Reticular dysgenesis	Decreased number of myeloid and lymphoid cells	Defective haematopoietic stem cells
Bare lymphocyte syndrome	Reduction in CD4+ T cell count	Failure to express class I and II MHC molecule on the cells
Severe Combined Immuno Deficiency Syndrome (SCID)	Marked reduction in T lymphocytes	Mechanisms vary
X-linked SCID		Defective T and B cell maturation
Autosomal recessive SCID		Defective T and B cell maturation
ADA deficiency SCID		Selective killing of T cells by metabolite that accumulates in the absence of Adenosine deaminase (ADA)
PNP-deficiency SCID		Same as above but in the absence of Purine Nucleoside Phosphorylase (PNP)
Wiskott Aldrich Syndrome (WAS)	Low levels of IgM Elevated levels of IgA and IgE Abnormal T cell with progressive dysfunction	Defective glycosylation of membrane glycoproteins (CD43) on lymphocytes

Reduction in Neutrophil counts

It is called **neutropenia** or **granulocytopenia**, where peripheral blood neutrophil count goes below $1500/mm^3$ or sometimes, complete absence of neutrophils (**agranulocytosis**) occurs. This may happen due to congenital defect or acquired. The congenital agranulocytosis may occur due to genetic defects in myeloid progenitor stem cells, which rarely differentiate beyond the promyelocyte stage. As a result, children born with this defect show severe neutropenia with neutrophil counts as low as $200/mm^3$. Such children constantly suffer from bacterial infections from the first month of life. Experimental evidence indicates that congenital agranulocytopenia causes decrease in the production of granulocyte colony stimulating factor (G-CSF), and therefore failure in differentiation of myeloid stem cells.

Radiation and drugs which act on fast dividing cells, especially neutrophils, whose turnover in the body is quite high due to innate immune response, can also cause Neutropenia. A autoimmune disease called Sjogren's syndrome or systemic lupus erythematosus leads to neutropenia, because the autoantibodies act on neutrophils and destroy them. Children who suffer from viremia or bacterimia may show transient neutropenia.

DEFECTIVE PHAGOCYTIC FUNCTIONS

An effective phagocytosis involves series of sequence of events that includes adherence of phagocytes to vascular endothelial cells, extravasation of phagocytes, chemotaxis, attachment to microorganisms, phagocytosis and ultimately killing of pathogen and digestion. Any defects in any of these functions will affect the defense mechanism and may led to immunodeficiency.

Adherence defects

Adherence of neutrophils and monocytes to the capillary endothelial cell near the site of infection will lead to the development of effective inflammatory response. Adherence of these cells will facilitate them to move into extravascular spaces, where an effective immune response develops. Lukocyte-adherence deficiency, an autosomal recessive trait, leads to inability of neutrophils, monocytes and lymphocytes to adhere to vascular endothelial cells, thus extravasation of these cells in to extravascular tissue spaces does not occur.

This autosomal defect also impairs CTLs and NK cells ability to adhere to their target cell and T_H cells fail to attach themselves to B cells, thereby leading to failure in cell-mediated immune response. Molecular basis of LAD is found to be due to defective β-chain synthesis of CD18, a membrane adhesion molecule of integrin family. In addition to this LAD results in a near total loss of ICAM-1, CR3 and CR4, which are receptors of complement degradation products.

Chemotactic defects

This disorder may be caused by defect in the neutrophil itself or due to complement component factors deficiency, such as C3a, C5a and C5b67. This disorder of neutrophils is also called as lazy – leukocyte syndrome, due to which, neutrophils fail to migrate to the area of infection.

Killing defects

This disease is inherited as X-linked recessive disorder, which is manifested in boys at early age, i.e. first 2 years of life. A milder autosomal form is also observed which occurs in both sexes. The disease is also called **chronic granulomatous disease (CGD)**, where phagocytes are unable to kill the pathogen, which has been phagocytosed. Live pathogen inside the phagocytes leads to granulomata in various organs. Neutrophils from CGD do not show respiratory bursts as observed in normal neutrophils (Explained in Chapter 2), no increase in utilization of hexose monophosphate shunt and no H_2O_2 production during phagocytosis. Such defective neutrophils are unable to kill bacteria that contain enzyme catalase. CGD is caused due to defect in gene encoding cytochrome b, which is necessary for NADP recycling. In this case, decrease in the level of pyridine nucleotides leads to decrease in H_2O_2 production, so that catalase –positive bacteria can survive inside the phagocytes.

HUMORAL DEFICIENCIES

Humoral immune response of an individual wholly rests on the status of B- lymphocytes. Failure in any stage of B cell formation or maturation or gene expression in B cells would lead to humoral deficiencies. Individuals suffering from B cell disorders usually suffer from recurrent bacterial infections but display normal immune response against viruses and fungal infections because T cell immune response in these patients is normal. Recurrent bacterial infection in humoral immunodeficiency patients is caused by encapsulated bacteria such as *Staphylococci, Streptococci and Pneumococci,* because clearance of these bacteria needs antibody and opsonization of bacterial wall, and promotion of cytolysis by complements. Severity of the disease depends on the degree of antibody deficiency.

X–linked agammaglobulinemia (XLA)

Children afflicted with this disease manifest recurrent bacterial infection at about 6 months, by which time passively acquired maternal antibody level has fallen. The gene for this defect has been mapped on the long arm of X chromosome, prevalent in male children. XLA causes failure in maturation of pre-B cells to mature B cells. Therefore, individuals suffering from XLA will have less than 0.1% B lymphocytes in their peripheral blood, which otherwise in the normal individuals is about 5 to 15%. XLA individuals also show extremely low concentration of serum immunoglobulins. At molecular level, it has been found that XLA patients pre-B cells will have immunoglobulin heavy chain genes rearranged but light chain genes remain in the germ line configuration.

X–linked hyper-IgM syndrome (XHM)

This disease is characterized by deficiency of IgG, IgA and IgE but remarkably high levels of IgM, which may reach up to 10 mg/ml, which otherwise in a normal person will be 1.5 mg/ml. It is an X-linked recessive disorder, prevalent in males but sometimes it is acquired also, which affects both male and female. XHM patients not only have higher number of IgM secreting plasma cells in their peripheral blood but also will have autoantibodies to neutrophils, RBCs and platelets. Pneumocystis carinii infects children afflicted with XHM constantly and the infection is very severe. At molecular level, its has been identified that XHM patients have a defect in the gene encoding CD40 ligand (CD40L) and this ligand is primarily expressed on T$_H$ cell membrane. B cells express CD40 on their membrane and the interaction of CD40 of B cell and CD40L of T$_H$ cell is essential for the activation of B lymphocytes. Absence of this costimulatory signal inhibits the B cell response to T-dependent antigens. CD40 and CD40L contact is found to be very essential for immunoglobulin gene class switching mechanism. Absence of this interaction in XHM does not allow class switch from IgM to IgG, IgA and IgE isotypes as well as failure in production of memory B cells. XHM individuals also fail to produce germinal centers during humoral response, for which CD40-CD40L contact is essential, which is lacking in XHM individuals

Common variable hypogammaglobulinemia (CVH)

This disorder has wide spectrum of defects and the patients suffering from this disorder develop recurrent bacterial infections between 15 and 35 years of age. They have severely low level of serum immunoglobulins. Some individuals show decrease in mature B cell number and the reason for this is defects in the differentiation process of mature B cells into immunoglobulin producing plasma cells. The disease has familial inheritance pattern but to date no definite genetic defect has been shown for CVH. In the CVH patients, production of antibodies may be affected at various levels, like defective heavy chain glycosylation, or defect in polyadenylation of the primary Ig transcripts or B cells may be lacking the receptors for cytokines that trigger differentiation of B cells into antibody secreting cells. Some CVH patients have defective T_H cells and some have excessive number of T cells. Those who have defective T_H cells cannot mediate B cell activation and differentiation and those who have excess T cells may show suppression of plasma cells from secreting antibodies.

Selective immunoglobulin deficiencies

When single or subclass immunoglobulin deficiency occurs, it is called selective immunodeficiency. Most common one is **selective IgA deficiency**. Individuals with this disease suffer from recurrent respiratory and gastrointestinal infections. It is well known that the major protective mechanism shown at the respiratory and gastrointestinal tract surface is by IgA and since it is lacking in IgA deficient patients, the infections are recurrent at these surfaces. Lack of IgA at GI tract or respiratory tract leads to penetration of antigens into the mucous lining of these surfaces, which may stimulate IgE production. At molecular level it has been identified that IgA deficient patients have defect in the maturation of IgA membrane bound B cells into immunoglobulin secreting plasma cells. In vitro studies have shown that defects in these patients are due to T cell mediated suppression of IgA production by plasma cells.

CELL -MEDIATED DEFICIENCIES

T cells control the entire cell-mediated and humoral immune response in an individual and any deficiency in T cell will affect both cell mediated and humoral immune response. Defects in humoral branch are primarily associated with infections from encapsulated bacteria and the defects in cell-mediated branch would result in infections by intracellular pathogens like *Candida albican, Pneumocystis carinii* and *Mycobacterium* and protozoan as well as viral and fungal infections. This indicates the importance of T cells in eliminating intracellular parasites. Viruses that are rarely pathogenic such as cytomegalovirus may become life threatening to these individuals. Decreased T cell counts will affect development of humoral immune response, which would lead to decreased antibody production.

DiGeorge syndrome (congenital thymic aplasia)

It is characterized by the absence of thymus and associated with it hypothyroidism, cardiovascular anomalies and increased incidence of infections. Children afflicted with this disease have an effective humoral immune response against bacterial infections but are highly susceptible to viral, protozoan and fungal infections. Sometimes, even the attenuated measles vaccine may be life threatening to these affected children. A complete evaluation of children affected by DiGeorge syndrome reveals:

- Severe decrease in total number of T cells.
- Absence of T_{DTH} skin-test (Montax reaction) reaction to common antigens.
- Decreased response of T cells to mitogen-PHA (phytohemagglutinins).
- Decreased response to MLR (mixed lymphocytic reaction) by allogenic cells.

Nude Mice

These mice have no hair follicles, hence they are hairless, and therefore, they are called as nude mice. It is developed due to autosomal recessive defect in development of thymus, which is lacking in these mice. They show varying degrees of cell-mediated immunodeficiency. The lack of cell-mediated immune response is best demonstrated in these mice by their ability to accept xenogenic grafts, which otherwise would be impossible in a normal individual with healthy cell-mediated immune response.

COMBINED IMMUNODEFICIENCIES

This is much more severe than the humoral or cell-mediated immunodeficiency because in this case both the branches of the immune system are defunct. Therefore, for the survival of the individual transplant of a healthy bone marrow from HLA-matched individual is the only alternative, otherwise death is ensured any time during the early life. At present *ex-vivo* gene therapy is available to treat these individuals and the success rate of this therapy is quite high (almost 95 to 98%).

Reticular dysgenesis

It is a fatal congenital disease, which afflicts the children and the disease is caused due to failure in differentiation of lymphoid and myeloid stem cells from the hematopoietic tissue. Individuals suffering from this disease will be lacking not only monocytes but also other granulocytes and, T and B cells. Onset of the disease is quite early. Therefore, children born with this disease have short life.

Bare–lymphocyte syndrome (BLS)

This disease is associated with deficiency in expression of class I or class II MHC molecules or both. Accordingly it is classified into three types:

- Type I involves defective class I MHC molecule expression
- Type II associated with defective class II MHC molecule expression
- Type III is associated the defective expression of class I and II MHC molecules.

Individuals afflicted from this disease suffer recurrent bacterial and viral infections and often death occurs by 5 years of age.

Type I BLS individuals have defects in TAP a transporter protein, which transports the antigenic peptides which are generated in the cytosolic processing pathway into endoplasmic reticulum for assembly with class I MHC molecule (Fig. 22.2). In the absence of antigenic peptide, the class I MHC α-chain fails to assemble with β2-microglobulin and therefore is not expressed on the plasma membrane of a cell.

In type II BLS afflicted individuals none of the three classes of class II MHC molecules from the DP, DQ, DR haplotypes are expressed. In addition, IFN-γ fails to induce class II MHC gene expression, which otherwise does in normal cells.

Severe combined immunodeficiency (SCID)

This disease is associated with increased susceptibility to bacterial, viral, fungal and protozoan infections due to insufficient number of T and B cells. Individuals are so much immunocompromised with this disease that even a nonpathogenic organism may lead to life threatening infection in these people. Children

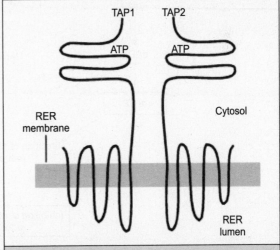

Fig. 22.2   Diagrammatic representation of TAP protein association with RER membrane

afflicted with this disease develop recurrent infections at 3 to 6 months of age. Oral Sabin polio vaccine or measles vaccine can cause progressive infection in these children and death. Molecular analysis of SCID revealed that, over half of all SCID cases are caused by X-linked recessive defects (XSCID). In the XSCID, defect lies in the gene encoding the γ subunit of number of cytokine receptors like IL-2R, IL-4R, IL-7R, IL-9R and IL-15 and part of IL-13R.

Adenosine deaminase (ADA) and Purine nucleoside phosphorylase (PNP) deficiency

It is caused by two autosomal recessive gene defects. In both cases the disease arises due to deficiency of enzyme of a major metabolic pathway of nucleotides and nucleosides (Fig. 22.3). Deficiency of ADA leads to accumulation of dATP and the deficiency of PNP leads to accumulation of dGTP and dATP. Both these nucleotides in excess are toxic to T and B cells, due to which, individuals with either of these deficiency suffer from depletion of B and T cells. For these patients up to 1990, only bone marrow transplant from HLA compatible donor was only the hope for survival. But in 1990, two children suffering from ADA deficiency SCID were successfully treated for the disease by **ex vivo gene therapy**. For this,

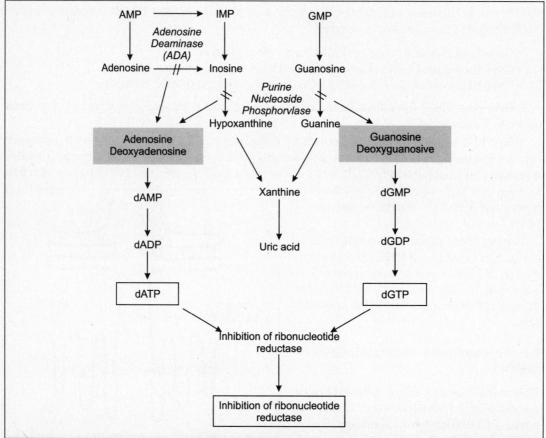

Fig. 22.3 Schematic presentation of molecular basis of severe combined immunodeficiency resulting from the defect in adenosine demainase (ADA) gene or purine nucleoside phosphorylase (PNP) gene deficiency.

peripheral blood lymphocytes and bone marrow progenitor cells from the patients were obtained and cultured. The cells were transfected with normal ADA gene by calcium phosphate precipitation method and the transfected cells are transfused back into the patients. Till today both the children are doing fine. More recently human chord blood was used for ADA gene transfection in to chord blood stem cells, which are pluripotent and do not cause untoward reaction in a patient if transfused because they have not yet developed their self-MHCs. A four year old infant treated in this manner is doing fine.

Wiskott – Aldrich syndrome (WAS)

It is yet another X-linked recessive immunodeficiency affecting male children. The disease is associated with severe compromization of mature T and B cells. Patients develop various types of complications, which includes thrombocytopenia, bloody diarrhea, eczema and susceptibility to bacterial infections. Unlike in the case of XHM, these patients have normal levels of IgG, excessive levels of IgA and IgE and very low levels of IgM. They fail to express blood group antigens and antibodies, and antibodies to polysaccharide antigens, hence more prone to infection by encapsulated pyogenic bacteria. T cell function tends to get worse in older patients and most WAS patients do not exhibit cutaneous DTH (delayed type hypersensitive) reaction. Lymphocytes of the WAS patients lack cell-membrane glycoprotein called sialophorin (CD43). Patients can survive with HLA compatible bone marrow transplants.

Exercise

1. Give an account of immunodeficiencies with reference to (15 marks each):
   (a) Phagocytic deficiencies
   (b) Humoral deficiencies
   (c) Cell-mediated deficiencies
2. Write notes on (5 marks each):
   (a) Defective phagocytic functions in relation to immunodeficiency
   (b) X-linked humoral immunodeficiencies
   (c) Severe combined immunodeficiency
   (d) Reticular dysgenesis and bare lymphocyte syndrome in cell-mediated immunodeficiencies
   (e) DiGeorge and Wiskott-Aldrich syndrome
   (f) Common variable hypogammaglobulinemia (CVH) and selective immunoglobulinemia in humoral deficiencies

Glossary

Acquired cell-mediated immunity: an immune state mediated by T cells and characterized by the development of activated macrophages.

Acquired immune deficiency syndrome (AIDS): a disease caused by the human immunodeficiency virus, which destroys key components of the immune system. As a result, infected individuals become very susceptible to infections and cancers.

Acquired Immunity: host defenses that are mediated by B and T cells following exposure to antigen and that exhibit specificity, diversity, memory and self/non-self recognition. See also **innate immunity.**

Activated macrophage: a macrophage in a stage of enhanced metabolic and functional activity.

Active Immunity: acquired immunity that is induced by natural exposure to a pathogen or by **vaccination.**

Acute inflammation: rapidly developing inflammation of recent onset. It is characterized by tissue infiltration by neutrophils.

Acute-phase protein: a protein secreted by hepatocytes whose levels in the blood rise rapidly in response to acute inflammation or infection.

Acute-phase response: the systemic effects, associated with an acute **inflammatory response**, that include production of hepatocyte-derived serum proteins, fever and increase in circulating leukocytes.

Adjuvant: a substance that, when given with an antigen, enhances the immune response to that antigen.

Adoptive immunity: the development of immunity as a result of the transfer of cells from an immunized animal to an unimmunized recipient.

Affinity maturation: the progressive increase in antibody affinity for antigen that occurs during an immune response.

Affinity: the binding strength between a single receptor site (e.g. one binding site on an antibody) and a ligand (e.g. an antigenic determinant). The association constant is a quantitative measure of affinity.

Agammaglobulinemia: the absence of gamma globulins in blood.

Agglutination: the clumping of particulate antigens by antibody.

Agglutinin: any antibody that causes visible clumping (agglutination) of particulate antigens. A haemagglutinin is an antibody that causes clumping of red blood cells.

Agretope: the region of a processed antigenic peptide that binds to an **MHC molecule**.

AIDS: the acronym for acquired immune deficiency syndrome. A disease caused by human immunodeficiency virus.

Albumin: strictly speaking, those serum proteins that remain in solution in the presence of half-saturated ammonium sulfate. In practice it is the name given to the major serum protein of 60 kD.

Allele: two or more alternative forms of a gene at a particular **locus** that confer alternative characters. The presence of multiple alleles results in **polymorphism**.

Allelic exclusion: the ability of a cell from a heterozygous individual to synthesize only one of two possible alleles.

Allergen: an antigen that provokes type I hypersensitivity (allergy).

Allergic contact dermatitis: an inflammatory skin condition occurring as a result of a type IV hypersensitivity reaction to skin cells modified by exposure to foreign chemicals.

Allergy: a **hypersensitivity** reaction that can involve various deleterious effects such as hay fever, asthma, **serum sickness**, systemic **anaphylaxis** or contact dermatitis.

Allogeneic (allogenic): genetically dissimilar individuals of the same species.

Allograft: a tissue or organ graft between two genetically dissimilar animals of the same species.

Allotype: genetically coded differences between the proteins of different individuals of a species.

Allotypic determinant: an antigenic determinant that varies among members of a species. The constant regions of antibodies possess allotypic determinants.

Alpha-feto protein (AFP): see **Oncofetal tumor antigen.**

Alternative complement pathway: activation of **complement** that is initiated by foreign cell-surface constituents; involves C3-C9, factors B and D, and properdin; and generates the **membrane-attack complex.**

Amyloid: an extracellular amorphous, waxy protein deposited in the tissues of individuals suffering from chronic inflammation or a myeloma.

Analog: an organ or tissue that has the same function as another but is of different evolutionary origin.

Anaphylatoxin: a complement fragment with the ability to stimulate mast-cell degranulation and smooth muscle contraction.

Anaphylatoxins: the **complement** split products C3a and C5a, which mediate **degranulation** of mast cells and basophils, resulting in release of mediators that induce contraction of smooth muscle and increased vascular permeability.

Anaphylaxis: a sudden, systemic, severe immediate hypersensitivity reaction occurring as a result of rapid generalized mast-cell degranulation.

Anergy: the failure to respond to an antigen in a sensitized animal.

Antibody: an immunoglobulin protein molecule synthesized on exposure to antigen that can combine specifically with that antigen.

Antibody-dependent cell-mediated cytotoxicity (ADCC): a cell-mediated reaction in which nonspecific cytotoxic cells that express **Fc receptors** (e.g. NK cells, neutrophils, macrophages) recognize bound antibody on a target cell and subsequently cause lysis of the target cell.

Antigen processing: degradation of antigens by one of two pathways yielding antigenic peptides that is displayed in association with MHC molecules on the surface of antigen-presenting cells or altered self-cells.

Antigen: a foreign substance that can induce an immune response often used as a synonym for **immunogen.**

Antigenic determinant: the site on an antigen that is recognized and bound by a particular antibody or T cell receptor; also called **epitope.**

Antigenic drift: a series of spontaneous point mutations that generate minor antigenic variations in pathogens and lead to strain differences.

Antigenic peptide: see **Antigen processing**.

Antigenic shift: sudden emergence of a new pathogen subtype possibly resulting from genetic reassortment leading to substantial antigenic differences.

Antigenic variation: progressive change in surface antigens exhibited by viruses, parasites, and some bacteria. This is an effective device used to evade destruction by the immune system.

Antigenicity: the ability of a molecule to be recognized by an antibody of lymphocyte.

Antigen-presenting cell: a cell that can ingest antigen, process it, and present this processed antigen to antigen-sensitive cells in association with MHC molecules.

Antigen-sensitive cell: a cell that can bind and respond to specific antigen.

Antiglobulin: antibody made against an immunoglobulin, usually by injecting immunoglobulin into an animal of another species.

Anti-idiotype antibody: a secondary antibody (Ab-2) that is specific for the **paratope** of a primary antibody (Ab-1) and thus mimics the **epitope** of the original antigen. It represents an internal image of the original antigen and thus might be effective as a vaccine, avoiding immunization with a pathogen.

Antiserum: serum that contains specific antibodies. Synonymous with immune globulin.

Antitoxin: antiserum directed against a toxin and used for passive immunization.

Apoptosis: morphologic changes associated with programmed cell death including nuclear fragmentation, blebbing, and release of apoptotic bodies, which are phagocytosed. In contrast to **necrosis**, it does not result in damage to surrounding cells.

Arthus reaction; a local inflammatory reaction due to a type III hypersensitivity reaction; it is induced by the repeated injection of antigen into the skin of an immunized animal.

Asthma: a type I hypersensitivity disease characterized by a reduction in airway diameter, leading to difficulty in breathing (dyspnea).

Atopy: a genetically determined pre-disposition to develop clinical allergies.

Attenuation: the reduction of virulence of an infectious agent.

Autoantibody: an antibody directed against an epitope of normal body tissues.

Autoantigen: a normal body component that acts as an antigen.

Autograft: tissue grafted from one part of the body to another in the same individual.

Autoimmune disease: disease caused by an immune attack against an individual's own tissues.

Autoimmunity: the process of mounting an immune response against a normal body component.

Autologous: derived from the same individual.

Autosomal: pertaining to all the chromosomes except the sex chromosomes.

Avidity: the functional binding strength between two molecules that (unlike **affinity**) reflects the interaction of the binding sites.

B cell: a lymphocyte that matures in the bone marrow and expresses membrane-bound antibody. Following interaction with antigen, it differentiates into antibody-secreting plasma cells and memory cells often used synonym for **B lymphocyte**

Basophil: a nonphagocytic granulocyte that expressed Fc receptors for IgE. Antigen-mediated cross-linkage of bound IgE induces **degranulation** of basophils.

B-cell co-receptor: a complex of three proteins (CR2, CD19, CD22, CD40 and TAPA-1) associated with the B-cell receptor. It is thought to amplify the activating signal induced by cross-linkage of the receptor.

B-cell receptor (BCR): complex comprising a membrane-bound immunoglobulin molecule and two associated signal-transducing Ig-α/Ig-β molecules.

BCG (Bacillus Calmette-Guerin): an attenuated form of *Mycobacterium bovis* used as a specific vaccine and as an adjuvant component.

β_2-**Microglobulin:** an invariant subunit that associates with polymorphic α chain to form **class I MHC** molecule, MHC genes do not encode it.

Benign tumor: a tumor that does not spread from its site of origin.

Blast cell: a cell that has large amounts of cytoplasm immediately prior to division.

Blocking antibody: an antibody that, by binding to a target cell, protects it from immune destruction.

Blood group: an antigen found on the surface of red blood cells. Blood group expression is inherited.

Bursa of Fabricius: a **primary lymphoid organ** in birds where B-cell maturation occurs. The bone marrow is the functional equivalent in mammals.

C (constant) gene segment: the 3' coding of a rearranged immunoglobulin or T cell receptor gene. There are multiple C gene segments in germ-line DNA, but as a result of gene rearrangement and, in some cases, RNA processing, only one segment is expressed in a given protein.

CAMS: see **Cell-adhesion molecules**.

Capping: the clumping of surface structures such as antigens or receptors in a small area on the surface of a cell.

Capsid: the protein coat around a virus.

Carcinoma: a tumor originating from cells of epithelial origin.

Carrier: an immunogenic macromolecule to which a hapten may be bound, so making the hapten immunogenic. T cells recognize this part of the molecule.

Carrier effect: dependence of a **secondary immune response** to a hapten on both the **hapten** and **carrier** used in the initial immunization.

Cascade reactions: an interlinked series of enzyme reactions in which the products of one reaction catalyze a second reaction, and so forth.

CD molecule: a cell surface molecule classified according to the internationally accepted CD (Cluster of Differentiation) system. They are identified by monoclonal antibodies.

CD3: a polypeptide complex containing three dimers: a $\gamma\epsilon$ heterodimer, a $\epsilon\delta$ heterodimer, and either a $\zeta\zeta$ homodimer or $\zeta\eta$ heterodimer. It is associated with a T-cell receptor and functions in signal transduction.

CD4: a monomeric membrane molecule, usually present on T_H cells, that acts as a coreceptor. It binds to the β_2 domain of **class II MHC molecules** and functions in signal transduction during T-cell activation.

CD8: a heterodimeric membrane molecule, usually present on T_C cells that act as a coreceptor. It binds to the α_3 domain of **class I MHC molecules** and functions in signal transduction during T-cell activation.

Cell line: a population of cultured tumor cells or normal cells that have been subjected to a chemical or viral **transformation**. Cell lines can be propagated indefinitely in culture.

Cell-adhesion molecules (CAMs): a group of cell-surface molecules that mediate intercellular adhesion. Most belong to one of four protein families: the **integrins, selectins,** mucin-like proteins, and **immunoglobulin superfamily**.

Cell-mediated cytotoxicity: destruction of target cells induced by contact with lymphocytes or macrophages.

Cell-mediated immune response: host defenses that are mediated by antigen-specific T cells and various non-specific cells of the immune system. It protects against intra-cellular bacteria, viruses, and cancer and is responsible for graft rejection. Transfer of primed T cells confers this type of immunity on the recipient. See also **Humoral immune response**.

Cell-mediated lumpholysis (CML): in vitro lysis of allogeneic cells or virus-infected syngeneic cells by T cells, can be used as an assay for CTL activity or class I MHC activity.

Cestode: a parasitic tapeworm.

Chemokine: any of several low molecular weight polypeptides with characteristic four cysteine residues that mediate **chemotaxis** for different leukocytes and regulate the expression and/or adhesiveness of leukocyte **integrins.**

Chemotaxis: the directed movement of cells under the influence of an external chemical gradient.

Chronic inflammation: slowly developing or persistent inflammation characterized by tissue infiltration with macrophages and fibroblasts.

Class I MHC molecules: heterodimeric membrane proteins that consist of non covalently associated α chain and β_2-**microglobulin,** both encoded in the **MHC**. They are expressed by nearly all nucleated cells and function in antigen presentation to $CD8^+$ T cells. The classical class I molecules are HLA-A, -B, and –C in humans.

Class II MHC molecules: heterodimeric membrane proteins that consist of a noncovalently associated α and β chains, both encoded in the **MHC**. They are expressed by **antigen-presenting cells** and function in antigen presentation to $CD4^+$ T cells. The classical class II molecules are HLA-DP, -DQ, and –DR in humans.

Class III MHC molecules: various proteins encoded in the **MHC** but distinct from class I and class II MHC molecules. They include some complement components, two steroid 21-hydroxylases, and tumor necrosis factor α and β.

Class switching: see **Isotype switching**.

Classical complement pathway: activation of **complement** that is initiated by antigen-antibody complexes; involves C1-C9; and generates the **membrane-attack complex**.

Clonal anergy: a proposed mechanism for rendering peripheral antigen-reactive lymphocytes functionally inactive.

Clonal deletion: the elimination of self-reactive T cells in the thymus.

Clonal selection: proposed mechanism whereby antigen binding to receptors (membrane antibody or T-cell receptor) on a lymphocyte stimulates the cell to undergo mitosis and develop into a **clone** of cells with the same **antigenic specificity** as the original parent cell.

Clone: cells arising from a single progenitor cell.

Clonotype: a clone of B cells with the ability to bind a single epitope.

Cluster of differentiation (CD): See CD molecule.

Coated pit: a structure employed to endocytose ligand attached to cell surface receptors while effectively re-cycling the receptors.

Coelomocyte: a phagocytic cell found in the coelomic cavity of invertebrates.

Colony-stimulating factors (CSFs): the group of factors that induces the proliferation and differentiation of hematopoietic cells and some other cells.

Colostrum: the secretion that accumulates in the mammary gland in the last weeks of pregnancy. It is very rich in immunoglobulins.

Combined immunodeficiency: a deficiency in both the T-cell and B-cell-mediated components of the immune system.

Complement: a group of serum proteins that is activated by factors such as the combination of antigen and antibody and results in a variety of biological consequences, including cell lysis and opsonization.

Complementarity-determining region (CDR): an area within the variable regions of antibodies and T-cell antigen receptors that binds to antigen and determines the molecule's antigen-binding specificity. Synonymous with hyper-variable regions.

Concanavalin A (ConA): a lectin extracted from the jack bean, which makes T cells divide.

Congenic: denoting individuals that differ genetically at a single genetic locus or region; also called coisogenic.

Constant domain: a structural domain with little sequence variability found in antibodies and TCR.

Constant (C) region: the nearly invariant portion of antibody heavy and light chains and of the polypeptide chains of the T-cell receptor.

Convertase: a protease that acts on a complement component to cause its activation.

Cortex: the outer region of an organ such as the thymus or lymph node.

Corticosteroid: steroid hormone released from the adrenal cortex that has profound effects on the immune system. Some corticosteroids may be synthetic in origin.

Co-stimulator: a molecule required to stimulate an antigen-sensitive cell simultaneously with antigen in order to initiate an effective immune response.

Co-stimulatory signal: additional signal that is required to induce proliferation of antigen-primed T cells and is generated by interaction of CD28 on T cells with B7 on antigen-presenting cells or altered self-cells. In B-cell activation, an analogous signal (competence signal 2) is provided by interaction of CD40 on B cells with CD40L on activated T_H cells.

Cross-reactivity: ability of a particular antibody or T-cell receptor to react with two or more antigens that possess a common **epitope.**

CTL: see **Cytotoxic T lymphocyte.**

Cutaneous basophil hypersensitivity: a form of delayed type hypersensitivity associated with an extensive basophil infiltration.

Cytokine: any of numerous secreted, low-molecular-weight proteins that regulate the intensity and duration of the immune response by exerting a variety of effects on lymphocytes and other immune cells.

Cytolysis: destruction of cells by immune processes.

Cytophilic antibody: immunoglobulin that has the ability to bind spontaneously to cellular Fc receptors.

Cytotoxic cell: a cell that can injure or kill other cells.

Cytotoxic T lymphocyte (CTL): an effector T cell (usually CD8$^+$) that can mediate the lysis of target cells bearing antigenic peptides associated with an MHC molecule. It usually arises from an antigen-activated T_C cell.

D (diversity) gene segment: that portion of a rearranged immunoglobulin heavy-chain gene or T-cell receptor gene that is situated between the V and J gene segments and encodes part of the hypervariable region. There are multiple D gene segments in germ-line DNA, but gene rearrangement results in only one occurring in each functional rearranged gene.

Degranulation: discharge of the contents of cytoplasmic granules by **basophils** and **mast cells** following cross-linkage (usually by antigen) of bound IgE. It is characteristic of type 1 **hypersensitivity**.

Delayed-type hypersensitivity (DTH): a type IV hypersensitive response mediated by sensitized T_{DTH} **cells,** which release various **cytokines** and **chemokines**. The response generally occurs 2-3 days after T_{DTH} cells interact with antigen. It is an important part of host defense against intracellular parasites and bacteria.

Dendritic cells: professional **antigen-presenting cells** that have long membrane processes. They are found in the lymph nodes, spleen, and thymus (follicular and interdigitating dentritic cells); skin (Langerhans cells); and other tissues (interstitial dendritic cells).

Desensitization: the prevention of allergic reactions through the use of multiple injections of allergen.

Diapedesis: the emigration of cells from intact blood vessels during inflammation.

Differentiation antigen: a cell-surface marker that is expressed only during a particular developmental stage or by a particular cell lineage.

Disulfide bonds: bonds that form between two cysteine residues in a protein. They may be either interchain (between two peptide chains) or intrachain (joining two parts of one chain).

Domain: an independently folded structural unit within a protein. See also **Immunoglobulin fold**.

Edema: abnormal accumulation of fluid in intercellular spaces, often resulting from a failure of the lymphatic system to drain off normal leakage from the capillaries.

Effector cell: a cell that is able to "effect" an immune response. These include T helper cells, cytotoxic T cells and plasma cells.

Electrophoresis: the separation of the proteins in a complex mixture by subjecting them to an electrical potential.

ELISA (enzyme-linked immunosorbent assay): an assay for quantitating either antibody or antigen by use of an enzyme-linked antibody and a substrate that forms a colored reaction product.

Endocytoses: process by which cells ingest extracellular macromolecules by enclosing them in a small portion of the plasma membrane, which invaginates and is pinched off to form an intracellular vesicle containing the ingested material.

Endogenous antigen: an antigen synthesized within body cells. An example of this is a virus protein.

Endogenous: originating within the organism or cell.

Endosome: a cytoplasmic vesicle formed by invagination of the outer cell membrane.

Endothelium: the cells that line blood vessels and lymphatics.

Endotoxins: certain lipopolysaccharide (LPS) components of the cell wall of gram-negative bacteria that are responsible for many of the pathogenic effects associated with these organisms. Some function as **super-antigens**.

Eosinophil: a granulocyte that functions in **antibody-dependent cell-mediated cytotoxicity,** particularly of parasites, and also has some phagocytic ability.

Eosinophilia: increased numbers of eosinophils in the blood.

Epithelioid cell: a macrophage that accumulates within a tubercle and resembles an epithelial cell in histological section.

Epitope: that an area on the surface of an antigen stimulates a specific immune response and against which that response is directed. Synonymous with antigenic determinant.

Epstein-Barr virus (EBV): the causative agent of Burkitt's **lymphoma** and infectious mononucleosis. It can transform human B cells into stable **cell lines**.

Equivalence: a measure of the proportion of antibody to antigen that yields the maximum precipitate in liquids and gels.

Erythema: redness of the skin caused by engorgement of capillaries during an **inflammatory response**.

Erythroblastosis fetalis: a type II hypersensitivity reaction in which maternal antibodies against fetal **Rh antigens** cause hemolysis of the erythrocytes of a newborn; also called hemolytic disease of the newborn.

Erythropoiesis: the generation of red blood cells.

Exocytosis: the export of material from a cell by the fusion of cytoplasmic vesicles with the outer cell membrane.

Exogenous antigen: a foreign antigen that originates at a source outside the body, for example, bacterial antigens.

Exon: a continuous segment of DNA that encodes part of a gene product; also called coding sequence.

Exotoxins: toxic proteins secreted by gram-positive and gram-negative bacteria; some function as **superantigens**. They cause food poisoning, toxic-shock syndrome, and other disease states. See also **Immunotoxin**.

Extravasation: movement of blood cells through an unruptured vessel wall into the surrounding tissue, particularly at sites of inflammation.

Exudate: fluid with a high content of proteins, salts, and cellular debris that accumulates extravascularly, usually as a result of inflammation.

Fab fragment: a monovalent antigen-binding fragment of an immunoglobulin molecule that consists of one light chain and part of one heavy chain. It is obtained by brief papain digestion.

Facultative intracellular organism: an organism that can, if necessary, grow within cells.

Fc fragment: a crystallizable, non-antigen-binding fragment of an immunoglobulin molecule that consists of the carboxyl-terminal portions of both heavy chains and possesses binding sites for Fc receptors and the C1q component of complement. It is obtained by brief papain digestion.

Fc receptor: a cell surface receptor that specifically binds antibody molecules through their Fc region.

Fc region: that part of an immunoglobulin molecule consisting of the C-terminal halves of heavy chains; it is responsible for the biological activities of the molecule.

Fibrinolytic: breakdown of fibrin.

First-set graft rejection: process whereby an **allograft** is rejected following first exposure to the alloantigens of the donor. Complete rejection usually occurs within 12-14 days.

Fluorescent antibody: an antibody chemically attached to a fluorescent dye.

Fluorochrome: a fluorescent dye, which can be conjugated with an antibody or other protein. Two common fluorochromes used to tag antibodies are fluorescent isothiocyanate (FITC), which emits a yellow-green color, and Rhodamine (Rh), which emits a red color. See also **immunofluorescence.**

Framework region: a relatively conserved sequence of amino acids located on either side of the hypervariable regions in the variable domains of immunoglobulin heavy and light chains.

Gamma (γ) globulin: a serum protein that migrates towards the cathode on electrophoresis. Gamma globulins contain most of the immunoglobulins.

Gel diffusion: an immunoprecipitation technique that involves letting antigen and antibody meet and precipitate in a clear gel such as agar.

Gene complex: a cluster of related genes occupying a restricted area of a chromosome.

Gene conversion: the exchange of blocks of DNA between different genes.

Gene locus: see **Locus**.

Gene segment: an exon that codes for a portion of a peptide chain.

Genes: a unit of DNA that codes for the amino acid sequence of a polypeptide chain.

Genome: the total genetic material contained in the haploid set of chromosomes.

Genotype: the combined genetic material inherited from both parents; also, the **alleles** present at one or more specific loci.

Germ line: the unmodified genetic material that is transmitted from one generation to the next through the gametes.

Germinal center: a region within lymph nodes and the spleen where B-cell activation, proliferation, and differentiation occurs.

Globulin: a serum protein precipitated by the presence of a half-saturated solution of ammonium sulfate.

Glomerulonephritis: pathological lesions in the glomeruli of the kidney.

Glycoprotein: a protein that contains carbohydrate.

G-protein: a GTP-protein that acts as a signal transducer for a cell surface receptor.

Graft-versus-host disease (GVHD): a reaction that develops when a graft contains immunocompetent T cells that recognize and attack the recipient's cells.

Granulocyte: any **leukocyte** that contains cytoplasmic granules, particularly the basophil, eosinophil, and neutrophil.

Granuloma: a localized nodular inflammatory lesion characterized by chronic inflammation with mononuclear (macrophage) cell infiltration and extensive fibrosis.

Granzyme: a family of proteolytic enzymes found in the granules of cytotoxic T cells, NK cells, Eosinophils.

Growth factor: a biologically active molecule that promotes cell growth.

Haplotype: the set of **alleles** of linked genes present on one parental chromosome; commonly used in reference to the **MHC** genes.

Hapten: a low-molecular-weight compound that is not immunogenic by itself but when coupled to a carried can elicit anti-hapten antibodies. Dinitrophenol (DNP) is a common hapten.

Heat shock protein: a protein synthesized by cells in response to physiologic stress.

Heavy chain: the larger polypeptide of an antibody molecule composed of one variable domain (V_H) and three or four constant domains (C_H1, C_H2, etc.)There are five major classes of heavy chains in humans, which determine the **isotype** of an antibody.

Helminth: a worm, many of them are parasites and so stimulate immune responses.

Helper T cell: a class of T cells that promotes immune responses by releasing cytokines such as interleukin-2 or interleukin-4.

Hemagglutination: the agglutination of red blood cells.

Hemagglutinin: see **Agglutinin**.

Hematopoiesis: formation and development of red and white blood cells.

Hematopoietic organ: an organ in which blood cells are produced.

Hematopoietins: family of proteins that includes many cytokines whose receptors share several conserved motifs.

Hemolytic disease: disease occurring as a result of the destruction of red blood cells by antibodies transferred to the young animal from its mother.

Hemolytic plaque assay: in vitro technique for detecting **plasma cells** based on their ability to lyse antigen-sensitized erythrocytes in the presence of complement, thereby forming visible plaques.

Herd immunity: immunity conferred on a population as a whole as a result of the presence of some immune individuals within that population.

Heterodimer: a molecule consisting of two different subunits.

Heterologous: originating from a different species; see also **Xenogeneic**.

Heterophile antibody: an antibody that reacts with epitopes found on a wide variety of unrelated molecules.

High-endothelial venule (HEV): an area of a capillary venule composed of specialized cells with a plump, cuboidal ("high") shape through which lymphocytes migrate to enter various lymphoid organs.

Hinge region: the portion of immunoglobulin heavy chains between the **Fc** and **Fab** regions. It gives flexibility to the molecule and allows the two antigen-binding sites to function independently.

Histamine: one of numerous mediators present in the cytoplasmic granules of basophils and mast cells. It is released during degranulation and causes increased vascular permeability and contraction of smooth muscle.

Histiocyte: a connective tissue macrophage.

Histocompatibility molecule: a cell membrane protein that is required to present antigen to antigen-sensitive cells.

Histocompatible: denoting individuals whose major histocompatibility antigens, which are encoded by the **MHC**, are identical Grafts between such individuals generally are accepted.

HIV (human immunodeficiency virus): a **retrovirus** that infects CD4$^+$ T cells and causes **acquired immunodeficiency syndrome (AIDS)**.

HLA (human leukocyte antigen) complex: term for the **MHC** in humans.

Homing receptor: a lymphocyte cell surface receptor that enables lymphocytes to bind to ligands on endothelial cells as a preliminary step to leaving the bloodstream.

Homodimer: a molecule consisting of two identical subunits.

Homolog: a part similar in structure, position, and origin to another organ.

Homologous: originating from the same species; also refers to similarity in the sequences of DNA or proteins.

Homology: the degree of sequence similarity between two genes (nucleotide sequences) or two proteins (amino acid sequences).

HTLV (human T lymphotrophic virus): a **retrovirus** that infects human CD4$^+$ T cells and causes adult T-cell leukemia.

Humoral: pertaining to extracellular fluid including the plasma and lymph.

Humoral immune response: host defenses that are mediated by antibody present in the plasma, lymph, and tissue fluids. It protects against extracellular bacteria and foreign macromolecules. Transfer of antibodies confers this type of immunity on the recipient. See also **Cell-mediated immune response**.

Humoral immunity: immunity that can be transferred in body fluids – antibody-mediated immunity.

Hypersensitivity: exaggerated immune response that causes damage to the individual. Immediate hypersensitivity (types I, II, and III) is mediated by antibody or immune complexes, and delayed-type hypersensitivity (type IV) is mediated by T_{DTH} cells.

Hypervariable region: a small area within an immunoglobulin or TCR variable region where the greatest variations in amino acid sequence occurs (see CDR or complementarity-determining region).

Hypogammaglobulinemia: low levels of gamma globulins in blood.

Idiotope: a single **antigenic determinant** in the variable domains of an antibody or T-cell receptor; also called idiotype determinant. Idiotypes are generated by the unique amino acid sequence specific for each antigen.

Idiotype: the set of antigenic determinants (**idiotopes**) characterizing each unique antibody or T-cell receptor.

Immediate hypersensitivity: an exaggerated immune response mediated by antibody (type I and II) or antigen-antibody complexes (type III) that manifests within minutes to hours following exposure of a sensitized individual to antigen.

Immune complex: a macromolecular complex of antibody bound to antigen, which sometimes includes **complement** components.

Immune elimination: the removal of an antigen from the bloodstream by circulating antibodies and phagocytic cells.

Immune globulin: an antibody preparation containing specific antibodies against a pathogen and used for passive immunization.

Immune response gene: an MHC class II gene, so called because it regulates the ability of an animal to respond to specific antigens.

Immune stimulant: a compound, commonly bacterial in origin that stimulates the immune system by promoting cytokine release from macrophages.

Immune surveillance: the concept that lymphocytes survey the body for cancerous or abnormal cells and then eliminate them.

Immunity: the state of resistance to an infection.

Immunization: the administration of an antigen to an individual to confer immunity.

Immunocompetent: denoting a mature lymphocyte that is capable of recognizing a specific antigen and mediating an immune response.

Immunodeficiency: disease conditions in which immune function is defective.

Immunodiffusion: another name for the gel-diffusion technique.

Immunodominant: describing the epitope on a molecule that provokes the most intense immune response.

Immunoelectrophoresis: a procedure involving sequential electrophoresis and immunoprecipitation; it is used to identify the proteins in a complex solution such as serum.

Immunofluorescence: technique of staining cells or tissue with **fluorescent antibody** and visualizing the section under a fluorescent microscope.

Immunogen: a substance capable of eliciting an immune response. All immunogens are **antigens**, but some antigens (e.g. haptens) are not immunogens.

Immunogenetics: that portion of immunology that deals with the direct effects of genes on the immune system.

Immunogenicity: the ability of a molecule to elicit an immune response.

Immunoglobulin (Ig): see **Antibody**

Immunoglobulin fold: characteristic **domain** structure present in immunoglobulins that consists of about 110 amino acids folded into two ? pleated sheets, each containing three of four anti-parallel ? strands, and stabilized by an intrachain disulfide bond forming a loop of about 60 amino acids.

Immunoglobulin superfamily: group of proteins that contain **immunoglobulin-fold** domains, or structurally related domains, including immunoglobulins, T-cell receptors, MHC molecules, and numerous other membrane molecules.

Immunological paralysis: a form of immunological tolerance in which an ongoing immune response is inhibited by the presence of large amounts to antigen.

Immunoperoxidase: an immunological test that uses antibodies chemically conjugated to the enzyme peroxidase.

Immunosuppression: inhibition of the immune system by drugs or other processes.

Inactivated vaccine: a vaccine containing an agent that has been treated in such a way that it is no longer capable of replication in the host.

Incomplete antibody: an antibody that can bind to a particulate antigen but is incapable of causing its agglutination.

Inflammation: the complex series of responses of tissues to injury. These responses generally enhance tissue defenses and initiate repair processes.

Inflammatory response: a localized tissue response to injury or other trauma characterized by pain, head, redness, and swelling. The response, which includes both localized and systemic effects, consists of altered patterns of blood flow, an influx of phagocytic and other immune cells, removal of foreign antigens, and healing of the damaged tissue.

Innate immunity: nonspecific host defenses that exist prior to exposure to an antigen and involve anatomic, physiologic, exocytic and phagocytic, and inflammatory mechanisms. See also **Acquired immunity**.

Integral membrane protein: cell surface proteins that are integral components of the cell membrane as opposed to proteins that are passively adsorbed to cell surfaces.

Integrins: a group of heterodimeric cell-adhesion molecules (e.g. LFA-1, VLA-4 and Mac-1) present on various leukocytes that bind to lg-superfamily CAMs (e.g., ICAMs, VCAM-1) on endothelium.

Interchain bond: a bond between two peptide chains, usually formed by a disulfide linkage between two cysteine residues.

Interdigitating cells: a form of dendritic cell found within lymphoid organs.

Interferons (IFNs): several glycoprotein **cytokines** produced and secreted by certain cells that induce an antiviral state in other cells and also help to regulate the immune response.

Interleukins (Ils): a group of **cytokines** secreted by leukocytes that primarily affect the growth and differentiation of various hematopoietic and immune-system cells.

Intrachain bond: a bond between two cysteine residues on a single peptide chain. Because disulfide bonds are short, its effect is to produce a loop in the peptide chain.

Intraepithelial lymphocyte: a small lymphocyte, probably a T cell, located among the epithelial cells in the intestinal wall.

Intron: noncoding sequence within a gene, which is transcribed into the primary transcript but is removed during processing and does not appear in mRNA.

In vitro: referring to experiments involving living cells or cellular components performed outside the intact organism.

In vivo: referring to experiments carried out in an intact, living organism.

Isoform: Different molecular forms of a protein that are generated by differential processing of RNA transcripts obtained from a single gene.

Isogeneic (syngeneic): genetically identical.

Isograft: graft between genetically identical individuals.

Isotype: an antibody class, which is determined by the heavy-chain constant-region sequence. The five human isotypes, designated IgA, IgD, IgE, IgG, and IgM, exhibit structural and functional differences. Also refers to the set of **isotypic determinants** that is carried by all members of a species.

Isotype switching: conversion of one antibody class (**isotype**) to another resulting from the genetic rearrangement of heavy-chain constant-region genes in B cells; also called class switching.

Isotypic determinant: an **antigenic determinant** within the immunoglobulin constant regions that is characteristic of a species.

J (joining) gene segment: that portion of a rearranged immunoglobulin or T-cell receptor gene that joins the variable region to the constant region and encodes part of the **hypervariable region**. There are multiple **J** gene segments in germ-line DNA, but gene rearrangement results in only one segment occurring in each functional rearranged gene.

J chain: a short peptide that joins two monomers in the polymeric immunoglobulins IgM and IgA.

Kappa (*K*) chain: see **Light chain**.

Kinins: group of peptides released during an **inflammatory response** that act as vasodilators, inducing smooth-muscle contraction and increased vascular permeability.

Knockout mouse: a form of **transgenic mouse** in which a normal gene is replaced with a mutant allele or disrupted form of the gene; as a result the animal lacks a functional gene product.

Kupffer cell: macrophages lining the sinusoids of the liver.

Lactenin: a bacterial factor in milk.

Lag period: the interval between administration of antigen and the first detection of antibody.

Lambda (λ) chain: see **Light chain**.

Langerhans' cell: a dendritic cell found in the skin. These cells are very effective antigen-presenting cells.

Lectin: a protein, usually of plant origin, that can bind specifically to a carbohydrate. Many lectins can induce lymphocytes to divide.

Leukemia: cancer originating in any class of hematopoietic cell that tends to proliferate as single cells within the lymph or blood.

Leukocyte: a white blood cell. This general term covers all the nucleated cells of blood.

Leukopenia: reduction in the number of circulating white blood cells.

Leukotriene: a vasoactive metabolite of arachidonic acid produced by the actions of lipoxygenase.

Ligand: a generic term for the molecules that bind specifically to a receptor.

Light chain: the smaller polypeptide of an antibody molecule composed of one variable domain (V_1) and one constant domain (C_1). There are two major types (kappa and lambda) of light chains in humans.

Locus: the location of a gene on a chromosome.

Looping out: a method of excising a segment of intervening DNA (intron) in order to join two gene segments (exons).

LPS (lipopolysaccharide): a group of substances present in the cell wall of gram-negative bacteria that are B-cell **mitogens**, can induce an inflammatory response, and also function as an **adjuvant**.

Lymph node: a small **secondary lymphoid organ** that contains lymphocytes, macrophages, and dendritic cells and serves as a site for filtration of foreign antigen and activation and proliferation of lymphocytes. See also **Germinal center**.

Lymph: a pale, watery, proteinaceous fluid that is derived from intercellular tissue fluid and circulates in lymphatic vessels.

Lymphadenopathy: literally, disease of the lymph nodes. In practice it is used to describe enlarged lymph nodes.

Lymphoblast: a dividing lymphocyte.

Lymphocyte trapping: the trapping of lymphocytes within a lymph node during the node's response to antigen.

Lymphocyte: a mononuclear leukocyte that mediates humoral or cell-mediated immunity. See also **B cell** and **T cell**.

Lymphokine: a cytokine released by lymphocytes.

Lymphokine-activated killer (LAK) cell: a lymphocyte activated by exposure to cytokines such as IL-2 in vitro.

Lymphoma: a cancer of lymphoid cells that tends to proliferate as a solid tumor.

Lymphopenia: abnormally low numbers of lymphocytes in blood.

Lymphopoiesis: the differentiation of lymphocytes from hematopoietic stem cells.

Lymphotoxin: a cytotoxic cytokine secreted by lymphocytes.

Lysogeny: state in which a viral genome (**provirus**) is associated with the host genome in such a way that the viral genes remain unexpressed.

Lysosomal enzyme: one of the complex mixture of enzymes, many of which are proteases found within lysosomes.

Lysosome: a small cytoplasmic vesicle found in many types of cells that contains hydrolytic enzymes, which play an important role in the degradation of material ingested by **phagocytosis** and **endocytosis**.

Lysozyme: an enzyme present in tears, saliva, and mucous secretions that digests mucopeptides in bacterial cell wall and thus functions as a nonspecific antibacterial agent.

Lysozyme: an enzyme present in tears, saliva, and neutrophils. It attacks the mucopeptides in the cell wall of gram-positive bacteria.

Macrophage: a large, leukocyte derived from a **monocyte** that functions in phagocytosis, antigen processing and presentation, secretion of cytokines, and antibody-dependent cell-mediated cytotoxicity.

Major histocompatibility complex: the gene region that contains the genes for the major histocompatibility molecules as well as for some complement components and related proteins. Also called **HLA complex** in humans.

Malignant tumor: a tumor whose cells have a tendency to invade normal tissues and spread by lymphatics or blood to distant tissue sites.

MALT (mucosal-associated lymphoid tissue): collective terms for **secondary lymphoid organs** located along various mucous membrane surfaces including Peyer's patches, tonsils, the appendix, as well as diffuse lymphoid follicles within the intestinal lamina propria.

Marginal zone: a diffuse region of the spleen, located between the **red pulp** and **white pulp**, that is rich in B cells and contains lymphoid follicles, which can develop into **germinal centers**.

Mast cell: a bone marrow-derived cell present in a variety of tissues that resembles peripheral-blood basophils, bears **Fc receptors** for IgE, and undergoes IgE –mediated **degranulation**.

Maternal antibodies: antibodies that originate in the mother but enter the bloodstream of her offspring either by transport across the placenta as in primates or by adsorption of ingested colostrum in other mammals.

Medulla: the region in the center of lymphoid organs such as the thymus or lymph nodes.

Megakaryocyte: a white blood cell that produces **platelets** by cytoplasmic budding.

Membrane-attack complex (MAC): the complex of complement components C5-C9, which is formed in the terminal steps of either the classical or alternative complement pathway, and mediates cell lysis by creating a membrane pore in the target cell.

Memory cell: clonally expanded progeny of T and B cells formed during the **primary immune response** following initial exposure to an antigen. Memory cells are more easily activated than **naive** lymphocytes and mediate a **secondary immune response** on subsequent exposure to antigen.

Memory response: the enhanced immune response that is triggered as a result of exposing a primed animal to antigen.

Mesangial cell: a modified muscle cell found within a glomerulus.

MHC molecules: proteins encoded by the major histocompatibility complex and classified as class I, class II, and class III MHC molecules.

MHC restriction: the characteristic of T cells that permits them to recognize antigen only after it is processed and the resulting antigenic peptides are displayed in association with either a **class I** or **class II MHC molecule**.

Microglia: macrophages resident within the brain.

Minor histocompatibility loci: genes outside of the MHC that encode antigens contributing to graft rejection.

Mitogen: any substance that makes cells divide.

Mixed-lymphocyte reaction (MLR): in vitro T-cell proliferation in response to cells expressing allogeneic MHC molecules, can be used as an assay for class II MHC activity.

Modified live virus: a virus whose virulence has been reduced so that it can replicate in the host but cannot cause disease in normal animals.

Molecular mimicry: the development by parasites of molecules whose structure closely resembles molecules found in their host. In this way the parasites may be able to evade destruction by the immune system.

Monoclonal: derived from a single cell.

Monoclonal antibody: homogeneous preparation of antibody molecules, produced by a hybridoma, all of which exhibit the same antigenic specificity.

Monocyte: a mononuclear phagocyte leukocyte that circulates briefly in the bloodstream before migrating into the tissues where it becomes a **macrophage**.

Monokine: a cytokine secreted by macrophages and monocytes.

Monomer: the basic unit of a molecule that can be assembled using repeating subunits.

Mononuclear cell: a leukocyte with a single round nucleus, for example, a lymphocyte or a macrophage.

Mononuclear-phagocytic system: the cells that belong to the macrophage family and their precursors.

Myeloid system: all the granulocytes and their precursors. These precursor cells are found in the bone marrow.

Myeloma: a tumor of plasma cells.

Naïve: denoting mature B and T cells that have not encountered antigen, synonymous with unprimed and virgin.

Natural antibody: an antibody against foreign antigens found in the serum of normal, unimmunized individuals. Most probably arise as a result of exposure to cross-reacting bacterial antigens.

Natural killer (NK) cell: a non-T, non-B large, granular lymphocyte (null cell) that has cytotoxic ability but does not express antigen-binding receptors. It exhibits antibody independent killing of tumor cells and also can participate in antibody-dependent cell-mediated cytotoxicity.

Necrosis: morphologic changes associated with death of individual cells or groups of cells, leading to disruption and atrophy of tissue. See also **Apoptosis**.

Negative feedback: a control mechanism whereby the products of a reaction suppress their own production.

Negative selection: a euphemism for the killing of cells that have the potential to react to self-antigens. It is a key mechanism in the prevention of autoimmunity.

Nematode: a roundworm.

Neoplasm: any new and abnormal growth, a benign or malignant tumor.

Network theory: the theory that the immune system is regulated by a network of idiotype and anti-idiotype reactions involving antibodies and T-cell receptors. See also **Anti-idiotype antibody**.

Neutralization: blockage of the activity of an organism or a toxin by antibody.

Neutropenia: low numbers of neutrophils in blood.

Neutrophil: a polymorphonuclear cell or granulocyte.

Neutrophilia: high numbers of neutrophils in blood.

NK cell: a natural killer cell.

Noncovalent bond: a chemical bond such as a hydrogen or hydrophobic bond that can reversibly link peptide chains. These play a key role in the binding of antigen with antibodies or with T-cell antigen receptors.

Normal flora: the microbial population consisting mainly of bacteria that colonize normal body surfaces. They play a key role in prevent invasion by pathogenic organisms.

Nucleocapsid: the key structural component of a virus, consisting of the viral nucleic acid and its protective capsid coat.

Nude mice: a mutant strain of mice that have no thymus and are hairless. This strain of mouse has proved very useful in immunological research.

Null cell: a small population of peripheral blood lymphocytes that lack the membrane markers characteristic of B and T cells. **Natural killer cells** are included in this group.

Oligosaccharide: chains of at least two covalently linked sugars.

Oncofetal tumor antigen: an antigen that is present during fetal development but generally is not expressed in tissues except by tumor cells. Alpha-feto protein (AFP) and carcinoembryonic antigen (CEA) are two examples that have been associated with various cancers.

Oncogene: a gene encoding a protein capable of inducing cellular **transformation** and **proliferation**. Oncogenes derived from viruses are termed v-onc, while their cellular counterparts (**proto-oncogenes**) are denoted c-onc.

Oncogenic virus: a virus that causes cancer.

Oncogenic: causing cancer.

Opportunistic pathogen: an organism that, although unable to cause disease in a healthy individual, may invade and cause disease in an individual whose immunological defenses are impaired.

Opsonin: a substance that facilitates phagocytosis by coating foreign particles.

Opsonization: deposition of opsonins on an antigen, thereby promoting a stable, adhesive contact with an appropriate phagocytic cell.

Ouchterlony method: a double immunodiffusion technique involving the diffusion of antigen and antibody within a gel resulting in formation of a visible hand of precipitate in the region of **equivalence**.

PALS (periarteriolar lymphoid sheath): see **White pulp**.

Paracortex: the region located between the cortex and medulla of lymph nodes in which T cells predominate.

Paratope: the site in the variable (V) domain of an antibody or T-cell receptor that binds to an epitope on an antigen.

Passive agglutination: the agglutination of inert particles by antibody directed against antigen bound to their surface.

Passive immunity: acquired immunity conferred by the transfer of immune products, such as antibody or sensitized T cells, from an immune individual to a nonimmune one. See also **Active immunity**.

Passive immunization: protection of one individual conferred by administration of antibody produced in another individual.

Pathogen: a disease-causing organism.

Pathogenesis: the mechanism of a disease.

Pathogenic organism: an organism that causes disease.

Perforin: a family of proteins made by T cells and NK cells that when polymerized can insert themselves into target-cell membranes and provoke cell lysis.

Peyer's patches: lymphoid nodules located along the small intestine that function to trap antigens from the gastrointestinal tract and provide sites where B and T cells can interact with antigen.

Phagocyte: a cell whose prime function is to eat bacteria (phagocytosis). These include macrophages and related cells, neutrophils, and eosinophils.

Phagocytosis: a process by which certain cells (phagocytes) engulf micro-organisms, other cells, and foreign particles.

Phagolysosome: A structure produced by the fusion of a phagosome and a lysosome following phagocytosis.

Phagosome: intracellular vacuole containing ingested particulate materials; formed by invagination of the cell membrane during **phagocytosis**.

Phylogeny: the evolutionary history of a species.

Phytohemagglutinin (PHA): a lectin derived from the red kidney bean. It acts as a T cell mitogen.

Pinocytosis: a type of **endocytosis** in which a cell ingests extracellular fluid and soluble materials contained within that fluid.

Plaque-forming cell: an antibody-secreting cell capable of secreting anti-red cell antibodies and so forming a plaque in a layer of red blood cells in the presence of complement.

Plaque-forming count (PFC): the number of plaques formed in the in vitro **hemolytic plaque assay**, which detects antibody-forming plasma cells.

Plasma cell: a fully differentiated B cell capable of synthesizing and secreting large amounts of antibody.

Plasma: the cell-free, fluid portion of blood, which contains all the clotting factors.

Plasmacytoma: a plasma-cell tumor.

Platelet: a small nuclear membrane-bound cytoplasmic structure derived from megakaryocytes, which contains vasoactive substances and clotting factors important in blood coagulation, inflammation, and allergic reactions; also called thrombocyte.

Point mutation: a mutation resulting from an alteration in a single base in a gene.

Pokeweed mitogen (PWM): a lectin derived from the pokeweed plant that stimulates both T and B cells to divide.

Polyclonal: pertaining to many different clones.

Polymorphism: inherited structural differences between proteins from allogeneic individuals as a result of multiple alternative alleles at a single locus.

Polymorphonuclear cell or granulocyte: a blood leukocyte possessing neutrophilic cytoplasmic granules and an irregular lobed nucleus.

Positive selection: the enhanced proliferation of cells within the thymus that can respond optimally to foreign antigen.

Precipitin: an antibody that aggregates a soluble antigen, forming a macromolecular complex that yields a visible precipitate.

Primary binding test: a serologic assay that directly detects the binding of antigen and antibody.

Primary immune response: the immune response resulting from an individual's first encounter with an antigen.

Primary immunodeficiency: an inherited immunodeficiency disease.

Primary lymphoid organ: an organ that serves either as a source of lymphocytes or in which lymphocytes mature.

Primary pathogen: an organism that can cause disease without first suppressing an individual's immune defenses.

Privileged site: a location within the body where foreign grafts are not rejected. A good example is the cornea of the eye.

Prostaglandin: a biologically active lipid metabolite of arachidonic acid produced by the actions of the enzyme cyclooxygenase.

Proteasome: a large multifunctional protease complex responsible for degradation of intracellular proteins.

Protein kinase: an enzyme that phosphorylates proteins.

Proto-oncogenes: genes that in normal cells encode various growth-controlling proteins. Under certain conditions, proto-oncogenes are converted into **oncogenes**.

Provirus: viral DNA that is integrated into host-cell genome in a latent state and must undergo activation before it is transcribed, leading to formation of viral particles.

Prozone: the inhibition of agglutination by the presence of high concentrations of antibody.

Pseudogene: nucleotide sequence that is a stable component of the genome but is incapable of being expressed. They are thought to have been derived by mutation of ancestral active genes.

Pyrogen: a fever-causing substance.

Radioimmunossay (RIA): a highly sensitive technique for measuring antigen or antibody that involves competitive binding of radiolabeled antigen or antibody.

Reagin: IgE antibody that mediates type I immediate **hypersensitivity**.

Receptor: a structure on cell membranes that binds specifically to ligands in the surrounding fluid.

Recombinant vaccine: a vaccine-containing antigen prepared by recombinant DNA technique.

Recombination signal sequences (RSSs): conserved nucleotide sequences that flank gene segments in germ-line immunoglobulin and T-cell receptor DNA and direct joining of segments during gene rearrangement.

Red pulp: portion of the spleen consisting of a network of sinusoids populated by macrophages and erythrocytes. It is the site where old and defective red blood cells are destroyed.

Respiratory burst: the rapid increase in metabolic activity that occurs in phagocytic cells while particles are being ingested.

Reticuloendothelial system: all the cells in the body that take up circulating colloidal dyes. Many are macrophages. This term is best avoided.

Retrovirus: a type of RNA virus that uses a reverse transcriptase to produce a DNA copy of its RNA genome. HIV, causing AIDS, and HTLV, causing adult T-cell leukemia, are both retroviruses.

Reverse transcriptase: an enzyme that reversely transcribes RNA to DNA. It is found in retroviruses such as HIV.

Rh antigen: any of a large number of antigens present on the surface of blood cells that constitute the Rh blood group. See also **Erythroblastosis fetalis**.

Rheumatoid factor: autoantibody found in the serum of individuals with rheumatoid arthritis and other connective-tissue diseases.

Rhogam: antibody against **Rh antigen** that is used to prevent **erythroblastosis fetalis**.

Rosette: the structure formed when several red blood cells bind to the surface of another cell in culture.

SALT, GALT, BALT, and MALT: abbreviations for skin-, gut-, bronchus-, and mucosa-associated lymphoid tissue, respectively.

Sarcoma: a tumor arising from cells of mesodermal origin.

Secondary binding tests: serologic tests that detect the consequences of antigen-antibody binding such as agglutination and precipitation.

Secondary immune response: an enhanced immune response that results from second or subsequent exposure to an antigen.

Secondary immunodeficiency: an immunodeficiency disease resulting from a known nongenetic cause.

Secondary infection: infections by organisms that can only invade a host whose defenses are first weakened or destroyed by other organisms.

Secondary lymphoid organ: an organ in which effector lymphocytes are located.

Second-set reaction: the rapid rejection of an organ or tissue graft by a previously sensitized host.

Secretory component: a protein found on intestinal epithelial cells that functions as an IgA receptor and, on binding to IgA, protects IgA against proteolytic digestion in the intestine.

Secretory IgA: dimeric IgA linked to the **secretory component**; it is present in mucous secretions.

Selectins: a group of monomeric cell-adhesion molecules present on leukocytes (L-selectin) and endothelium (E- and P- selectin) that bind to mucin-like CAMs (e.g., GlyCam, PSGL-1).

Sensitization: the triggering of an immune response by exposure to an antigen.

Septic shock: a disease that results from the massive release of cytokines such as TNF as a result of infection with large numbers of gram-negative bacteria.

Serum: the clear yellow fluid that is expressed when blood has clotted and the clot contracts.

Serum sickness: a type III hypersensitivity reaction that develops when antigen is administered intravenously; resulting in the formation and tissue deposition of large amounts of antigen-antibody complexes. It often develops when individuals are immunized with antiserum derived from other species.

Signal transduction: the transmission of a signal through a receptor to a cell by means of a series of linked reactions.

Skin test: a diagnostic procedure that induces a local inflammatory response following intradermal inoculation of an antigen or allergen.

Somatic mutation: gene mutation occurring in non germ-like cells.

Specificity: a term that describes the ability of a test to give true-positive reactions.

Spleen: secondary lymphoid organ where old erythrocytes are destroyed and blood-borne antigens are trapped and presented to lymphocytes in the PALS and marginal zone.

Splice: the joining of two DNA or RNA segments.

Stem cell: a cell that can give rise to many differentiated cell lines.

Substrate modulation: a method of controlling enzyme activity seen in the complement system in which a protein cannot be cleaved by a protease until it first binds to another protein.

Superantigen: a molecule that, as a result of its ability to bind to certain TCR variable regions, can cause T cells to divide. It is distinguished from a mitogen by its specificity for T cells bearing these variable regions. Mitogens make all T cells divide.

Superfamily: a grouping of molecules that share certain distinguishing common structures. Thus the members of the immunoglobulin superfamily all contain characteristic immunoglobulin domains.

Supressor cells: a lymphocyte (usually a T cell) that is claimed to suppress the response of other cells to antigen. Their existence is disputed.

Syncytium (*plural*: synctia): the fusion of many cells into one large cytoplasmic mass containing multiple nuclei. This is usually the result of viral action.

Syndrome: a group of symptoms that together are characteristic of a specific disease.

Syngeneic: denoting genetically identical members of the same species.

T cell: a lymphocyte that matures in the thymus and expresses a T-cell receptor, CD3 and CD4 or CD8. Several distinct T-cell subpopulations are recognized.

T cytotoxic (T_C) cell: generally a $CD8^+$ class I MHC-restricted T cell, which differentiates into a **CTL** following interaction with altered self-cells (e.g., tumor cells, virus-infected cells).

T helper (T_H) cell: generally a $CD4^+$ class II MHC-restricted T cell, which plays a central role in both humoral and cell-mediated immunity and secretes numerous cytokines when activated.

T lymphocyte: a lymphocyte that has undergone a period of processing in the thymus and is responsible for mediating cell-mediated immune responses.

T-cell receptor (TCR): antigen-binding molecule expressed on the surface of T cells and associated with **CD3**. It is a heterodimer consisting of either an α and β chain or a γ and δ chain.

T_{DTH} cell: generally a $CD4^+$ lymphocyte derived from a T_H cell that mediates **delayed-type hypersensitivity**.

T_H1 subset: subpopulation of activated $CD4^+$ T cells that secrete characteristic cytokines and function primarily in cell-mediated responses by promoting activation of T_{DTH} cells, macrophages, and T_C cells.

T_H2 subset: subpopulation of activated $CD4^+$ T cells that secrete characteristic cytokines and function primarily in the humoral response.

Thoracic duct: the major lymphatic vessel that collects the lymph draining the lower portion of the body.

Thromboxane: lipid inflammatory mediator derived from arachidonic acid.

Thy-1: glycoprotein that is the earliest appearing surface marker of the T-cell lineage.

Thymectomy: surgical removal of the thymus.

Thymocyte: a developing lymphocyte in the thymus.

Thymus: a primary lymphoid organ, located in the thoracic cavity, where T-cell maturation occurs.

Thymus-dependent antigen: an antigen that requires the assistance of helper T cells to provoke an immune response.

Thymus-independent antigen: an antigen that can provoke an antibody response without help for T cells.

Titer: a measure of the relative strength of an antiserum. The titer is the reciprocal of the last dilution of an antiserum capable of mediating some measurable effect such a precipitation or agglutination.

Titration: the measurement of the level of specific antibodies in a serum by testing increasing dilutions of the serum for antibody activity.

Tolerance: state of immunologic unresponsiveness.

Tolerogen: a substance that induces tolerance.

Toxic shock: a disease resulting from the uptake of large amounts of staphylococcal superantigen.

Toxoid: nontoxic derivatives of toxins used as antigens.

Transcription: the conversion of a DNA nucleotide sequence into an RNA nucleotide sequence by complementary base pairing.

Transduction: the conversion of a signal from one form to another.

Transfection: experimental introduction of foreign DNA into cultured cells, usually followed by expression of the genes in the introduced DNA.

Transformation: change that a normal cell undergoes as it becomes malignant, also, permanent, heritable alteration in a cell resulting from the uptake and incorporation of foreign DNA into the genome.

Transgene: a cloned foreign gene present in an animal or plant.

Transgenic mouse: a mouse carrying a transgene, which has been introduced and stably incorporated into germ-line cells so that it can be passed on to progeny. See also **Knockout mouse**.

Translation: the conversion of the RNA nucleotide sequence into an amino acid sequence in a ribosome.

Transporter protein: proteins that bind fragments of endogenous antigen and carry them to newly assembled MHC class I molecules in the endoplasmic reticulum.

Trematode: a helminth known as a fluke. These include important human parasites such as schistosomes.

Tubercle: a persistent inflammatory response to the presence of mycobacteria in the tissues.

Tuberculin: an extract of tubercle bacilli that is used in a diagnostic skin test for tuberculosis.

Tumor antigens: cell-surface proteins present on the surface of tumor cells that can induce a cell-mediated immune response. Some are found only on tumor cells; others are also found on normal cells.

Tumor necrosis factor: a macrophage or lymphocyte-derived cytokine that can exert a direct toxic effect on neoplastic cells.

Tyrosine kinase: an enzyme that phosphorylates tyrosine residues in proteins. They play a key role in signal transduction.

V (variable) gene segment: the 5' coding portion of rearranged immunoglobulin and T-cell receptor genes. There are multiple V gene segments in germ-line DNA, but gene rearrangement results in only one segment occurring in each functional rearranged gene.

Vaccination: intentional administration of a harmless or less harmful form of a pathogen to induce a specific immune response that protects the individual against later exposure to the same pathogen.

Vaccine: a suspension of living or inactivated organisms used as an antigen to confer immunity.

Variable region: that part of the immunoglobulin or TCR peptide chains where the amino acid sequence shows significant variation between molecules.

Vasculitis: inflammation of blood vessel walls.

Virgin lymphocyte: a lymphocyte that has not previously encountered antigen.

Virion: a virus particle.

Virulence: a measure of the infectious ability of a pathogen.

Western blotting: a common technique for detecting a protein in a mixture in which the proteins are separated electrophoretically and then transferred to a polymer sheet, which is flooded with radiolabeled or enzyme-conjugated antibody specific for the protein of interest.

Wheal and flare reaction: characteristic type I hypersensitivity response that occurs in the skin involving a sharply delineated swelling of the skin (wheal) with surrounding redness (flare).

White pulp: portion of the spleen that surrounds the arteries, forming a periarteriolar lymphoid sheath (PALS) populated mainly by T cells.

Xenogeneic: denoting individuals of different species.

Xenograft: a graft between two animals of different species.

Index

ABO blood group
   antigens, 17
   typing, 110,
Accessory molecules, 179, 180
   in T-cell activation, 179
   in T-cell mediated toxicity, 180
Acetylcholine (ACh) receptor
   in myasthenia gravis, 347
Acquired immune response, 27
   cell-mediated, 33
   antigen presenting cells, 36
   B lymphocytes, 34
   T lymphocytes, 34
   cellular interactions, 36
Activation of immune responses
   humoral, 146
   cell-mediated, 162
Acute graft rejection, 300
   role of humoral immunity in, 300
   role of cell-mediated immunity in, 299, 300
   in kidney, 300
ADA *See* Adenosine deaminase
ADCC *See* Antibody-dependent cell-mediated
   cytotoxicity
Adenosine Deaminase (ADA)
   in severe combined immunodeficiency, 362
Adenoviruses
   effect on class I MHC expression, 264
Adhesion molecules, 197
   CD2, 179, 181, 182
   ICAM-1, ICAM-2, 180, 197
   Ig superfamily, 173
   integrin family, 197
Adjuvants, 68
Affinity

antibody, 101
   defined, 101
   determination, 102, 103
   effect of antigen dose on, 68
Affinity maturation, 153
   in humoral immune response, 153
   relationship to antigen dosage, 68
   somatic mutation in, 136
AFP (alpha-fetoprotein), 333
Alpha defensins, 15
African trypanosome, 270, 273
   Antigenic shift, 273
Agammaglobulinemia, 359
   common variable hypogammaglobulinema, 359
   pooled gammaglobulins for
   selective agammaglobulinemia, 360
   X-linked hypogammaglobulinemia (Burton's), 359
Agar gel diffusion, 103
Agglutination, 110
   detecting antigen-antibody reactions, 110
Agretope, 182
Agranulocytosis, 357
Allelic exclusion
   of antibodies, 131
   of T-cell receptors, 175
Allergens, 279, 286
Allergy, 286
   anaphylaxis, 277-289
   atopy, 286
   clinical manifestations, 277-289
   definition of, 286
   immunotherapy of, 289
   See also Immediate hypersensitivity, 277
   allergic asthma, 287
   eczema, 288

food allergies, 288
Alloantigens, 64, 182
Allogenic grafts, 299, 300
Allograft. *See also* Graft
  transplantation
  of bone marrow, 308, 312
  graft rejection, 299
    acute rejection, 300
    mechanisms of, 304
    role of CD4$^+$ and CD8$^+$ in, 304-306
    role of cytokines in, 227, 229, 305
  of organs, 307
Alloreactivity of T cells, 183
Allotypes, 90
Alpha-fetoprotein (AFP), 333
Alternating pathway of complement, 17, 18, 237
Altered peptide ligands, 169, 317
Altered self-cells, 326
  cancer-cells as, 326
Altered-self model, 183
Alveolar macrophages, 43
Anaphylatoxins, 285, 286
Anaphylaxis, 285
  localized (atopy), 286
  systemic. 285
Anatomic barriers, 14
Anemia
  autoimmune hemolytic, 346
  pernicious, 347
Anergy *see also* Clonal anergy
Ankylosing spondylitis, 346
  MHC alleles in, 350
Antagonism, of cytokines, 266
Antagonists
  antagonistic peptides, 353
  autoantibodies, 352
Antibody(ies), *see also*
Immunoglobulins and humoral response
Antibody- dependent cell-mediated cytotoxicity
  (ADCC), 201, 275, 305
  in antibody- mediated cell destruction, 201, 275
  eosinophils in, 201, 275
  macrophages in, 201, 305
  natural killer cells in, 201, 275, 305
  neutrophils in, 201, 305
Antigen(s), 63

agretope, 182
allergens, 279, 286
antigenic shift, 273
antigen-mediated regulation, 207
bacterial, 267-270
B-cell activation by, 146-153,
binding
CDR's and, 88
conformational changes from, 65
to MHC, 78, 79
to T-cell receptor, 173
blood group, 17
CD (cluster of differentiation), 40
circumsporozoite, 270-272
cross-reactions, 69, 70, 102
endogenous, presentation of, 193-195
epitopes, 69, 182
  conformational determinants, 65
  immunodominant, 64
exogenous, presentation of, 191-193
factors affecting immunogenicity, 64-67
adjuvants, 68
chemical composition and heterogeneity, 65
dosage, 67
foreignness, 64
molecular size, 65
heterogeneity, 65
conformation, 65
charge, 66
accessibility, 66,
genetic constitution of individuals, 67
MHC, role of, 67, 78, 79
route of administration, 67
susceptibility to antigen processing, 65
haptens, 69
histocompatibility, 72
identity, nonidentity, partial identity, 105
immunogenicity versus antigenicity, 63
lymphocyte activation by
mitogens, 203
processing *see* Antigen processing
recognition of *see* Antigen recognition
Rh antigen, 111, 291
Self-antigens, 64, 143-146, 158-162-173
T-cell activation by, 158-167
thymus-dependent (TD), 146

thymus- independent (TI), 146
tumor antigens *see* Tumor antigens
Antigen-antibody complexes,
  in autoimmunity, 352
  in B-cell activation, 143-148
Antigen-Antibody (Ag-Ab) interactions 101
  affinity, 101, 102
  agglutination reactions, 110
    bacterial, 110-111
    hemagglutination, 110
    inhibition of, 111
    passive, 111
  avidity, 111
  cross-reactivity, 69, 70, 102
  enzyme-linked immunosorbent assay (ELISA), 116-117
  immunoelectrophoresis
    countercurrent, 109
    rocket, 105
    two-dimensional, 106
  immunofluorescense, 116
  precipitation reactions, 103-110
  antibody excess, region of, 103, 104
  antigen excess, region of, 103, 104
  in fluids, 110
  in gels, 103-110
  immunodiffusion reactions, 104
  Mancini method, 105
  Ouchterlony method, 103
  Radioimmunoassay, 114
  Specificity of, 102
  Strength of, 102-104
  Western blotting, 119
Antigenic commitment, of B-cells, 146-153
Antigenic determinants, 69 See also
Antigenicity
  Defined, 63
  Haptens and, 69
  Versus immunogenicity, 63
Antigenic modulation, 264, 343
Antigenic peptides, 79, 80
Antigenic specificity, 69, 102
Antigen presentation, 189
  cells that function in, 189, 190
  class I MHC-associated, 78, 190-193
  class II MHC-associated, 79, 193-195

defined, 189
Antigen-presenting cells (APC's), 36, 190
  B cells as, 34, 36 40
  in cancer immunotherapy, 339
  class I and II MHC expressed, 78, 79
  defined, 36
  in delayed-type hypersensitivity, 294, 295
  dendritic cells as, 48
  macrophages as, 43-45
  nonprofessional, 190
  professional, 190
  role of, 190
Antigen processing, 65
  cytosolic pathway, 190
  early evidence for, 189
  endocytic pathway, 193-195
  endogenous antigen, 63, 189, 193-195
  exogenous antigen, 189, 191-193
Antigen recognition
  by B-cells, 40, 143-155
  by T-cells, 42, 155-172
    MHC-restricted, 190
Antihistamines, 289, 290
Anti-idiotypic antibodies, 207, 340
  in immune regulation, 207
  as possible vaccines, 258
  in tumor immunotherapy, 340
Anti-inflammatory agents corticosteroids, 210, 310
Anti-isotype antibody, 90
Anti-TAC antibody, 311, 354
APC's *see* Antigen presenting cells
APL see also altered peptide ligand, 169, 317
Apoptosis *see also* Programmed cell death, 160
Arthus reaction, 292
Aspergillus fumigatus, 16
Asthma, 287
  allergic, 286
  and anaphylaxis, 284-286
  early and late response, 287
  intrinsic, 287
Athymic (nude) mice, 360
Atopic dermatitis, 288
Atopic urticaria, 288
Atopy *see also* Allergy
  Localized anaphylaxis, 286
Attenuation of organisms, for vaccines, 245, 248

Autoantibodies, 352
  Goodpasture's syndrome, 347
  Grave's disease, 347
  Hashimoto's thyroiditis, 346
  hemolytic anemia, 346
  rheumatoid arthritis, 348
  systemic lupus erythematosus, 348
  thrombocytopenia, 351
Autocrine action, by cytokines, 214
Autograft, 298
Autoimmune hemolytic anemia, 346
Autoimmunity, 345
  Association with MHC, 351
  $CD4^+$, role in, 351
  and defects in antigen processing, 351
  defined, 345
  diseases, organ specific, 345-347
    Goodpasture's syndrome, 347
    Grave's disease, 347
    Hashimoto's thyroiditis, 346
    hemolytic anemia, 346
    insulin-dependent diabetes mellitus, 347
    myasthenia gravis, 347
    pernicious anemia, 347
  diseases, systemic, 348
    multiple sclerosis, 348
    rheumatoid arthritis, 348
    Systemic lupus erythematosus, 348
    environmental, 349
  genetic factors, 348
  mechanisms of, 349-352
  inappropriate class II MHC expression, 350
  molecular mimicry, 350
  polyclonal B-cell activation, 351
  role of heat shock proteins, 350
  T-cell receptors and V genes in, 352
  T_H1/T_H2 balance, role in,
  treatment of, 353-388
  current therapies, 353, 354
  experimental approaches, 354
  monoclonal antibodies, 354
  peptide blockage of MHC, 353
  T-cell vaccination, 353
  tolerance induction by oral antigens, 354
Autologous transplantation, 298
Avidity, of antigen-antibody binding, 101, 102

Azathioprine (Imuran), 309

B7, 41, 167, 168, 171
B220, 41
Bacillus Calmette-Guerin (BCG), 30, 248
  attenuated, vaccine for tuberculosis, 30, 248
  in cancer immunotherapy, 337
Bacteria, 248
  cell wall antigens, 29, 249-251
  diphtheria, 29, 247
  exotoxins, 29, 252
  humoral response to
  infection, 268, 269
    extracellular, 267
    intracellular, 267
  molecular mimicry, 350
Bacterial septic shock, 232
Bacterial toxic shock, 232
Bare-lymphocyte syndrome, 80, 361
Basal light zone, 153
Basophils, 47, 281
  in type-I hypersensitivity, 281
B-cells, 40, 50, 52, 143-153
  activation of, 143-148
    B-cell coreceptor complex, 145-147, 183-187
    origin of activating signals, 146
    role of CD40/CD40L, 152, 187, 188
    role of T_H cells, 151
    by thymus-dependent antigens, 146
    by thymus-independent antigens, 146
    transduction of activating signals, 147
    in vivo sites for, 152
  affinity maturation, 153
  antigen-dependent phase, 143
  antigenic commitment, 151, 153, 154
  antigen-independent phase, 143
  antigen presentation by, 151, 152
    in T-cell activation, 170
  clonal selection, 168
  development
    overview, 144-150
    regulation of, 154
  differentiation of, 153
    affinity maturation, 153
    antigen selection of high-affinity centrocytes, 152-153

class switching, 154
plasma cells or memory B cells, 154
role of cytokines, 152
somatic hypermutation in, 154
in vivo sites for, 152
effector B cells, 40, 50, 152, 153
immature, 143, 145
immunocompetent, 143, 146
immunodeficiencies of, 359
in lymph nodes, 52
maturation of, 143-146
bone marrow environment, 143
Ig-gene rearrangements, 143, 144
negative selection, 145, 146
pre-B cell receptor, 143, 144
rescue by editing light-chain genes, 143-145
selection of immature self-reactive B cells, 145
mature, 144
memory B cells, 50, 154, 155,
generation of, 154-155
membrane markers of, 155
properties of, 154, 155
molecules on membrane of, 50
naive, 143, 154
proliferation of (clonal expansion), 146, 152, 153
in humoral response, 152-153
negative selection of mature self-reactive B cells, 145
in vivo sites for, 152
regulation of development, 154
T$_H$ cells, collaboration with,
transcription factors, in development of, 146, 151, 152
B-cell coreceptor complex, 145-147, 150, 183-187
B-cell receptor (BCR), 183
in B-cell activation, 147-150
formation of, 143, 144
Beta sheet peptides, 15
BCG *see* Bacillus Calmette-Guerin
Bcl-2, 211
Blocking antibody, 289, 312
Blood *see also* ABO blood group
ABO blood-group antigens, 17
transfusion reaction, 290
typing blood cells, 17
B lymphocytes, See B cells

Bone marrow, 50
B cell maturation in 143-144
in severe combined immuno-deficiency disease, 361
stromal cells, 144
transplantation of, 308, 312
Bordatella pertussis, 268, 269
Bradykinin, 24, 284
Breast milk, immune benefits of, 14, 15

Candida albicans, 16, 243
C1-C9 complement components. *See* Complement system
Calnexin, 193
Cathelicidins, 16
CAM's. *See* Cell Adhesion Molecules
Cancer, *See also* Tumors
immune response to, 326-327, 334-336
immune surveillance theory, 336
immunotherapy, 337-343
adjuvants, 68, 337
cytokine therapy, 342-343
enhancement of APC activity, 339
interferons, 343
TIL cells, 339
manipulation of co-stimulatory signal, 339
monoclonal antibodies, 340, 341
tumor-cell vaccines, 336-342
tumor necrosis factors, 340, 342
tumor antigens. *See* Tumor antigens, 327-334
Carcinoembryonic antigen (CEA), 333
Carcinomas, 326
Carriers, hapten, 69-70
Cascade reaction, 234
CD (cluster differentiation) antigens, 40
CD2, as accessory membrane molecule, 179, 181, 182
CD3, 42, 178
ITAM motif in, 147, 149, 179
role in signal transduction, 147, 149, 179
structure of, 179
TCR-CD3 membrane complex, 162, 178
CD4, 42, 155, 156-162
in antigen recognition and T-cell activation, 156-160
binding to class II MHC molecules, 179-182
as coreceptor, 179

expression of, 156-159
structure of, 180
in thymic selection of T-cells, 156-159
CD4⁺ T cells *See also* T helper cells
in cell mediated immunity, 45, 156-162
CD4⁺8⁺ (double positive state), 156-159
CD8, 42, 155, 156-162
in antigen recognition and T-cell activation, 156-160
binding to class I MHC molecule, 179-182
as coreceptor, 179
expression of, 156-159
functions of, 180
structure of, 180
in thymic selection of T cells, 156-159
CD8⁺ *See also* T cytotoxic cells
in cell mediated immunity,
CD19, 184, 186
CD21, 41, 186
CD22, 183, 186,
CD25, 156
CD27, 160
CD28, 42, 167, 168, 179, 182
in T-cell activation, 168, 183
CD30, 160
CD32 (FceR II), 183
CD35 (CR1), 41
CD40, 186-188
CD40/CD40L, 186-188
in B cell activation, 188
and class switching, 154
CD44, 156
CD45, 42
CD45R, in T cell activation, 167-170
CD81, 184
CD117, 160
CDR's *See* Complementarity determining regions,
CEA (Carcinoembryonic antigen), 333
Cell adhesion molecules, 197
effector T cells, 197
Immunoglobulin superfamily, 173
integrin family, 197
interactions of, 197
in lymphocyte extravasation, 23
selectin family, 197
Cell lysis, by complement, 240, 241, 224
Cell mediated immunity, 197

CD4+ T cells in, 197
CD8+ T cells in, 198
clonal proliferation of T cells, 167
delayed-type hypersensitivity *See also* Delayed-type hypersensitivity, 294, 295
direct cytotoxic response *See also* Cytotoxicity; Cytotoxic T lymphocytes, 198
effector responses in, 198-200
generation of the response, 198
to intracellular pathogens, 198
in viral infections, 261
Centroblast, 152
Centrocytes, 152, 153
high-affinity, selection by antigen, 152, 153
Cercariae, 275
CGD (Chronic Granulomatous Disease), 356, 358
Chaga's Disease, 232
Chemokines, 214, 220-222
C-C subgroup, 221
C-X-C subgroup, 221-222
as mediators of inflammation, 222
Chemotactic defects, 358
Chemotaxis, 243
Chronic Granulomatous disease (CGD), 356, 358
CIITA, an MHC trans activator, 80
Circulating dendritic cells, 48
Circumsporozoite (CS) antigen, 270-272
c-Kit, 216, 217
Class I MHC molecules *See* Major histocompatibility complex
Class Ib MHC molecules *See* Major histocompatibility complex
Class II MHC molecules *See* Major histocompatibility complex
Class III MHC molecules *See* Major histocompatibility complex
Class (isotope) switching, among immunoglobulin genes, 136
CLIP (class II-associated invariant chain peptide), 195
Clonal anergy, 169
Clonal deletion, of immature B cells, 314
Clonal expansion, of TH cells, 167
Clonal selection theory of, 314
Cloning vectors, 253, 254
Clostridium tetani, 28
Cluster of differentiation (CD), antigens, 40

Colony- stimulating factors (CSF's), 216
  granulocyte (G-CSF), 218
  granulocyte-macrophage (GM-CSF), 216
  macrophage (M-CSF), 217
  multilineage (Multi-CSF or IL-3), 216
Colostrum, 27
Combinatorial joining, 133
Common variable hypogammaglobulinemia (CVH), 357, 359
Competence signals, 146
  effective, 146-150
  signal-1, 146
  signal-2, 146
Complement system, 234-244
  activation of, 235
  alternative pathway, 17, 18, 237
    components involved in, 235-241
    initiators of, 235
  amplification step, 248
  biological roles, 241-243
    cell lysis, 240, 241
    inflammatory response, 242, 243
    opsonization, 241
    solubilization of complexes, 242
    viral neutralization, 237
  bound C5b, 236
  C3 convertase, 237
  C5 convertase, 262
  classical pathway, 235
    initial-stage components, 235
  deficiencies and diseases, 243, 244
  "innocent-bystander" lysis, 240
  membrane-attack complex (MAC), 240, 243
  in cell lysis, 242
  components involved in formation of, 235
  structure of, 235
  poly C-9 complex, 241
    decay-accelerating factor (DAF), 17
    Factor H, 17, 237
    Factor I, 17, 237
    membrane cofactor protein (MCP), 17
Complementarity-determining regions (CDR's), 88
  and antigen binding, 88
  in immunoglobulins, 88
Complement fixation test, 112
Congenital thymic aplasia *See* DiGeorge syndrome

Constant (C) region, 86-89
  of antibody heavy chains, 87, 88
  of antibody light chains, 86
  domains of
  kappa sequence, 86
  lambda sequence, 86
Coomb's test, 111
Coreceptors, 145-147, 150, 178-180, 183-187
Cornea transplants, 307
Cortex of lymph node, 52, 53
Cortex of thymus, 49, 50
Corticosteroids, 210
  as anti-inflammatory agents, 210, 310
  in graft survival, 310
Cortisone, for Type I hypersensitivity, 290
Co-stimulatory signal, 167
  blocking of, for graft survival, 312
  in cancer immunotherapy, 344
  lack of, and tumor growth, 344
  in T_H-cell activation, 167, 168
Cross-reactivity
  of antigen-antibody reactions, 69, 70, 102
  of haptens, 69
Cross- regulation, by cytokines, 283
CSF. *See* Colony-stimulating factors
CTL's *See* Cytotoxic T lymphocytes
CTL precursors (CTL-P's), 199, 339
CTLA-4, 167, 168, 338
Curschmann's spirals, 288
Cutaneous-associated lymphoid tissue, 61
Cyclophosphamide, 309
Cyclosporin A, 310
  in graft survival, 310
  negative side effects, 310
  to treat autoimmunity, 311
Cytokines *See also* Interleukins,
  antagonism, 215
  antagonists, 215
  in antiviral defense, 229
  autocrine action by, 214
  in B-cell differentiation, 154
  in cancer immunotherapy, 342
  in delayed-type hypersensitivity, 295
  bacterial toxic shock, 232
  Chaga's disease, 232
  effect on MHC expression, 80

in graft rejection or survival, 305
as inflammatory mediators, 228-232
in neural or endocrine responses, 208-210
overproduction, toxic syndromes from, 234
paracrine action by, 214
pleiotropic action by, 215
properties of, 215
redundant, 215
secretion by T_H subsets, 222
synergism, 215
in Type I hypersensitivity, 281, 284
Cytomegalovirus (CMV), 265, effect on MHC
expression, 265
Cytosolic processing pathway, 191-193
assembly of peptides with class I MHC, 192, 193
overview, 191
peptide generation by proteasomes, 191-197
peptide transport from cytosol to RER, 192
Cytotoxicity, cell-mediated
in allograft rejection, 305
antibody-dependent, 201, 305
CTL-mediated, 198, 199, 305
NK cell- mediated, 220, 302
Cytotoxic T lymphocytes (CTL's), 198, 199, 305
in altered self-cell elimination, 334, 335, 339
in antiviral defense, 262, 263
in cell-mediated cytotoxicity, 198, 199
phase 1: generation of CTL's, 198
phase 2: destruction of target cells, 199
CTL- target cell conjugate,
in graft rejection, 305
intracellular antigen elimination by, 262, 263
MHC restriction of, 190

D (diversity) gene segment, 127
DAF (decay-accelerating factor), 17
DAG, 148, 149, 164
Decay accelerating factor (DAF), 17
Defensins, 15, 16
Degranulation of mast cells and basophils, 47, 97, 279, 281
intracellular events leading to, 283
receptor cross linkage, 97, 279
Delayed- type hypersensitivity (DTH), 294-296
activated macrophages in, 294-296
in allograft rejection, 304, 305

antigen-presenting cells in, 294
in autoimmunity, 346, 347
cytokines involved in, 295
detection of, 296
effector phase, 295
endothelial cells in, 295
granulomatous reaction, 295
sensitization phase, 294
skin test reaction, 296
T_{DTH}- mediated (Type IV), 294-296
T_H1 cells in, 294
in tuberculosis, 245
Dendritic cells, 48
as antigen-presenting cells, 48
follicular dendritic cells, 48
interdigitating dendritic cells, 48
interstitial dendritic cells, 48
Langerhans cells, 48
veiled cells, 61
Dermis, 61
Determinant-selection model, 81
Diabetes mellitus
insulin-dependent (IDDM) *See* insulin dependent
diabetes mellitus, 347
Diapedesis, 23
DiGeorge syndrome, 357
Diphtheria
exotoxin, 29, 247
toxoid vaccine for, 29, 252
Direct plaque-forming cells (PFC) assay, 120
Diversity
of antibodies, generation of, 127-139
of T-cell receptor, 174-178
Diversity (D) gene segment, 127-139
DNA
vaccines, 254
exons and introns, 128, 129
in immunoglobulin genes, 127-139
in immunoglobulin gene transcription, 138-139
leader sequence, 138
rearrangement of
in immunoglobulin genes, 126-132
in T-cell receptor genes, 174-178
recognition signal sequences, 139-141
Domains
in immunoglobulins, 87

of MHC molecule, 75, 80
of T-cell receptor, 174-178
Double-negative thymocytes, 156
Double-positive state (CD4⁺8⁺), 156
Dryer and Bennett model, of Ig genes, 123
DTH. *See* Delayed-type hypersensitivity

EAE. *See* Experimental autoimmune encephalomyelitis, 353
Early genes, 162
EBV (Epstein- Barr virus), 243, 265, 336
Eczema, allergic, 288
Edema (swelling), 24, 288
Edmonston-Zagreb strain, 249
E. coli, 251
Effector cells *See also* Effector response
    B cells, 40, 50, 52, 143-153
    in cell-mediated immunity, 197
    T-cells, 197
        activation requirements, 162- 167
        cell-adhesion molecules, 197
        effector molecules, 198-200
        functions of, 42, 160
        properties of
        T_H1, T_H2 subsets, 42, 228-232
Effector response
    in cell-mediated branch, 197-199
    in humoral branch, 204
    regulation of, 206
ELISA (enzyme- linked immunosorbent assay), 116
Elispot assay, 120
Encephalomyelitis, experimental autoimmune (EAE), 353
Endocrine action, by cytokines, 216
Endocytic processing pathway, 193-195
    assembly of peptides with class I MHC, 192
    class II MHC transport to endocytic vesicles, 193-195
    overview of peptide generation, 191
Endocytosis, 19, 45
Endogenous antigens *See also* cytosolic pathway, 191-193
Endosomes, 19, 45
Enhancer sequences
    in immunoglobulin genes, 139
Enterobacter aerogenes, 232

Enzyme- linked immunosorbent assay. *See* ELISA
Eosinophil chemotactic factor (ECF), 282
Eosinophils, 47, 274
    in antibody-dependent-cell-mediated cytotoxicity, 201, 305
    in asthma, 287, 288
    in late-phase reaction, 288, 289
Epidermis, 61
Epinephrine, in treatment of anaphylaxis, 290
Epithelial cells, in thymic selection, 159-161
Epitopes *See also* Antigens
    B-cell epitopes, 183-187
    T-cell epitopes, 173-183
    antigen processing, 190
    immunodominance, 69
    trimolecular complex: TCR/peptide/ MHC, 180, 181
Epstein-Barr virus (EBV), 243, 265, 336
Escherichia coli, 251
Exocytosis, 19
Exogenous antigen, *See also*
    endocytic pathway, 193-195
Exons
    in immunoglobulin genes, 126-137
    in T-cell receptor genes, 176-178
Exotoxins, 29, 247
Experimental autoimmune encephalyelitis (EAE), 353
    myelin basic protein in, 353
    T-cell vaccination for, 353
    T_H role in, 353
Extravasation, 29, 274
    defined, 29
    of lymphocytes *See also* lymphocytes, extravasation of
    of neutrophils, 29, 274

Fab fragments, 86
Factor B, in compliment system, 17, 18, 237
Factor D, in compliment system, 17, 18, 237
Factor H, in compliment system, 17, 18, 237
Factor I, in compliment system, 17, 18, 237
Fc fragment, crystalline, 86
Fc receptors, 92, 98, 279, 281
    in Type I hypersensitivity, 281
FcgRII (CD32), 183

Flourescein, 116
Follicular dendritic cells, 48
Framework regions (FRs), 88
Freund's adjuvants, complete and
    incomplete, 68

Gamma-globulin, 85
Gell and Coomb's classification of
    hypersensitivity, 277
Gene therapy,
    with engineered stem cells,
    for SCID, 362
Germinal center, 51-54
    formation of, 51-54
    in lymph node structure, 51-53
    in somatic hypermutation, 136, 145
    in splenic structure, 53-54
Germ line, 123
Germ-line model, of Ig genes, 123
Glomerulonephritis, and
complement deficiencies, 243
GM-CSF, *See* granulocyte-macrophage colony
    stimulating
Goiter, 346
Goondpasture's syndrome, 347
Graft rejection, *See also* Transplantation, 298
    allograft, defined, 299
    autograft, defined, 298
    cell-mediated responses, 304-306
    clinical manifestations,
        acute rejection, 300
        chronic rejection, 300
        hyperacute rejection, 300
    first set rejection, 299
    immunologic basis of, 299-301
    immunosuppressive therapy, general, 308
        corticosteroids, 310
        cyclosporin A, FK506, 310
        rapamycin, 310
        mitotic inhibitors, 309
        total lymphoid irradiation, 309
    immunosuppressive therapy, specific, 311
        blocking co-stimulatory signal, 312
        donor-cell microchimerism, 312
        monoclonal antibodies, 311
    isograft defined, 299

mechanism in, 304, 305
    effector stage, 305
    passenger leukocytes, 305, 306
    sensitization stage, 304
role of MHC in, 301-303
second set rejection, 299
tissue typing, 301, 302
    major histocompatibility antigens, 301
    minor histocompatibility antigens, 82, 83, 301
xenograft defined, 299
Graft versus host disease (GVHD),
    in bone marrow transplantation, 302
    natural killer cells, 302
Granulocyte, 45
Granulocyte colony-stimulating
    factor (G-CSF), 218
    and congenital agranulocytosis, 357
Granulocyte macrophage colony-
stimulating factor (GM-CSF), 216
    secretion by T_H subsets, 222
Granulocytopenia, 357
Granuloma, 295
Granzymes, 199
Grave's disease, 347
    autoantibodies, role in, 352
    long-acting thyroid-stimulating antibodies, 352
Growth factor, *See also* Cytokines,
GVH, *See* Graft versus-host disease

Haemophilus influenzae, 29, 269, 249-251
Haemolin, 6
Haplotypes, MHC, 73
Haptens, 69
    and antigenicity, 69
    cross-reactions of, 70
    defined, 69
    hapten carrier conjugate, 69
    humoral response to, 69-71
    as immunodominant determinant, 69, 70
Hashimoto's thyroiditis, 346
Hay fever, 286
HCG pregnancy test, 111
Heart transplants, 308
Heat-shock proteins, 22,
    in autoimmunity, 350
    molecular mimicry of, 350

Heavy (H) chains of
  immunoglobulins, *See* Immunoglobulins, heavy
  chains
Helminthic infections,
  See also Schistosomiasis,
Hemagglutination test,
  Passive, 111
Hemolytic anemia,
  autoimmune, 347
  drug induced, 346
Hemolytic disease of newborn, 291
Hemolytic plaque assays, 120
Herpes simplex, 253, 254
Heteroconjugate antibodies, 341
Hinge region, 89
  flexibility, 89
  in immunoglobulin heavy chains, 89
Histamine, 24, 282
Histatins, 16
Histiocytes, 72
Histocompatibility, 72
Histocompatibilitiy antigens, 72
Histocompatibilitiy genes, *See also*
  major Histocompatibity Complex, 72, 73
HLA complex (in humans), *See*
  also Major Histocompatibity Complex, 72, 73
HLA-DM, 195
HLA-typing, 301-303
Holes-in-the-repertoire model, 81
Hormones
  in T-cell maturation in thymus, 160-163
Human immunodeficiency virus (HIV). 263-265
Human T-lymphotropic virus –1
(HTLV-1), 332
Humoral immune response, 204
  affinity maturation, 153
  B-cell activation, 143-148
  class switching in, 154
  contact-dependent help and CD40-CD40L interaction, 188
  Elispot assay, 120
  hemolytic plaque assays, 120
  to extracellular pathogens, 268
  generation of, 204
  to hapten-carrier conjugates, 69
  immediate hypersensitivity, 290, 291

lag phase, 204
primary response, 204
role of T_H cells in, 151
secondary response, 204
T-B conjugate formation, 151, 152
viral neutralization, 261-263
in vivo site for induction of, 152
Humoral deficiencies, 359
Hypersensitivity, 277
  defined, 277
  delayed type. *See* Delayed-type hypersensitivity,
  immediate. *See* Immediate hypersensitivity,
Hypervariable (HV) regions, 88

IDDL. *See* Insulin -dependent diabetes mellitus
Identity of antigens, 63-67, 105
Idiotope, 91, 92, 207
Idiotypes, 91, 92, 207
  and network theory, 207
In regulation of immune response, 207
IFNs. *See* Interferons
Ig. *See* Immunoglobulins
Ig-α/ Ig-β heterodimer
IgA. *See* Immunoglobulin A
IgD. *See* Immunoglobulin D
IgE. *See* Immunoglobulin E
IgG. *See* Immunoglobulin G
IgM *See* Immunoglobulin M
IL1- IL. *See* Interleukins
Immature B-cells, 143, 144
Immediate hypersensitivity, 277, 290, 291
  antibody-mediated cytotoxic (type II), 201, 305
    drug induced hemolytic anemia, 346
    hemolytic disease of newborn, 291
    transfusion reactions, 290
  Gel and Coomb's classification, 277
  IgE mediated (Type I), 97, 278-284
    allergens, 279, 286
    anaphylaxis, 285
    atopy, 286
    components, 282-284
    consequences of, 284, 285
    cytokines, role of, 284
    degranulation, mechanism of, 279
    IgE-binding Fc receptors, 279
    late-phase reaction, 288

mast cells and basophils, 281
    mediators of, 282-284
    reagenic antibody (IgE), 97, 278-284
    therapy for, 289, 290
Immune complex-mediated (Type III)
    Arthus reaction, 291
    complement proteins in, 292
    generalized reactions, 292
    localized reactions, 292
    serum sickness, 292
    in SLE and rheumatoid arthritis, 348
Immune complexes, 242
    deposition of, 243
    formation of, 101, 242, 243
    illness associated with, 348
    in regulation of immune response, 207
    solubilzation of, by complement, 242
    in Systemic Lupus Erythematosus, 348
    in Type III hypersensitivity, 291
Immune response
    cell- mediated. *See* Cell-mediated immunity
    humoral. *See* Humoral response
Immune responsiveness, 69
    MHC, and, 72-75
Immune surveillance theory, 336
Immunity
    acquired (specific), 27
    cell-mediated. *See* cell-mediated immunity,
    humoral. *See* humoral immune response
    innate (nonspecific), 13-26
    mucosal, 14, 54-60
    neonatal, 14
    protective, 13-26
    to tumors, 326, 327, 334-336
Immunization. *See also* vaccines
    active, 29-31
    passive, 27, 29
Immunoassays, sensitivity of, 114
Immunodeficiencies, 355-363
    cell-mediated deficiency
        DiGeorge syndrome, 357, 360
        Nude mice, 360
    combined deficiencies
        bare lymphocyte syndrome, 361
        reticular dysgenesis, 361

severe combined immunodeficiency (SCID),
    361, 362
        Wiskott-Aldrich syndrome, 363
        X-linked severe combined immunodeficiency
        (XSCID), 359
    complement deficiencies, 243
    congenital, 361
    humoral deficiencies, 359
        common variable hypogammaglobulinemia
        (CVH), 359
        selective IgA deficiency, 359
        X-linked agammaglobulinemia (XLA), 359
        X-linked hyper IgM syndrome, 359
    phagocytic deficiencies, 355
        adherence defects, 358
        chemotactic defects, 358
        killing defects, 358
        neutropenia, 357, 358
Immunodiffusion reactions
    double (Ouchterlony's method), 103
    radial (Mansinis method), 105
Immunodominance, 64, 69
Immunodominant determinant, 64, 69
Immunodominant epitopes, 64, 69
Immunoelectrophoresis, 109
    countercurrent, 108
    rocket, 105
    two-dimensional, 106
Immunofluorescence, 116
    direct staining, 117
    indirect staining, 118
Immunogen. *See also* Antigens
Immunogenicity versus antigenicity, 63
    defined, 63
    factors influencing, 64-67
Immunoglobulins (Ig), 92, 93
    antigen binding site, 88
    antigenic determinants on
        allotypic, 90
        idiotypic, 91
        isotypic, 90
    Classes
        IgA. *See* Immunoglobulin A
        IgD. *See* Immunoglobulin D
        IgE. *See* Immunoglobulin E

IgG. *See* Immunoglobulin G
IgM. *See* Immunoglobulin M
complementarity determining regions, 88
constant (C) region, 88-89
diversity, generation of, 127-139
domains, 88
    Constant region domain structure, 88, 89
immunoglobulin fold, 87
variable region domain structure, 88
expression and gene rearrangement, 126-132
framework regions, 88
heavy (H) chains sequencing, 87
hinge region, flexibility at, 89
hypervariable regions, 88
isotypes, 90
light (L) chains sequencing, 86
membrane bound, 89, 97
pathogen elimination, mechanisms of, 267, 274
secreted, 15, 58, 94-97
structure, 85-89
synthesis of, 138, 139
variable (V) region, 88
viral neutralization by, 261
Immunoglobulin A (IgA), 15, 58, 94-97
in colostrum, 15
in defense against bacteria, 94-97
in defense against viruses, 94-97
in mucosal immunity, 58, 94-97
polio vaccine, 31, 248
poly-Ig receptor, 97
secretory component, 96, 97
secretory IgA, 94-97
selective IgA deficiency, 360
structure of, 95
Immunoglobulin D (IgD)
structure, 97-98
and IgM coexpression of, 97
and function of, 97-99
Immunoglobulin E (IgE), 97
in allergic reaction, 97, 278-289
determining serum level of, 114, 115
Fc receptors for, 92, 98, 279, 281
identification of, 114, 115
IL-4 in synthesis of, 225
immediate hypersensitivity, 278-289
As mediator of degranulation, 97, 279, 281

Prausnitz- Kustner (PK) reaction, 280, 281
helminth infection, 274
Immunoglobulin G (IgG)
as an opsonin, 44, 92, 241
as blocking antibody, 289, 312
in complement activation, 92
in delayed transfusion reactions, 291
Fc receptor binding, 92, 351
in neonatal immunity, 27, 92
in rheumatoid arthritis, 348
in secondary response, 204
subclasses, 92
in Type I hypersensitivity, 278, 279
Immunoglobulin genes, 127-139
allelic exclusion, 131
class switching, 136
diversity, generation of, 127-139
    association of heavy and light chains, 135
    combinatorial joining, 133, 135
    junctional flexibility, 134
    multiple germ-line genes, 133
    N-region nucleotide addition, 135
    P-nucleotide addition, 135
    somatic hypermutation, 136
expression of, 138
genetic models, 123
    Dryer and Bennet two-gene model, 123
    germ-line model, 123
multigene organization of
    heavy-chain multigene family, 125, 133
    kappa-chain multigene family, 124, 133
    lambda-chain multigene family, 125, 133
rearrangements, 126-130
    enzymatic joining of gene segments, 129
    mechanism, 128-130
    productive and non-productive, 131
    recombination signal sequences, 128
recombination-activating genes (RAG-1, RAG-2), 130, 175
RNA processing, 138
IgM and IgD, 138
membrane versus secreted immunoglobulin, 139
polyadenylation signal sequences, 138, 139
    somatic hypermutation, 136
    synthesis, assembly, secretion of immunoglobulins, 139, 140

transcription of, 139
  effect of DNA rearrangement, 129
  regulation of, 138-140
Immunoglobulin M (IgM), 93, 94
  agglutination, role in, 93, 94
  in complement activation, 93, 94
  high valency, 94
  and IgD, co-expression of, 99, 145
  isohemagglutinins, 93, 94
  J (joining) chain, 93
  in mucosal immunity, 93
  pentameric, 93, 94
    in primary response, 204
    in response to TI antigens, 146
    as rheumatoid factor, 348
    X-linked hyper-IgM syndrome, 359
Immunoglobulin superfamily, 173
  cell-adhesion molecules, 197
Immunologically privileged sites, 307
Immunologic memory, 210-213
  initial generation, 210
  during primary response, 210
    turnover and lifespan, 211
    migratory property, 211
  factors controlling survival of memory cells, 212
    role of specific antigen, 212
    cell to cell communication, 212
    B cells in T cell memory, 212
    CD4⁺ and CD8⁺ cells in memory, 213
    CD4⁺ cells in B cell memory, 213
Immunologic unresponsiveness. *See* Tolerance
Immunoreceptor tyrosine-based activation motif
    (ITAM), 147, 149, 179
Immunostimulating complexes (ISCOMs), 256-258
Immunosupression, 308-310
  Chagas' disease, 232
  for graft acceptance, 308-310
  by hydrocortisone, 310
  by viruses, 264-266
Immunosuppressive therapy, 311
  for transplantation, 311-314
Immunotherapy
  of cancer, 337-343
  of Type I hypersensitivities, 289
Immunotoxins, 256
  preparation of, 256

  in tumor immunotherapy, 337-343
Incomplete antibodies, 111
Indirect hemolytic plaque assay, 120
Infections
  bacterial, 267-268
    evasion of host defense, 269
    extracellular, 267
    immune response to intracellular, 267
    tuberculosis. *See also* M*ycobacterium tuberculosis*
  death due to, 268
  helminthes (*Schistosoma*), 273
    malaria, 272
    Trypanosoma, 273
  viral. *See also* Viruses
    cell-mediated response, 261
    evasion of host defense, 264
    neutralization by antibody, 261
Inflammation, defined, 22
Inflammatory response, 22, 279-285
  acute response, 23
    role of IFN-g and TNF-a, 219, 229
  complement system in, 243
  cytokines in, 219, 228-230
  extravasation in, 22
  fever response, 22
  mediators of, 22, 228-230
    chemokines, 220-222
    Cytokine inflammatory
      mediators, 228-230
    lipid inflammatory
      mediators, 284
    neutrophils, role in, 22
Innate immunity, 13-26
  anatomic barriers, 14, 15
  endocytosis, 19
  inflammatory response, 22
  phagocytosis, 20
  physiological barriers, 16
"Innocent-bystander" lysis, 240
Insulin-dependant diabetes mellitus (IDDM), 347
  heat-shock proteins and molecular mimicry in, 22,
    350
Integrins, 197
  adhesion defect (LAD), 358
Interdigitating dendritic cells, 48

Interferons (IFNs), 21, 218, 229
  in antiviral defense, 21, 218, 229
  in cancer immunotherapy, 218, 229, 337-343
  effect of MHC expression, 218, 229
  functions of, 21, 218, 229
  interferon alpha, 21, 218
  interferon beta, 21, 218
  interferon gamma, 21, 229
    in autoimmunity, 347, 351, 352
    effect on IgE production, 278-284
    effect on macrophages, 43
    in inflammatory response, 22, 219, 229, 279-285
    In response to mycobacterium, 268
    stimulation of NK cells by, 229
Interleukin(s)
  interleukin-1 (IL-1), 220
    in bacterial septic shock, 232
    biological functions of, 220
    expression of cell adhesion molecules by, 220
    in inflammatory response, 220, 229
    in toxic shock syndrome, 232
  interleukin-2 (IL-2), 223
    biological functions of, 223
    in clonal proliferation of T-cells, 167, 223
    in CTL-mediated cytotoxicity, 199-201
    expression by activated T-cell, 167, 168
    role in T_H cell activation, 167, 168
  interleukin-3 (IL-3), 216
    biological functions of, 216,
    Secretion of T_H subsets, 216,
  interleukin-4 (IL-4), 223
    biological functions of, 223
    in class switching, 223
    in IgE synthesis, 224
  in regulating Type I response, 223-227
  in T_H – subset response, 223-227
  interleukin-5 (IL-5), biological functions of, 230
  interleukin-6 (IL-6), 220
    biological functions of, 220
    in inflammatory response, 220
    in myeloma proliferation, 220
  interleukin-7 (IL-7), biological
    functions of, 218
  interleukin-10 (IL-10)
    biological function of, 230
  interleukin-12 (IL-12)

biological functions of, 232
  stimulation of NK cells by, 232
  in T_H –subset response, 232
Interstitial dendritic cells, 48
Intestinal epithelial lymphocytes (IEL), 56
Intracellular pathogens, 267, 273
Intraepidermal lymphocytes, 56
Intraepithelial lymphocytes (IELs), 56
Introns, in immunoglobulin genes, 126-139
Invariant (Ii) chain, 194
Islets of Langerhans. *See* pancreatic islets
Isograft, 298
Isohemagglutinins, 17
Isotope switching. *See* class switching
Isotypes (classes), 90
ITAM (immunoreceptor tyrosine-based activation
  motif). 147, 149, 179

J (joining) chain, 93
J (joining) gene segment, 127-139
Junctional flexibility, 134
  in antibody diversity, 127-139
  in T-cell receptor diversity, 174-178

Kaposi's sarcoma, 336
Kappa sequence, 86, 124
Keratinocyte, 61
Keyhole limpet hemocyanin (KLH), 59
Kidney transplants, 307
Klebsiella pneumoniae, 232, 24
Kupffer cells, 43

LAD (Leukocyte-adhesion deficiency), 358
LAK (Lymphokine-activated killer cells), 339, 342
Lamina propria lymphocytes (LPL), 56
Lamina propria T cells (LTL), 56
Langerhans cells, 61
  in delayed-type hypersensitivity, 294
  Dendritic cells in graft rejection, 304
Late-phase reaction, in Type I hypersensitivity, 288
Lazy leukocyte syndrome, 356
LCMV(Lymphocytic choriomeningitis) virus, 262-264
Lectins, 237
Lectin pathway, 237
  in complement activation, 237
Leishmania majo, 270, 271
Leukocyte-adhesion deficiency (LAD), 358

Leukotrienes, 284

LFA-1, T-cell accessory membrane molecule, 179, 181, 182

Light (L) chains, of immunoglobulins. *See* immunoglobulins, light chains

Lipopolysaccharide (LPS), 24, 68, 146, 268
  in bacterial cell wall, 24, 268
  in resistance to complement-mediated lysis, 270
  as TI-1 antigens, 146

Liposomes, 256, 257

Listeria monocytogenes, 44, 226, 269

Liver transplants, 308

Long-acting thyroid-stimulating (LATS) antibodies, 347

LPL (Lamina propria lymphocytes), 56

LPS. *See* Lipopolysaccharides

LPT (Lamina propria T cells), 56

Lymph, 51

Lymphatic system, 51

Lymphatic vessels, 51

Lymph nodes, 52
  B-cells in, 52-54
  germinal centers, 52-54
  helper T-cells, 52-54
  humoral response in, 52-54
  lymphocyte proliferation in, 52-54
  primary follicle, 52-54
  secondary follicle, 52-54
  structure, 53

Lymphoblasts, 51, 52

Lymphocytes. *See also* T-cells; B-cells
  activation of, 143-148, 158-167
  effector and memory lymphocytes, 152-155, 170
  naive lymphocytes, 152, 157

Lymphocyte choriomeningitis virus (LCMV), 262-264

Lymphoid cells, 51, 52

Lymphoid follicles, 51-54

Lymphoid organs, 51-56
  primary, 49
  secondary, 51

Lymphokine-activated killer (LAK) cells, 339, 342
  in tumor immunotherapy, 342

Lymphokines, 214

Lysosomes, 14, 19, 21, 44

Lysozymes, 14, 19, 21, 44

MAC. *See* Membrane-attack complex

Macrophage(s), 19, 44
  activation of, 19, 44, 219, 220, 335
  in acute-phase inflammatory response, 23, 279-285
  as antigen presenting cells, 36, 190
  antimicrobial and cytotoxic activities, 19,
    oxygen-dependant killing, 19
    oxygen-independent killing, 20
  in antitumor immunity, 335
  in complement protein biosynthesis, 36, 235
  in delayed-type hypersensitivity, 294, 295
  differentiation from monocyte, 44
  effect of IFN-g on, 229
  fixed or free, 44
  interaction with T_H cells, 158-167
  names and locations of, 43
  phagocytosis, 20, 44
  secretion of factors, 44

Macrophage colony-stimulating factor (M-CSF), 44, 217

Macrophage inflammatory protein, 44, 221

Major and Minor histocompatibility complex. *See also* MHC restriction
  in acquired immune response,
  as antigen-presenting structures, 75, 76, 189-195
  in autoimmunity, 353
  in bare lymphocyte syndrome, 80, 361
  in cancer, 335, 343
  cellular distribution of, 80
  class I MHC, 75
    alpha chain, 75
    in antigen presentation of T_c
    cells, 75, 198, 199, 305
    association with a_2-microglobulin, 75
    cellular expression of, 80
    in cytosolic pathway, 191
    genes, 73, 77
    interaction with peptides, 75
    map of, 73, 77
    peptide binding cleft in, 75
    structure of, 75, 76
  class II MHC
    alpha beta chains, 75, 76
    in antigen presentation to T_H cells, 79
    association with invariant chain, 193

cellular expression of, 80
deficiency of, in bare lymphocyte syndrome, 80, 361
domains, 75, 76
in endocytic pathway, 193-195
genes, 73, 77
interaction with peptides, 79
map of, 75, 76
peptide-binding cleft in, 76
structure of, 75, 76
class III MHC, 79
complement components, 73
genes, 73
heat-shock proteins, 75
map of, 73
steroid 21-hydroxylase enzymes (21-OHA, 21-OHB), 79
tumor necrosis factor, 79
genes, 73
detailed genomic map of, 73, 86
haplotypes, 73
and immune responsiveness, 79, 80
determinant-selection model for, 81
holes-in-the-repertoire model for, 81
in infectious diseases, 81
MHC regions, location and function, 80
organization and inheritance of, 82-84
peptide binding by, 76
polymorphism of, 73-75, 79
regulation of MHC expression, 80
effect of cytokines and interferons, 81, 218, 229
effect of viruses, 264, 265
Malaria, 272
Circumsporozoite (CS) antigen, 272
immune response to, 272
vaccines, 272
MALT (mucosal-associated lymphoid tissue), 54, 55
Mancini assay, 105
Marginal zone of spleen, 54
Mast cells, 47, 97, 279, 281
degranulation of, 47, 97, 279, 281
in Type I hypersensitivity, 279, 281
in innate immunity, 24
Mature B cells, 144
MBP. *See* Myelin basic protein
M cells, 55

MCP (monocyte chemotactic protein, 221
Measles
vaccine for, 29, 31, 246, 247
Medulla of lymph node, 52-54
Medulla of thymus, 49, 50, 315-322
Melanomas
TATAs (antigens) on, 328
Membrane-attack complex (MAC), 240, 243
Membrane-bound immunoglobulin (mIg), 89, 97
in B-cell activation, 144-147
Membrane co-factor protein (MCP), 17
Memory cells
B-cells, 154-155, 204-205
formation of, in immunization, 204-205
T-cells, 170
Memory response, 210-213
Methotrexate, 309
Methyl cholanthren, as carcinogen, 328
MHC. *See* Major histocompatibility complex
MHC restriction, 182, 190
of T-cell receptor, 182, 190
in T-cell recognition of antigen, 182, 190
Micelles, 257
Microchimerism, in graft acceptance, 312
β_2-Microglobulin, 75, 77
mIg. *See* Membrane-bound immunoglobulin
Migration-inhibition factor (MIF), 295,
Minor histocompatibility loci, 82-84
minor H antigens as peptides, 82
graft rejection, 82
immunodominance, 83
identification, 83
genes, 83
minor H peptide encoded by, 83
mitochondrial genome, 83
Y-chromosome, 83
autosomal genes, 84
MIP (macrophage inflammatory protein), 44, 221
Mitogens
lectins, 203
lipopolysaccharides, 24, 68, 146, 268
polyclonal activators, 203, 205
Mitotic inhibitors, 309
Mixed-lymphocyte reaction (MLR), 203
Molecular chaperones, 192
Molecular mimicry, 350

Monoclonal antibodies, 311, 340, 341, 354
anti-idiotype, 340
in cancer immunotherapy, 340, 341
to treat auto-immune disease, 354
Monocyte(s), 43
Monocyte chemotactic and activating factor (MCAF), 295
Monokines, 21
Mononuclear phagocytic system, 43
Mucosal associated lymphoid tissue (MALT), 54, 55
Mucous membranes, 55
Mucous, 14, 15, 55
Multilineage colony stimulating factor (Multi-CSF or IL-3), 216
Multiple sclerosis (MS), 348
Myasthenia gravis, 347
Mycobacterium tuberculosis, 30, 44, 270, 296
and chronic DTH, 296
evasion of host defense, 270
inflammatory response to, 296
tuberculin skin test, 296
vaccine for, 30, 248
M. avium, 44, 270
M. bovis, 30, 248, 252, 270
M. leprae, 44, 270
Myelin basic protein (MBP)
In experimental autoimmune encephalomyelitis, 353
Molecular mimicry of, 350

Naive B-cells, 143
Naive T-cells, 156-159
Natural Killer (NK) cells
in cell- mediated cytotoxicity, 200-201
in innate, 22
characteristics of, 200
in Graft verses host reaction, 302
IL-12 stimulation of, 200
interferon stimulation of, 200, 229
lineage of, 200
mechanism of killing by, 201
receptors, 201
in tumor immunity, 327, 339, 343
in viral immunity, 22
Negative selection
of autoimmune self reactive B-cells, 152
of mature self reactive B-cells, 152
in Thymus, 160
Neisseria gonorrhoea, 44, 97, 243, 251, 252, 269
N. meningitides, 232, 250, 251, 269
Neoplasm. *See also* Tumors
Network theory, 207
Neuroendocrine regulation, 208-210
Neutropenia, 257
Neutrophils
in asthma, 287, 288
in chronic granulomatous disease (CGD), 358
extravasation, 29, 274
in innate immunity, 29
in late-phase reaction, 288, 289
role in inflammation, 29, 288
NK cells. *See* Natural Killer cells
Nippostorngylus brasiliensis, 226
N-nucleotides, 135
Non-classical MHC genes, 73, 77
Non-identity of antigens, 105
Non-self /self discrimination, 1
Non-specific immunity. *See* innate immunity
Normal flora, 2
Nude (athymic) mice, 360
Null cells, 43

Oncocerca lienalis, 275
Oncofetal tumor antigens, 333
Oncogenes, 331
encoding of tumor antigens by, 331
viral, 331
One-turn signal sequences, 128
One-turn/two turn joining rule, 129
Opsonins, 44, 92, 241
Opsonization
by antibody, 44, 92, 241
by complement system, 241
Ouchterlony immunodiffusion, 103
Origin of immune system in
invertebrate, 4
vertebrates, 7

PAF (platelet-activating factor), 288
Paneth cells, 16
Paracortex of lymph node, 52, 53
Paracrine action by cytokines, 214

Parasites. *See also* Schistosomiasis
  helminth infections, 273
  immune response to, 273
Parenteral administration of immunogen, 67
Partial agonist peptides, 169
Partial identity of antigens, 105
Passenger leukocytes, 304
Peptide binding cleft
  in class I MHC, 75
  in class II MHC, 76
Perforin, 199, 201
Peripheral gd T-cells, 171
Pernicious anemia, 347
Peyer's patches, 55
Phagocytes, 19, 44
Phagocytosis, 20, 44
  cells involved in, 19, 44
  complement proteins in, 19, 241
  in innate immunity, 19
  phagocytic deficiencies, 355
Phagolysosomes, 19, 44, 45
Phagosomes, 19, 44, 45
Physiologic barriers, 16
Phytohemagglutinin (PHA), 203
Pili, 252
Pinocytosis, 19
P-K reaction, 280, 281
Plasma cells, 154, 155
Plasmodium chaubadi, 272
Plasmodium falciparum, 270, 272, 276,
P. Malariae, 272
P. vivax, 272
Platelet activating factor (PAF), 288
Pleiotropic action by cytokines, 215
Pneumococcal pneumonia *See Streptococcus
  pneumoniae*
P-nucleotides, 135
Pokeweed mitogen (PWM), 205
Polio vaccine, 29, 30, 245, 249
Polyadenylation signal, 138, 139
Poly-A sites, 138, 139
Poly-C9 complex, 241
Polyclonal activators, 203, 205
Polyclonal antibody response, 85,
Poly-Ig receptor, 97
Polymorphism of MHC, 74

Polymorphonuclear leukocyte (PMN), 44, 45
Polysaccharides
  as immunogens, 29, 249, 250
  as vaccines, 29, 249, 250
Positive selection
  of B-cells, 154
  of T-cells in thymus, 160
Postcapillary venules of lymph node, 51
Pre-B cell (precursor B-cell), 143
Pre-B cell receptor, 143
Precipitins, 103
Precursor B-cells (pre-B cells), 143
Pregnancy test, 110
Pre-Ta, 158
Pre-T cell receptor (pre-TCR), 158
  effects of signal transduction by, 159
  structure of, 158
Primary follicle, 51, 52
Primary immune response, 204
Primary lymphoid organs, 49
Primary lysosomes, 19, 44, 454
Primary mediators, in Type I hypersensitivity, 282, 283
Pro-B cell (progenitor B cell), 143
Progenitor cells
  progenitor B-cell (pro-B cell), 143
  progenitor T-cell, 158
Programmed cell death, 160
Progression signals
  induced by T_H-cell cytokines, 167, 168
Proliferation of B-cells, 146
  in humoral immune response, 146
    of lymphocytes, in lymph nodes, 51, 52, 53
Promoter sequences
  associated with MHC genes, 73, 77
  in immmunoglobulin genes, 139
Properdin
  in complement system, 18, 237
  deficiency disorder, 244
ProPo (Prophenol oxidase), 5
Prostaglandins, 284
Proteasomes, 191
Protective immunity, 27
Proteins as immunogens, 65
Protein kinases (PTKs), 147, 162
Protozoan diseases
  African sleeping sickness, 274

malaria, 272
Prozone effect, 110
Pseudomonas aeruginosa, 251
Pseudopodia, 44, 45
Purified protein derivative (PPD), 205
Purine nucleoside phosphorylase (PNP), 362
    deficiency in SCID, 361, 362
PWM (Pokeweed mitogen), 205

Radial immunodiffusion, 105
Radioallergosorbent test (RAST), 114
Radioimmunoassay (RIA), 114
Radioimmunosorbent test (RIST), 114
RAG-1, RAG-2 (recombination-activating genes), 130, 175,
Rapamycin, in graft survival, 310
Reactive oxygen intermediates (ROIs), 19
Reaginic antibody, 97
Receptor-mediated endocytosis, 19
Recognition, 1
Recombination-activating genes (RAGs), 130, 175,
Recombination signal sequences (RSSs), 128
Red pulp, of spleen, 54
Regulation of immune effector response, 206
    antibody-mediated suppression, 207
    antigen-mediated, 207
        Idiotype: network theory
        By immune complexes, 207
        Neuroendocrine, 208
RER (Rough Endoplasmic reticulum), 192
Respiratory burst, 20
Response, 1
Reticular dysgenesis, 361
Rh antigen, 111, 291
Rheumatoid arthritis
    Rheumatoid factors, 348
    Role of heat-shock proteins, 350
Rhodamine, 116
Rhogam, 291
RIA. *See* Radioimmunoassay
RNA processing, 138, 139
Rocket immunoelectrophoresis, 105
Rough endoplasmic reticulum (RER), 192
Rubella, 30, 246, 247, 287

Salmonella typhi, 251, 254, 268
Sarcomas, 326

Schistosoma haematobium, 274
S. japonicum, 274
S. mansoni, 275
Schistosomiasis, 275
    cell-mediated DTH reaction to
    cercariae, 275
    immune response to
    schistosomules, 275
SCID *See* Severe combined immunodeficiency
    syndrome
Secondary follicle, 51, 52
Secondary immune response, 204
Secondary lymphoid organs, 51, 52
Secondary lysosomes, 19, 44, 45
Secreted immunoglobulin (sIg), 94-97
Secretory component, 96, 97
Secretory IgA, 94-97
Selective IgA deficiency, 360
Self-antigens, 64, 143-146, 158-162
Self-MHC restriction. *See* MHC restriction
Self/nonself discrimination, 1, 72
Self-reactive B cells. *See* Negative selection
Self-reactive lymphocytes, 145, 159
Self –tolerence, 160, 313
    of T- cells, 160
Sensitization, 294
Sequencing studies, of immunoglobulins. *See* Immuno-
    globulins, sequencing studies
Serotonin, 284
Serum sickness, 292
Severe combined immunodeficiency disease (SCID),
    361
    ADA-deficiency SCID, 362
    gene therapy for, 362
    PNP-deficiency SCID, 362
    X-linked SCID, 362
Sheep red blood cells (SRBCs), 112
Shigella sonnei, 251
S. flexneri, 251
Signal joint, 125, 126
Signal peptide, 125, 126
Silencer sequences, in immunoglobulin genes, 139
Single-positive CD4$^+$ thymocytes, 156-158
Single-positive CD8$^+$ thymocytes, 156-158
Skin
    as anatomic barrier, 14

SLE. *See* Systemic lupus erythematosus

Slow-reacting substance of anaphylaxis (SRS-A), 284

Smallpox
> eradication of, 245
> vaccine for, 245

Solid matrix-antibody-antigen (SMAA) complexes, 256

Somatic hypermutation
> in antibody diversity, 136, 145
> in immunoglobulin genes, 136, 145
> suggested mechanism, 136-140

Somatic-variation model, of Ig genes, 123

Specific immunity. *See* acquired immunity

Specificity, of immune recognition, 32, 69, 70

Spleen, 54
> marginal zone, 54
> periarteriolar lymphoid sheet, 54
> red pulp of, 54
> white pulp of, 54

"Split products", of complement system, 235-237

Spondylitis, ankylosing, , 346

Sporozoites, 272

SRBCs (Sheep red blood cells), 130-112

SRS-A (Slow-reacting substance of anaphylaxis), 284

STATs (signal transducers and activators of transcription), 167

Stem-cell factor (SCF), 143, 144

Streptococcus pneumoniae, 250, 269
> evasion of host defense, 269
> vaccine for, 250

Stromal cells
> role in B-cell maturation, 143, 144
> role in T-cell maturation, 156-157

Superantigens, 71, 170
> exogenous and endogenous, 71, 170
> and negative thymic selection, 170
> in T-cell activation, 170
> toxins acting as, 170

Surrogate light chain, 144

Switch sites, 136

Systemic lupus erythematosus (SLR), 348, 352
> complement deficiencies in, 352
> immune complexes, role in, 352

TAP (transporters associated with antigen processing), 192, 361

Target cells
> in antigen presentation, 191
> destruction of
>> By ADCC, 201, 275, 305
>> By CTLs, 199

TATAs. *See* Tumor-associated transplantation antigens

T-B conjugate formation, 151

T-cell(s), 42, 43, 155-160
> accessory membrane molecules, 179, 180
> activation. *See* T-helper cells, activation of
> alloreactivity of, 183
> antigen-committed, 158
> clonal selection cross-functional T-cell lines, 155, 314
> cytotoxic (Tc). *See* T-cytotoxic cell deficiency of
> development, in thymus, 42, 43, 155-160
>> double negative cells, 156-158
>> double positive cells, 156-158
>> progenitor T cells, 158
>> single-positive CD4 $^+$ thymocytes, 156-158
>> single-positive CD8 $^+$ thymocytes, 156-158
> differentiation of
>> co-stimulatory differences among antigen-presenting cells, 167, 168
> effector cells. *See* T helper cell
> in humoral response, 146, 151
> in hypersensitivity, 282-284
> maturation, 156
> membrane molecules, 179-183
> memory T cells, 170
> MHC restriction of antigen recognition, 182, 190
> naive, 157
> peripheral gd T-cells, 171
> distribution of, 171, 172
>> function of, 171, 172
>> ligands recognized by, 172
> self-tolerence, development of, 160-162, 323
> thymic selection, 160-162
>> negative, 160
>> positive, 160
>> role of epithelial cells, 160-162

T-cell receptor (TCR), 173-183
> accessory membrane molecules, 179-183
> alloreactivity of T cells, 182
> altered-self model, 182
> diversity, generation of, 174-178

alternative joining of D gene segments, 177
combinatorial joining of gene segments, 176-178
junctional flexibility, 176
N-region nucleotide addition, 177
P-region nucleotide addition, 177
$\alpha\beta$ heterodimer, 175, 177
$\gamma\delta$ heterodimer, 175, 177
immunoglobulin superfamily, 174
self-MHC restriction of
altered-self model, 182
dual-receptor model, 182
structure of, 178
domains, variable and constant, 175-177
TCR-CD3 membrane complex, 178
TCR genes, 174-177
allelic exclusion, 175
generation of TCR diversity, 177
organization and rearrangement of, 174-177
structure of rearranged genes, 177
variable-region rearrangements, 174-175
TCR-peptide-MHC complex, 180
affinity of TCR for peptide-MHC, 180, 181
influence of peptide on topology of, 180, 181
interactions in formation of, 180, 181
TCR recognition of peptide-MHC
TCR. *See* T-cell receptor
T cytotoxic (Tc) cells, 42, 198
activation of, 198
and generation of CTLs, 199
antigen recognition by, 199
in antiviral defense, 261
Class I MHC restriction of, 190
T_{DTH}-mediated (Type IV) hypersensitivity, 294-296
Tetanus
toxin, antiserum to, 28
T_H1 response, 42, 214, 222
T_H2 response, 42, 214, 222
T helper (T_H) cells, 42, 151-154, 162
accessory molecules, 179-183
and activation of, 162
altered peptide ligands as
antagonists, 169
clonal expansion or clonal anergy, 169
co-stimulatory signal, 167, 171
gene expression, 174-177
role of TCR-CD3, 178

superantigen-induced T-cell
activation, 71, 170
in autoimmunity, 352
In B-cell activation, 151
Class II MHC restriction of, 190
In humoral response, 151
In somatic hypermutation, 136, 145
T_H1, T_H2 subsets, 42, 214, 222
cytokine secretion by, 214, 222
in hypersensitivity reactions, 294-296
Thoracic duct, 51
Thymocytes, 49, 50, 156-160
double-negative, 156
double-positive, 156
Thymus
cortex, 49, 50
medulla, 49, 50
Negative selection in, 160
Nurse cells, 50
Positive selection in, 160
Programmed cell death, 160
Role in immune function, 49, 50
Selection of T cells, 160, 161
Stromal cells, 156-160
T-cell maturation in, 156
Thymus-dependent (TD) antigens, 146
Thymus-independent (TI) antigens, 146
Thyroid-stimulating hormone (TSH), 297
TILs (Tumor-infiltrating lymphocytes), 339
Tissue typing, 301
Titre, serum antibody, 204, 205
TI (thymus-independent) antigens, 146
T lymphocytes. *See* T cells
TNF. *See* Tumor necrosis factor
Tolerence, immunologic. *See also* Self-tolerence, 311
Induced, for graft acceptance, 311- 313
Induction by oral antigens, 59, 354
Tonsils, 55
Toxic shock, syndrome toxin-1 (TSST-1), 170
Toxins. *See also* Immunotoxins
Toxoid vaccines, 28, 252
Transformation of cells, 328
malignant transformation, 328-331
retrovirus-induced, 331
Transfusion reactions, 290

Transplantation. *See also* Graft rejection; Graft-versus-host disease
of bone marrow, 302
for severe combined immunodeficiency disease, 361
immunological basis of graft rejection, 299
of organs
and MHC matching, 301-303
Trypanosoma cruzi, 232, 243, 273
T. gondi, 270, 271
antigenic shifts in, 273
Variant surface glycoprotein
(VSG) of, 273
TSTAs (Tumor-specific transplantation antigens), 328-329
T supressor (Ts) cells
postulated, 42
Tuberculosis. *See Mycobacterium tuberculosis*
Tumor(s). *See also* Cancer
benign, 326
classification of, 326, 327
evasion of immune system, 343, 344
antigenic modulation, 343
immunologic enhancement of tumor growth, 343
lack of co-stimulatory molecules, 344
reduction in class I MHC, 344
immune response to
immune surveillance theory, 336
macrophages, role of, 335
NK cells, role of, 335
immunotherapy. *See* Cancer immunotherapy
malignant, 326
oncogenes, 331
Tumor antigens, 327
characterization of, 328
chemically or physically induced, 328, 329
oncofetal, 333
tumor specific antigens for identification of, 328
tumor associated, 333
tumor specific virally induced, 331
Tumor-infiltrating lymphocytes (TIL), 339
Tumor necrosis factor (TNF), 219
in bacterial septic shock, 232
biological functions of, 219
in cancer immunotherapy, 342
TNF-a
antitumor activity of, 342

in toxic shock syndrome, 232
Tumor-specific transplantation antigens (TSTAs), 328
Tumor-suppressor genes, 331
Two-dimensional immunoelectrophoresis, 106-107
Two-turn sequences, 128, 129

Ubiquitin, 191

Vaccination
boosters, 28, 29, 248
recommended schedule for children, 30, 246
T-cells, in autoimmunity, 353
Vaccine(s)
active immunization, 28, 29
antiidiotype vaccines, 258
attenuated (avirulent), 245, 248
classification of, 245
designing of, 245-258
development of, 245-258
DNA vaccines, 254
inactivated (killed), 248
for measles, 28, 29, 247
multivalent subunit vaccines, 251
passive immunization, 28, 29
for polio, 28, 29
polysaccharide vaccines, 249-251
recombinant antigen vaccines, 252
recombinant vector vaccines, 252
for rubella, 28, 29
synthetic peptide vaccines, 251
toxoid vaccines, 28, 29, 252
tumor-cell vaccines, 336-342
whole organism vaccines, 247
Vaccinia virus, 252-254
recombinant, 252-254
as vector vaccine, 252-254
Variable(V) regions
domain of, 86, 87
of immunoglobulin heavy chains, 87
of immunoglobulin light chains, 86
of T-cell receptors, 173
Variant surface glycoprotein (VSG), of trypanosomes, 273
Vasodilation, 22, 279, 282-284
V(D)J recombinase, 129
Vector vaccines, 252-254

Veiled cells, 61
Vibrio cholera, 28, 29
Viral oncogenes, 331
Virus(es)
    antigenic variation, 264
    complement-mediated lysis of, 261
    complement-mediated neutralization of, 264
    cytokine antagonist production by, 266
    effect on MHC expression, 264
    evasion of host defense, 264

V pre-B sequence, 143
VSG. *See* Variant surface glycoprotein

Western blotting, 119
Wheal and flare reaction, 286
White pulp of spleen, 54
Wiscott-Aldrich syndrome (WAS), 363

Xenogenic antigens, 63
X-linked agammaglobulinemia (XLA), 359
X-linked hyper-IgM syndrome (XHM), 359

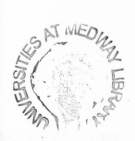